Maori Health and Government Policy 1840–1940

Ana Robinson
Senior Social Work Practitioner

Maori Health and Government Policy 1840–1940

Derek A. Dow

VICTORIA UNIVERSITY PRESS
in association with the
Historical Branch, Department of Internal Affairs

VICTORIA UNIVERSITY PRESS
Victoria University of Wellington
PO Box 600 Wellington
http://www.vup.vuw.ac.nz

ISBN 0 86473 366 6

First published 1999

Printed by Publishing Press Ltd, Auckland

Contents

Abbreviations

AJHR	*Appendix to the Journals of the House of Representatives*
ATL	Alexander Turnbull Library, Wellington
CHO	Chief Health Officer
CMS	Church Missionary Society
GBPP	*British Parliamentary Papers: Papers Relating to New Zealand*
HBA	Hospital Boards Association
LSA	Licentiate of the Society of Apothecaries
MD	Doctor of Medicine
MHR	Member of the House of Representatives
MOH	Medical Officer of Health
MOsH	Medical Officers of Health
MRCS	Member of the Royal College of Surgeons of England
NA	National Archives, Wellington
NMO	Native Medical Officer
NZBMA	New Zealand Branch of the British Medical Association
NZJH	*New Zealand Journal of History*
NZMJ	*New Zealand Medical Journal*
NZPD	*New Zealand Parliamentary Debates*

Preface

Some five years ago Crown Forestry Rental Trust historian David Armstrong sought guidance from Linda Bryder and myself, as medical historians, about the issues which needed to be addressed in relation to the history of Maori health since 1840. In late 1996 I was invited by the Trust to write a history of government policy towards Maori health, to be overseen by the Historical Branch.

The original scoping study envisaged a project covering the period 1840 to about 1910, on the assumption that my history of the New Zealand Department of Health, published in 1995, provided an adequate framework for twentieth century developments. I was certain from the outset, however, that this offered only a skeletal outline and it would be more appropriate to extend the study to 1940. The commissioning bodies agreed and the scope was enlarged.

I am grateful to both the Trust and the Branch for their faith in assigning this task to a non-Maori non-New Zealander. Hopefully any disadvantage in terms of background knowledge has been outweighed by the ability to bring a fresh perspective and a non-partisan approach to what is potentially a highly politicised issue. In this respect I have been delighted and fortified by the response to seminar presentations given to a number of Maori audiences during the past two years.

The dearth of publications dealing with the history of Maori health, referred to in the Bibliographical Essay at the end of the book, made this a daunting task. I am grateful to all those who gave advice and comfort as required. In the early stages Chief Historian Jock Phillips and John Martin, as supervising historian, offered encouragement and a critique of the draft chapters. These high standards have been maintained by Claudia Orange, who succeeded Jock to become Acting Chief Historian. Claudia's expertise in Maori history provided several shrewd insights which helped reshape and strengthen the text. Bill Oliver also read the entire manuscript in detail, picking up on a number of suspect interpretations and demonstrating a rare ability to cut through any tendency to verbosity. Bronwyn Dalley read a late draft of the manuscript, and proofread the text. The final polishing and cutting was provided by the copy editing of David Green, whose meticulous attention to detail proved invaluable.

Finally, my thanks go to my partner, Linda Bryder, whose own interest in Maori health, and wider knowledge of colonial health issues, provided stimulation and a new sense of purpose any time the story threatened to flag.

Derek A. Dow
University of Auckland
June 1999

Introduction

In May 1842 a Mr Lester of Auckland sought information from the Colonial Secretary on how to deal with Mokia, a Maori who had fallen ill at his residence. By the time Colonial Surgeon John Johnson received permission from Governor William Hobson to attend the patient, he had recovered. It was perhaps just as well that Mokia had no need of the doctor's help, for Johnson was not fluent in the Maori language. He urged the Governor to overcome the desultory and unsatisfactory nature of existing arrangements in Auckland by providing a medical centre and an interpreter. The response was not encouraging. A marginal addendum to Johnson's letter noted that no action could be considered at present, partly as a result of the 'destruction' of public offices.[1] This was not the first occasion on which such representations had been made to the government; the response, however, was indicative of the difficulties and frustrations faced by those who sought to promote Maori health in the century following the signing of the Treaty of Waitangi.

This history of health care for Maori covers the period from 1840 to 1940, a time span chosen to reflect the passage of a critical phase in the history of government policy. The health benefits ushered in by the 1938 Social Security Act marked the end of the subsidised doctors who had served many Maori communities since the mid nineteenth century. This legislation also removed the financial impediments which had hindered the integration of hospital services for Maori and Europeans. This is arguably a more important watershed than 1900, the year which saw the inception of the Department of Public Health and the passage of the Maori Councils Act.

The text has been broken down into four distinct periods. The first of these, from 1840 to 1869, examines the origins of the New Zealand hospital system and the Native Medical Officers. The second deals with developments from the conclusion of the New Zealand Wars until the Public Health Act of 1900. The third covers the two decades stretching from the foundation of the Department of Public Health to the end of World War I, an era which saw the emergence of the first Maori health professionals.[2] The final period opens with the creation of a separate Division of Maori Hygiene in 1920, embraces the changes introduced by the first Labour government, and concludes with New Zealand again embroiled in world conflict.

The primary focus of this book is upon policy initiatives, illustrated by frequent reference to individual circumstance or practice. The ad hoc evolution of New Zealand's health system during this century ensured that no one policy or set of standards was adopted nationwide. The piecemeal character of change continued to affect development after 1940.[3]

Four major themes form the backbone of the present analysis. The first relates to the administration and funding of Maori health. This involved the departments of Native Affairs, Justice, Education and, after 1900, Health. The evaluation of these core elements incorporates the impact of financial constraints and the relationship between politicians and officials. The second strand running through the book is the association between Maori and hospitals. This explores such matters as chronological and geographical variance in Maori bed occupancy, the acceptance or rejection of Western medicine, and the attitudes of hospital management towards Maori patients. Much of the data is inconclusive, for reasons explained in the text.

A third recurring theme is the role of the subsidised medical officer; this assesses the numbers involved in this work, their qualifications, and the calibre of recruits. The workload and remuneration of doctors in specific localities are considered. A clear indication of the enormous disparities in the provision of health care for Maori, and the impact of political rather than professional considerations, emerges from this evaluation. The fourth pivotal topic is infection control and the associated public health issues grouped under the umbrella of sanitation. The threat posed by typhoid and tuberculosis encouraged officials to examine preventive strategies such as vaccination, isolation and hospitalisation. Health education played a vital role in this field. The book describes some of the contributions made by departmental officials, schoolteachers and Maori Councils.

A number of other issues are dealt with in rather less detail. The role of missionary medicine in the 1840s and 1850s is outlined, as it helped set the scene for the later official intervention. Concern about the poor health status of Maori children is referred to in passing throughout the text. The concluding chapter contains a more detailed appraisal of measures adopted by the Health Department during the inter-war years. This includes the work of the school medical and dental services, the response of government to high infant mortality, and its cooperation with external agencies such as the Plunket Society and Women's Institutes. The book concludes with an account of health research initiatives prior to 1940.

There are, inevitably, significant omissions. Because this book is specifically concerned with health policies as an activity of government, and does not address the question of the outcomes of those policies, that dimension of health history is not explored. That topic would require a separate but parallel study, for which this book would provide an essential basis. However, it should be added that the absence of reliable data for the period under review would severely restrict any conclusions. Mental health has also been omitted from this study since it appears that few Maori were treated by Western doctors prior to 1940.[4] Another notable but deliberate omission from the present study is the impact of land sales and land alienation on Maori health. The thesis that land loss had a disastrous impact on health was first propounded in the New Zealand context by Keith Sorrenson in his 1955 MA thesis.[5] His approach was soon adopted by health professionals and health historians; in 1991 Ian Pool described Sorrenson's argument as 'a piece of classical historical demographic research'.[6] Pool's reiteration of this theme was cited in the preface to the Public Health Commission's *Strategic Plan for Maori Health* (1995).[7] The concept also permeates many of Mason Durie's writings, though without acknowledgement of Sorrenson's work.[8] However, the idea that there was an association between land alienation and poor health had no discernible impact upon the thinking of policy makers before 1940, and it is therefore not examined in this book.

Finally, a conscious decision was made to omit any consideration of the Treaty of Waitangi, which was rarely mentioned in discussion of health issues before 1940. Several speakers at a meeting of North Auckland Maori Councils held at Kaikohe in 1938 referred to the fact that the 1900 Maori Councils Act had been implemented at the request of Maori 'to carry out in some measure, the spirit of the Treaty of Waitangi'.[9] It was not until 1985, however, that the Board of Health's standing committee on Maori health recommended that the three articles of the Treaty should be 'regarded as the foundation for good health in New Zealand'.[10] A decade later this view had gained widespread acceptance. The Public Health Commission stressed in 1995 that 'Any discussion on Maori public health must begin with reference to the Treaty of Waitangi. The Treaty is recognised as the founding document of New Zealand.'[11]

Dr Michael Watt, Director-General of Health from 1930 to 1947, commented after his retirement that Maori health had been a 'veritable terra incognita' until the 1930s.[12] This present book, building upon the work of Raeburn Lange, Mason Durie and others, attempts to fill part of that gap by appraising official endeavours to meet Maori health needs during the first hundred years of European administration in New Zealand.

I
'A Tolerably Efficient System' 1840–1870

The provision of western medical services for Maori prior to 1846 was haphazard. Much of the responsibility fell upon the missionary bodies, a small contingent of colonial surgeons[1] and an equally restricted number of philanthropic doctors. Europeans were initially keen to extend institutional care to Maori, who in turn were eager to avail themselves of such opportunities. Within a relatively short time, however, both races appear to have drawn back from this partnership. Western health care for Maori became dependent on a patchy distribution of subsidised doctors, funded by the central government, with some continuing assistance from missionaries and Native Department officials. Again, the goodwill apparent at the outset became somewhat tempered over time, due in large part to a combination of racial tension and funding difficulties. While little attention was given to the sanitary improvement of Maori settlements in this period, the European community suffered similarly. Nevertheless, more extensive health care provision was made for Maori between 1840 and 1870 than has been generally recognised.

'The means of doing so': funding Maori health

In February 1846 the Colonial Secretary informed the Chief Protector of Aborigines that Governor George Grey intended '*altogether to remodel* the

Protectorate Department and to expend such portion as the Colony can afford of the larger sum that Establishment has hitherto cost annually, upon schools hospitals and other institutions for the Natives'.[2] As part of this reform the colony's resident magistrates would oversee expenditure on Maori health.

Earl Grey, the British Secretary of State for the Colonies, regarded Grey's proposal of hospitals for Maori as 'extremely gratifying', and encouraged the Governor to extend the scheme 'whenever the means of doing so may render it practicable'.[3] Fiscal constraint was to play a major part in determining the extent to which Grey and others were able to implement this ideal.

Several years elapsed before Grey could place Maori health care on a sounder footing. In 1850 he attempted to introduce Civil List payments for 'native purposes', a plan defeated by the opposition of settlers.[4] Grey achieved partial success two years later. Under the New Zealand Constitution Act 1852, which introduced responsible central and provincial governments, a fixed amount of £7,000 per annum was earmarked for Maori purposes in the Civil List budget, which remained in the control of the Governor.[5] This sum was intended to cover the cost of medical care, pensions, and rations for the indigent. The figure remained unchanged for almost a century and was from time to time the focus of spirited debate, accompanied by allegations of parsimony or misappropriation. While the scheme is said to have been tightly monitored, many of the 'recipients of compassionate allowances' had their grants renewed year after year.[6]

The potential for conflict in the handling of the Native Civil List was recognised almost from its inception. In 1854 William FitzHerbert, Provincial Secretary for Wellington, drew attention to the 'inadequacy of existing machinery for native medical treatment'. Reminding the Colonial Secretary that considerable funds had been set aside for 'Native purposes', he commented on the lack of any clear division of responsibility between the central and provincial authorities.[7] The conflict between local and central bodies would exercise the minds of generations of officials.

George Grey left New Zealand in December 1853 before he could implement the new Civil List allocation, and his replacement, Sir Thomas Gore Browne, did not arrive until September 1855. Browne made Maori policy an imperial rather than a colonial responsibility, but the purse strings were controlled by the colonial politicians, apart from the £7,000 set aside under the Constitution Act. Grey's return in 1861 to serve a second term as Governor brought further challenges to the existing system. The Native Department was initially under Grey's control, but he soon relinquished this function to ministers at their urgent request. By May 1863 he had had second thoughts, complaining that officers in the Native Department had never recognised the Governor as their head, and that the requirement to obtain ministerial agreement for any expenditure prevented him from acting quickly.[8]

Grey's letter was part of an extensive correspondence, concerned almost entirely with military rather than civil responsibilities, which led to the creation of a separate ministerial portfolio for Native affairs in 1863 and the appointment of William Rolleston as the first Under-Secretary in June 1865; the title Native Department was adopted the following year.[9]

Calculating the actual level of expenditure on Maori health is no easy task. The presentation of the government's annual accounts in the nineteenth century changed with bewildering frequency and items sometimes migrated from one category to another. Matters were further complicated with the creation of a separate set of accounts for expenditure under the Native Purposes Appropriation Act 1862. In 1862/3 almost £25,000 was expended under this heading, of which £3,192 was allocated for 'Medical Attendance on Natives'. With the exception of a miserly £58 for Canterbury, the entire sum was apportioned to the North Island.[10]

This seems to indicate a marked increase on the previous year's 'Civil List: Native Purposes' expenditure which totalled £2,137, principally for hospital expenses but with a modest amount for medical attendants.[11] In 1864 and 1865, however, the government accounts give no breakdown of Civil List medical expenditure, although £32,000 was spent under the 1862 Act on unspecified 'local charges'. By 1866 the Civil List £7,000 had reappeared on the books, described as the 'Amount transferred to Permanent Charges in reduction of expenditure chargeable on Native Purposes Appropriation Act'.[12] The following year's disbursement showed an outlay of £1,419 on hospitals and medicines, together with an allocation to medical officers which ranged from £1,160 (Auckland) through £687 (Wellington), £300 (Hawke's Bay), £89 (Canterbury), £51 (Chatham Islands) and £32 (Southland) to a meagre £25 (Nelson and Marlborough).[13]

In 1870 the Government tabled a 'Return of Expenditure Under Civil List Acts, for Five Years Ended 31 May 1870'. The 'Second Division' listed funds allocated to Native Purposes. No figures were shown for 1867/8 but the cost of medical officers in 1868/9 and 1869/70 was given as £802 and £968 respectively from a total outlay of £6,581 and £5,311.[14]

It thus appears that funding for Maori health was erratic in the 1860s, perhaps as a result of the dislocation and upheavals of war. These inconsistencies almost certainly had an effect at the local level. Some communities were probably immune from the effects of these fluctuations while others would have been vulnerable to any variation. Planning and implementing any kind of coherent health policy in these circumstances must have been impossible. Nevertheless, there were some significant developments in health care for Maori during this period.

'Medicines and other matters': missionary contributions

Missionary medicine was not part of official provision for Maori in the early years of European settlement. Yet the services provided by missionaries, in the absence of other medical assistance, helped shape the reaction of Maori to Western medicine. Few missionaries were fully trained in this discipline, but a number had a smattering of knowledge which enabled them to provide rudimentary care to family and colleagues in their isolated mission communities. This also allowed them to afford physical relief as well as spiritual succour to the Maori among whom they worked.

No medical personnel accompanied the earliest missions. Despite this, Maori attended mission stations in the expectation of receiving treatment for various disorders.[15] In New Zealand as elsewhere, missionaries used whatever knowledge they could glean from textbooks, or from classes attended before leaving Britain.

In 1834 the American Board of Commissioners appointed Peter Parker as its first missionary doctor, thereby introducing a new and important element to the missionary enterprise.[16] During the same year, William Marshall visited New Zealand briefly as naval surgeon aboard HMS *Alligator*. In his account of the trip, published in 1836, he advocated clerical appointees with qualifications in both theology and medicine.[17] New Zealand missionaries made 'constant and repeated calls' for medical missionaries to be sent out from Britain. The responses of the two major

2 STATEMENT OF SUMS EXPENDED UNDER

AMOUNT EXPENDED FOR 1862-63, IN "MEDICAL ATTENDANCE ON NATIVES."

	£	s.	d.
Arrears, being payment to Gundry's Estate for Medicines supplied to Natives during the past six years	209	7	1
Bay of Islands	203	0	6
Mongonui	73	0	7
Wangarei and Kaipara	93	19	0
Waiuku	291	12	4
Thames	21	18	6
Raglan and Lower Waikato	213	12	0
Upper Waikato	326	16	0
East Cape	89	1	6
Bay of Plenty	116	9	5
Taupo	26	3	5
New Plymouth	374	14	11
Whanganui	446	19	9
Wellington and West Coast	443	0	3
Napier	204	3	4
Canterbury	58	6	8
	£3,192	5	3

The £3,192 expended on medical attendance of Maori in 1862/3 included just £58 for South Island inhabitants. *AJHR, 1863, E-8, p.2*

missionary bodies were quite different. The Wesleyans refused to countenance appointing medical missionaries,[18] but the Church Missionary Society (CMS) responded by appointing a doctor, Samuel Ford, to give medical treatment and advice to Bay of Islands Maori, 'and to look for no other remuneration than simple subsistence'. He was also charged with providing care for the missionary families, but attendance on European inhabitants was not to interfere with healing and teaching his Maori flock.[19] Ford arrived in August 1837 and quickly gained the confidence of local Maori. He appears to have been asked to purchase land and hold it in trust for them, a role attributed to the fact that he was 'no doubt highly esteemed' at a time when the indigenous population was faced with 'uncustomary plagues' and 'fatal epidemics' to which tohunga had no answer. There is little evidence of Ford's effectiveness as a physician which, given the contemporary state of medical knowledge, was unlikely to have been great.[20] Ill health compelled him to resign in 1841.

Jean Kehoe has suggested that George Selwyn, Anglican Bishop of New Zealand from 1841 to 1868, was unique in bringing medical men to New Zealand 'for the express purpose of working among the Maori'. She identified only two: 'Butts' and Arthur Purchas.[21] Henry Butt, who qualified MRCS 1840, was appointed in 1842 as a catechist, and after ordination as deacon and priest became Archdeacon of Wairau in the late 1860s. Medicine probably played no more than a subsidiary role in his career. Purchas became medical officer to the Anglican St John's College Hospital in Auckland in 1846, four years after he obtained the MRCS LSA. Within a short time he was ordained, and he had sole charge of Onehunga parish for the next 28 years. Once again, medical work was secondary to his other duties. In 1862 Purchas declined to act as medical commissioner for a proposed 'native hospital' at Te Awamutu on the grounds that this was inconsistent with his clerical duties.[22]

One missionary stood out above all others in the delivery of medical care to Maori in the two decades after 1840. William Williams completed a surgical apprenticeship in Southwark, London before commencing his training for the mission field. He was sent in 1826 by the CMS to Paihia, where he conducted a mission school and studied the Maori language. In 1849 Williams and his wife Jane were transferred to the Poverty Bay mission. The published letters and journals of their life and work over the next decade afford some penetrating insights into the relationship between Maori people and Western medicine.[23]

From the moment of his arrival Williams regularly treated sick Maori while pursuing his evangelical vocation. On 29 October 1841 he wrote: 'Natives began to come about for medicines and other matters'. Williams frequently visited both neighbouring and more distant settlements to examine patients and distribute medicine. Sick Maori also travelled to the mission station for attention; the journals suggest that significant numbers awaited his arrival home from preaching tours or visits to mission headquarters in Auckland. His journal entry for 18 September 1843 typifies this role: 'Occupied the whole morning in administering medicine.'[24]

Jane Williams was equally in demand, especially during her husband's absences. Her journal entries tend to supply greater detail than those of her husband. On 8 June 1840, for instance, she recorded 'An unusual number of applicants for physic, which with my school, occupied the greater part of the day.' Again, on 19 August 1852 she wrote to William's sister: 'They [Maori] are now very anxious for medicine and English food when they are ill and will sometimes ask for physic *for fear* they should be so.'[25] Such linkage of health and education was widespread in early colonial New Zealand. A committee was set up by the Presbytery of Otago in 1858 'to

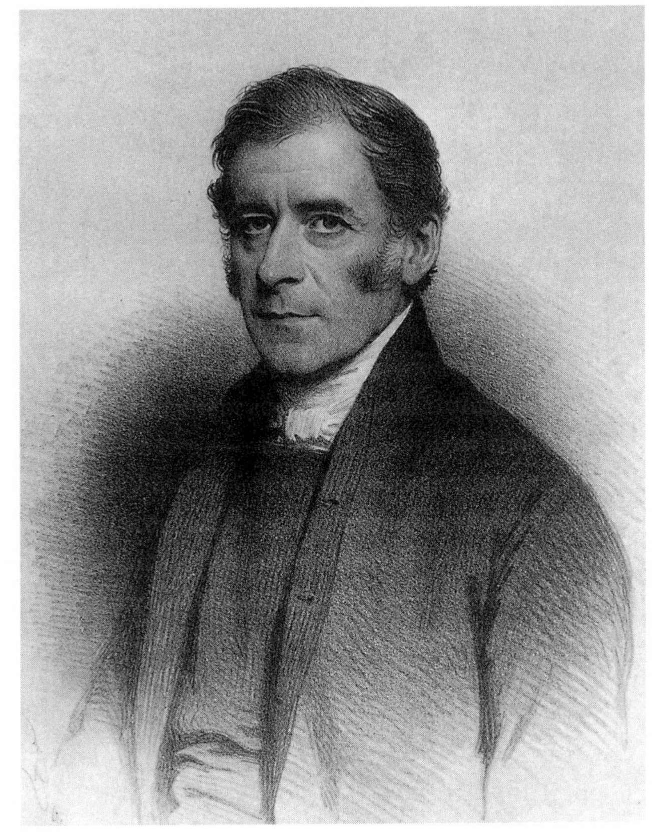

William Williams (1800–78) did not acquire a formal qualification after completing his medical studies. He chose instead to complete an Oxford BA as preparation for service with the Church Missionary Society.
ATL, D-P020006-C

devise a scheme for alleviating the physical and moral condition' of Maori; its report envisaged the creation of an industrial school to offer training in agricultural and domestic skills, but the proposal was not implemented.[26]

Other missionaries with little or no knowledge of medicine were drawn into providing clinical as well as spiritual care. William Colenso, a printer by profession, was employed by the CMS in New Zealand from 1834 to 1852. After his ordination in 1844 he assumed the role of healer. He regarded this medical work as a worthwhile and necessary part of his pastoral role, not least in providing an antidote to the influence of tohunga. It was a high-risk venture, for the failure of Western medicine could and did lead to the rejection of the spiritual message.[27]

James Stack, who came to New Zealand as a Wesleyan missionary in 1824 before transferring to the CMS nine years later, spent much of his time during the 1840s visiting and prescribing for the sick. The instruments and medicines stored in his bedroom are suggestive of a more interventionist approach than the mere distribution of the ever-popular Epsom salts. Again, the risks to the reputation of the missionary and his message were considerable, with Stack fearful on one occasion that the prospective death of an injured chief might be attributed to his unskilful treatment.[28]

While Maori generally appreciated the care bestowed upon them by the missionaries, some remained suspicious. In October 1843 William Williams recorded a visit to a chief whose daughter had recently died: 'He said that the death of his daughter was occasioned by the medicine Mr. Baker had given her, that there was some of it left and if we would drink it & nothing happened to us he should know that it was not the medicine. It was not an agreeable ordeal to be subjected to but having ascertained from Mr. Baker that it was a simple bitter I took a draught of it & Mr. Stack drank the remainder.'[29]

As a result of such activities a number of mission stations doubled as de facto hospitals. Thomas Chapman, the CMS missionary in Rotorua, noted in his diary for 4 April 1845 that he often had up to five patients on the station, 'as if it were an Hospital'. The disruption this caused was more than offset by the opportunity to demonstrate the 'practical lessons of Christianity'. Such a rationale lay at the heart of medical missionary enterprise around the world. By early 1859 Chapman had settled permanently at Maketu for health reasons; many of his Maori parishioners viewed his headquarters as 'a hospital and rest home'.[30] Chapman was aided and abetted in this work by William Davis, Colonial Surgeon at Auckland, who in March 1850 received permission from the Colonial Secretary to furnish him with medicines from the Auckland Hospital stocks.[31]

The alliance, however loose, between missionaries and government agencies was an important factor in determining the shape and extent of medical provision for Maori. During a parliamentary debate on the subject in 1855 Thomas Forsaith (Northern Division) paid tribute to the missionary contribution: 'There was no tribe of importance that had not a mission-station adjacent, where medical aid could always be obtained.'[32] Later evidence from government officials supported this assertion. In 1861 Governor Grey called for reports from officials around the North Island. W. Baker's first dispatch on 3 January 1862 as Resident Magistrate for the

East Cape reported that 'Since the reduction of the Missionary body in the Diocese of Waiapu the Natives have been deprived of medical attention, and several instances of death by poisoning have been the result of their attempts to administer relief.'[33] Grey's plan to appoint some twenty district surgeons was presumably intended to compensate for such withdrawals.

In a young colony with limited medical provision, the missionary presence had helped create an expectation among Maori that Western medicine had a contribution to make to their welfare. In 1837 John Watkins informed a United Kingdom parliamentary select committee that the Maori 'used to esteem me as the Surgeon of the Missionaries; the Missionaries are the only People there to give one any Consequence'.[34] Writing in 1863, Dr J.B. Tuke concluded that from his experience and observation of Maori character, 'none of the forms of missionary enterprise are so likely to succeed, and be of lasting benefit, as the medical mission.'[35] The expansion of European settlement and the introduction of subsidised medical attendants for Maori from the late 1850s rendered the medical mission virtually redundant.[36] Yet for almost 40 years it had played a major role in health care for Maori and paved the way for their partial acceptance of Western medicine.

'Of paramount importance': Maori and hospitals

By the 1840s most sizeable British towns possessed one or more general hospitals. These were intended for the indigent sick and supported by voluntary subscriptions and donations from the better off, who were not themselves eligible for treatment. State hospital care was restricted to the lowest stratum of society, those classed as paupers, and provided in workhouses or poorhouses. New Zealand's small settler population in the early 1840s was ostensibly screened to restrict immigration to the healthiest members of society and to prevent any influx of paupers. There was little incentive to erect hospitals in the colony. Nevertheless, some planners recognised the need to make provision for illness. An 1840 draft plan for the town of Wellington incorporated four public bath-houses and separate colleges for physicians and surgeons. It also contained four possible sites for a hospital. This plan, drawn up in London, was more suited to a metropolitan centre than a fledgling colonial outpost; it was never implemented.[37]

Samuel Marsden, who had founded the inaugural CMS settlement, apparently planned to establish a hospital in 1826. He also hoped to recruit a qualified doctor to 'establish a medical school where "intelligent" Maoris would be educated in the rudiments of medicine and surgery'.[38] Neither suggestion came to fruition. A decade later, William Marshall of HMS *Alligator* floated the idea of setting up 'local hospitals at the several mission stations'.[39] Although Samuel Ford arrived in 1837 with high hopes of accomplishing this aim, nothing came of his plans.[40]

Some writers have claimed there was a hospital in Auckland by 1841, intended for use by Maori, seamen, and Europeans approved by the Colonial Secretary.[41] However, the British Army surgeon Arthur Thomson, who was based in Auckland from 1847 to 1858, declared that in the early 1840s there were no hospitals in New Zealand for the sick or insane, and that 'as disease was rare, several medical emigrants, finding their professional talents useless, turned store-keepers'.[42] One of them was John Logan Campbell, later dubbed the Father of Auckland. Shortly after his arrival in August 1840 Campbell set up a temporary tent hospital for two Maori injured in a gunpowder explosion, although there is nothing in his memoirs to suggest he regarded this as anything other than a short-term expedient.[43]

The lack of official action in the early years of the colony prompted at least three further private initiatives. Lady Martin, wife of the colony's first Chief Justice, established a hospital for Maori in Auckland in 1842. Originally housed in a cluster of rough huts and a tent made of blankets, it later occupied a three-roomed dwelling. On occasion patients came from as far afield as Thames. This hospital closed in 1856 when ill health forced William Martin's retirement.[44]

A few months before Logan Campbell's arrival in the colony John FitzGerald, who had docked in Wellington as a ship's surgeon and was soon afterwards appointed coroner and port health officer, called for a hospital to serve the increasing European population and to provide 'the benefits that such an institution might extend to the natives who certainly have a claim on the cause of humanity for it is truly deplorable the frightful ravages disease has among them'.[45] Three years later the Colonial Secretary expressed his gratification at the steps taken by FitzGerald to establish a 'native hospital' in Wellington.[46] Little is known about this institution, although in 1843 the Bishop of New Zealand complained to the Colonial Secretary, on whose behalf he appears to have administered health matters, that the funds received from the Native Reserves were insufficient to meet both hospital requirements and FitzGerald's expenses as Native Medical Officer.[47]

FitzGerald's venture was bedevilled from the outset by underfunding. On 24 June 1844 he wrote to the Secretary of the colony's Southern District seeking supplies for the Maori hospital since the Bishop could no longer provide them. The official response was not encouraging. A marginal note by 'AS' (Dr Andrew Sinclair, Colonial Secretary since January 1844) noted that 'However laudable may be the purpose for which Dr F applies for these articles the want of means in the hands of Govt prevents compliance with the request.' The praise which had been heaped on FitzGerald in 1843 by Sinclair's predecessor, Willoughby Shortland, was thus revealed as empty rhetoric.[48]

Events in Auckland largely mirrored those in Wellington. It has already been seen that the case of a Maori who had fallen ill at the residence of Mr Lester led Colonial Surgeon John Johnson to propose the construction of a dispensary. This would have six beds and be staffed by an assistant and a nurse, with an interpreter in daily attendance. Four weeks later Johnson received a reply from the Colonial Secretary regretting that the government lacked the means to erect a 'hospital for Natives . . . until sufficient funds are procurable from the native reserves'.[49] Spurred by this incident, Shortland, whose brother was a recently qualified doctor employed as Sub-Protector of Aborigines for Tauranga, chaired a meeting in Auckland to discuss such a hospital. His hopes were dashed by public concern about the propriety of tending European and Maori patients in the same institution.[50]

One of those who noticed these proceedings was Samuel Martin, a Glasgow medical graduate turned Auckland newspaper editor. Martin proposed that 'well behaved and moral medical men should be settled in various districts in charge of hospitals, to which the natives should have free admission'.[51] There is no evidence that his suggestions were acted upon; in 1845 he returned to Britain, where he petitioned Parliament about the New Zealand Company's ill-treatment of Maori.[52]

At Wanganui the Revd Richard Taylor, who had taken over the CMS mission station, established a Maori hospital at Putiki in 1844. As he recorded in his diary: 'It will be near my house and will enable me to attend more closely to my sick.'[53] Taylor had moved to Wanganui from the CMS's main mission centre at Waimate, where a hospital had recently been opened with Christopher Davies, a nephew of William Williams, appointed in 1843 as surgeon in charge. By 1846 this had been transferred to Auckland, where it was renamed St John's College Hospital and its catchment area extended to Taranaki and Wherowhero (Poverty Bay). Two 'native teachers' were taken to the hospital. Unfortunately, both men died, one in the hospital and the other following his return home. An attempt to extort payment for one of the deaths on the grounds that it had been caused by the treatment meted out in Auckland was repulsed.[54]

Sarah Selwyn described St John's Hospital as a place where the missionaries could 'make some Maoris comfortable and feed them up'.[55] That reputation may have been shaken in mid 1847, when an outbreak of typhoid fever saw every house at St John's pressed into hospital use. Seventeen victims, both Maori and Pakeha, were hospitalised. One, the second son of William Williams, died.[56]

This outbreak does not seem to have deterred Maori from making use of Pakeha hospitals. One of the first fruits of Governor Grey's intention to provide medical care was an unseemly squabble in the Rotorua region. Dr Johnson's comment during a visit to the locality in January 1847 that Tikitere would be an excellent site for the hospital proposed for the hot springs region spread 'like wildfire'. Disputes between rival land claimants caused the scheme to be dropped.[57]

Grey's motives in promoting hospitals have been widely debated over the years. In 1969 the Health Department described how the first four hospitals—Auckland and Wellington in 1847, New Plymouth in 1848 and Wanganui in 1851—were opened 'for the treatment of sick and destitute Europeans, and free treatment for all Maoris.'[58] Other commentators have challenged this interpretation. Alan Ward argued in the early 1970s that Grey favoured individual chiefs or tribes, especially those who had supported land sales, when making provision for social or welfare institutions such as hospitals.[59]

Malcolm Nicholson and Jean Kehoe typify a later generation of historians who argue that hospitals were constructed as part of the technology of empire, and as one of the tools to amalgamate indigenous peoples without stationing a large body of troops to subjugate them. Michael Belgrave added a different slant, claiming that 'The lack of segregation between Maori patients . . . and Europeans was an indication of the degradation associated with admission rather than enlightened attitudes to race.'[60] An editorial on the opening of Auckland Hospital in 1847, however, suggests that contemporary attitudes differed from those ascribed by Belgrave. The new institution, according to the *New Zealander*, 'will fix in the minds of the natives an impression that we are their sincere friends, disposed, really and practically to secure them and to ameliorate their condition'.[61]

Grey himself, in a dispatch dated 4 February 1847, was in no doubt as to the purpose of and necessity for the proposed state hospitals. Acknowledging that the government had not yet erected any hospital, school, place of shelter or church for Maori, he claimed that the four planned hospitals, three of which were currently under construction, would 'fully provide for the medical wants of the important districts in which they are situated'. Medical staff had already been appointed to two of these; they comprised men qualified by 'education, manners, and position in society' to gain the regard and esteem of the indigenous people. The hospitals would, he assured the Secretary of State for the Colonies, 'produce very beneficial effects on the native race'.[62]

Fourteen months later, Grey brought the Secretary of State up to date with attempts to establish hospitals upon a 'European' model as a means to civilise the Maori.[63] The first of Grey's hospitals had opened in Wellington on 15 September 1847. Within a week Dr FitzGerald had conducted New Zealand's first surgical operation under general anaesthetic on the Waikanae chief Hiangarere. This was a high-risk strategy, since the failure of this novel procedure might well have deterred other Maori. Fortunately the operation was a success.[64] This episode was part of a conscious strategy by FitzGerald, who in 1841 had successfully amputated the arm of a relative of another chief. His report on this earlier case indicated his anxiety that it go well, 'in order that it might inspire the Natives with confidence in our art, with which they are yet but imperfectly acquainted'. FitzGerald also regarded the willingness of the patient to undergo the operation as proof of the rapid progress of civilisation among Maori, who in earlier years would have died rather than submit to amputation.[65]

Maori willingness to utilise the hospitals was evident from the outset. In Wellington, 23 of the 31 inpatients admitted by January 1848 were Maori. During 1848 the number of inpatients evened out, with 42 Europeans and 43 Maori, at a time when the local Maori population outnumbered Europeans by more than three to one. This reversal was temporary. Maori admissions in 1849 and 1850, at 167 and 283 respectively, comprised nearly 90 per cent of all inpatients, and more than 92 per cent of outpatients in each of the four years to 1851 were Maori (in 1850 all were Maori).[66]

Almost all the patients at New Plymouth during 1848 were Maori. The first annual report of the Medical Superintendent, Dr Wilson, noted that some Maori resorted to the 'knavish trick of feigning illness to remain', a ploy which he overcame by cutting the rations of those identified as malingerers.[67] However, there appears not to have been the same predominance of Maori patients at Auckland Hospital, where in 1848 they comprised only 158 of the 276 inpatients. When it came to outpatients, the pattern was more akin to that elsewhere, with 376 Maori

The first Wellington Hospital was a modest two-storey brick building, intended to house twelve patients. It was replaced by a 40-bed unit in 1853. *Audiovisual unit, Wellington Hospital*

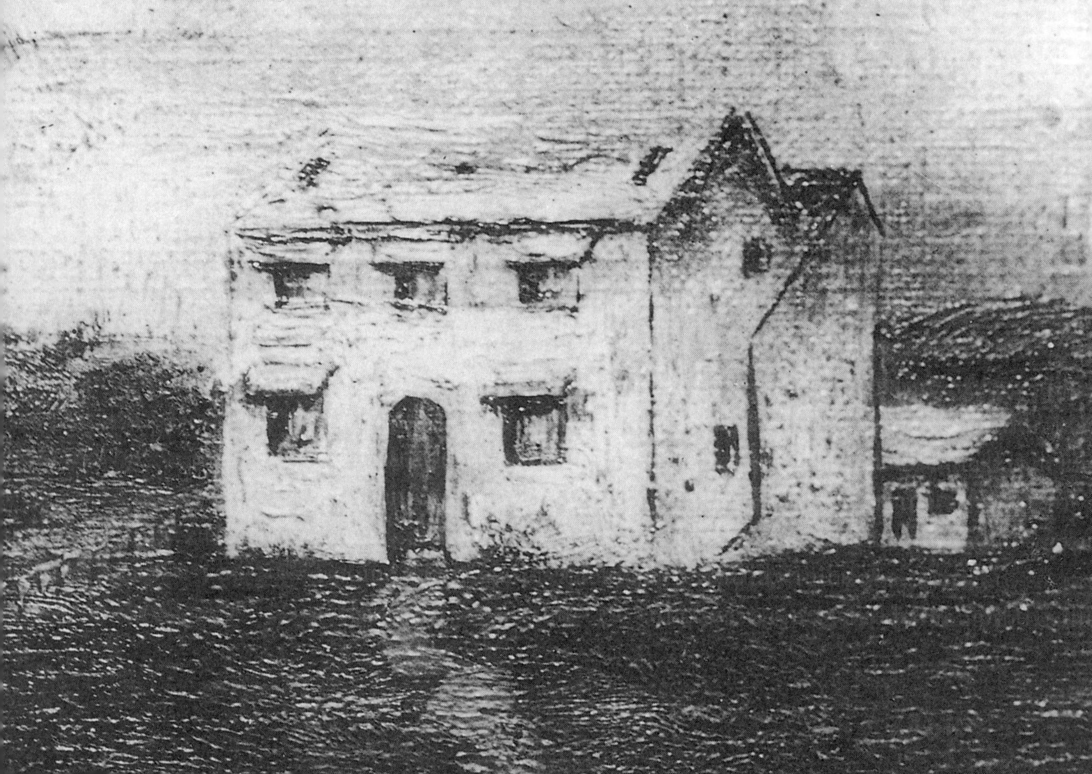

and just twelve Europeans.[68] By 1850, Pakeha inpatients in Auckland outnumbered Maori by 2:1.[69]

Wanganui Hospital opened after the other three. The delays associated with its construction indicate the difficulties which were to inhibit the colony's hospital system. Taylor had urged Grey to take action a month after an epidemic at Putiki in December 1847. Although it has been claimed that Grey left immediately to select a site for a new hospital, the failure to engage a contractor meant that money set aside for the hospital was used for other purposes such as roads.[70] An earthquake in Wellington led to a change of plans, and instructions that the building should be made of wood, not brick as originally envisaged. The subsequent failure to proceed was blamed on the lack of government staff in Wanganui itself, and the distance from Wellington officialdom.[71] As a result of these delays, the hospital did not open until April 1851. In a move reminiscent of the beginnings of St John's College Hospital, the first patient was the head teacher of Taylor's Putiki school, a victim of tuberculosis of the glands.[72] In its first three months 179 patients were admitted, of whom 159 had been discharged by the time Dr George Rees, who had been associated with Taylor's earlier venture, submitted his first report on 29 July 1851.[73]

The table of admissions supplied by Rees in this report related to the 'Natives' Hospital, the subjects being aboriginal'. Within a short time the institution had ceased to conform to this description. A quarter of the patients were Pakeha in the first three months of 1852, a ratio maintained in 1853, when there were 153 Maori and 47 European inpatients.[74]

Any analysis of admission patterns must take account of more than numbers. The instructions from Earl Grey had been to establish hospitals in areas with substantial Maori populations.[75] In the event they were established in or near European settlements. It seems this initially did not deter Maori from seeking aid, for one striking feature of the early hospital returns is the extensive catchment areas they reveal. In March 1848 Dr Johnson drew attention to the fact that many of Auckland Hospital's patients were Maori visitors to the town, some employed in quarrying and road construction. At the end of the year he reported that patients had come from as far afield as Rotorua, Tauranga, Waikato, Taupo and Hokianga. Seven different tribes were represented among the eight Maori patients who died in 1848; the other was identified simply as a 'native policeman'.[76]

A similar outreach occurred at Wellington. The first printed return of the inpatients admitted before 24 January 1848 noted ten different tribal affiliations for the 23 Maori admissions. FitzGerald later examined the records of 41 Maori admitted during 1848. One had journeyed for 238 miles to seek attention, while no fewer than six patients had travelled the 48 miles from Otaki.[77] Before Wanganui opened its doors some local Maori travelled to New Plymouth Hospital to be treated by Dr Wilson.[78]

The status of the patients also had a bearing on the success of the venture. In January 1850 FitzGerald noted that Wellington's inpatients during the previous year included some of the most influential coastal chiefs, the clear implication being that this would foster the hospital's reputation.[79] It is difficult to determine when, and to what extent, this initial enthusiasm declined. Fatalities among hospital patients was one potential deterrent, although the incidence was significantly lower than that recorded for contemporary British hospitals.[80] Between October 1847 and December 1848 just three of Wellington's 64 Maori inpatients died, and for the calendar years 1849–51 the figure was thirteen deaths (from 660 cases). This was considerably lower than the mortality rate for outpatients, reported by Fitzgerald to be almost 10 per cent for 1851.[81]

Contemporary accounts are ambiguous about the effect of these deaths on Maori perceptions. Some reports suggest that they had little impact. In July 1854 a select committee of the Wellington Provincial Council investigated the management of Wellington Hospital. It compared New Zealand's publicly funded hospitals with their British equivalents, which were supported almost entirely by voluntary contributions, and concluded that the New Zealand system had arisen in part from the needs of a 'large native population, just emerged from barbarism, and requiring aid, which, without free institutions, they could only claim at the hands of the Executive Government'. The committee warned the central government that because of this obligation it would not be practicable to close the existing hospital until some alternative was in place to treat the many Maori who used it.[82]

In Auckland, concern about a possible prejudice in the 'native mind' against the hospital prompted the Colonial Surgeon to ask George Kissling, a CMS missionary and former headmaster in Sierra Leone, to conduct an investigation. Kissling reported in 1852 that all fifteen deaths during the previous year, including those of six Maori, had been unavoidable. Although Maori had been treated in hospital with 'a care and anxiety almost amounting to parental affection', many were adversely influenced by these deaths.[83] At New Plymouth the demise of one Maori in 1857 led to the hospital being classed as tapu and becoming primarily an outpatient service. According to Peter Wilson, surgeon in charge, this had far-reaching repercussions, with Wanganui suffering the 'same diminution' in patient numbers.[84] This decline occurred in spite of Rees' best efforts to ensure the hospital's success. Richard Taylor had recorded in 1851 that Rees was anxious to discharge mortally afflicted patients to their own homes so their deaths would not impact upon the hospital's reputation.[85] Three years later Rees urged the Wanganui chiefs to send patients to hospital at the onset of disease and not, as commonly happened, when death was imminent. He promised to treat as many as possible as outpatients rather than admit them.[86]

The first Auckland Hospital was located near the Domain and contained six wards, capable of accommodating about 50 patients. In 1849 the Colonial Surgeon, William Davis, criticised its location because of the lack of an adequate water supply and the distance from the town. *ATL, D-P145001-A (Charles Heaphy, 1850s). Reproduced by permission of Auckland Museum*

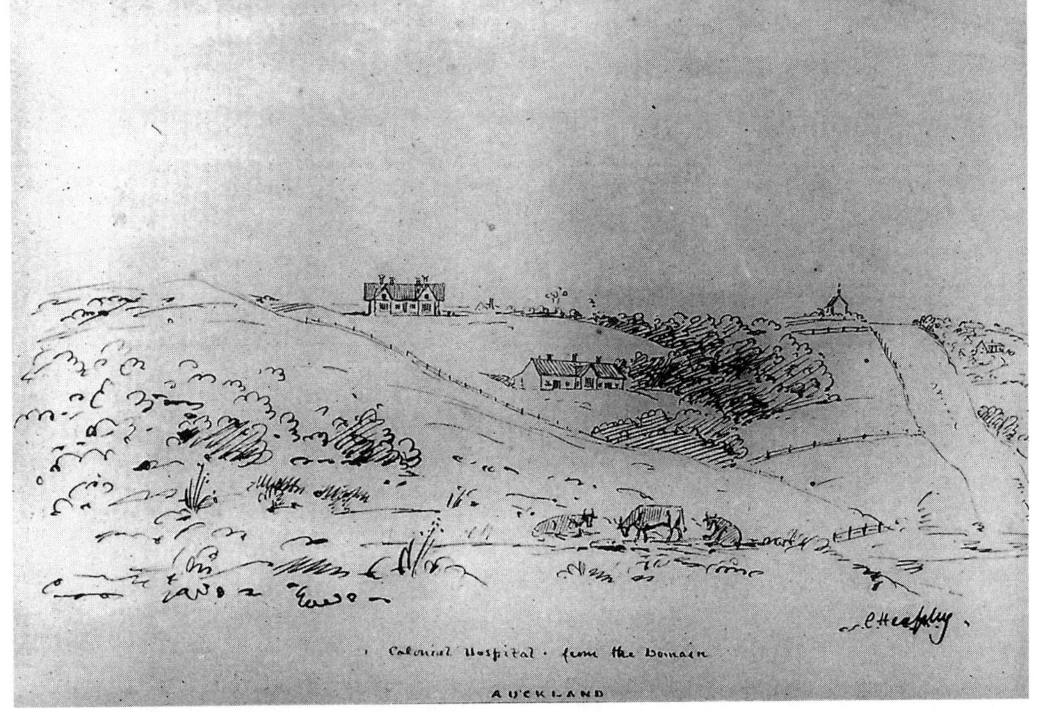

The relationship between Maori, hospitals and government became more complex after the introduction of provincial government following the passage of the New Zealand Constitution Act. A parliamentary debate in 1854 on transferring hospital funding from central to provincial governments raised a number of fundamental issues about health care for Maori.[87] Samuel Revans (Wairarapa and Hawke's Bay) 'was sure that the hospital system was wrong. It was wrong in principle. The Natives ought to be attended at their own homes.' David Monro (Waimea), a doctor turned sheepfarmer, took an almost diametrically opposed view. He believed the social status of Maori entitled them to be regarded as 'objects of charity', and that the advantages of access to hospital treatment would be appreciated: 'He thought the Natives would consider the establishment of hospitals as a kind action on the part of the white men.' Three days after this original discussion the subject was again brought forward by Alfred Ludlam (Hutt), who wished the funding of Maori hospital patients in the different provinces to be a first charge on the £7,000 reserved for Native purposes in the Civil List. Parliament voted for the management of hospitals to be transferred to the provincial governments, with the expense divided 'between the General and Provincial Governments in proportion to the European and Native patients treated'.[88]

For the financial year 1854/5, the central government agreed to spend just over £36,000 on the civil establishment. £2,070 of this constituted grants in aid 'to defray the expenses of treating Native Patients'. The distribution was £650 (Auckland), £550 (Wellington), £420 (Wanganui), £250 (New Plymouth), £100 (Nelson), and £50 each to Otago and Canterbury. For the following year this sum was reduced to £1,400, with Wanganui and New Plymouth removed entirely; they were still to receive grants in aid, but the estimates no longer specified that these were for Maori patients.[89] The colony's statement of expenditure for 1858/9 included less than £1,200 for 'medical treatment of natives in hospitals', with Wanganui (£473) and New Plymouth (£303) heading the list.[90] Further analysis of the complexities of the colonial accounts is required to obtain a clearer picture of the level of commitment to Maori health care.

Only a few thousand Maori lived in the South Island. In November 1850 Governor Grey surprised Dunedin residents by granting £400 for the erection of a public hospital because of his concern about the health of local Maori; there seems to have been no settler agitation for a hospital. Maori subsequently sought free treatment from the Colonial Surgeon, Dr Robert Williams, claiming that Grey had sent them. The position was supposedly regularised in 1853, but little more than two years later the central government refused to cover the cost of the scheme. On this occasion the shortfall was met from his own pocket by Governor Gore Browne. A.C. Strode, Dunedin's Resident Magistrate, subsequently stressed that the hospital was a 'most useful and desirable institution for Pakeha and Maori', but the entire episode was indicative of the unwillingness of local authorities to accept responsibility for Maori health.[91]

Pressure on hospital facilities was intensified by the desire of an ever-increasing European population to utilise these services. In 1840 Maori had outnumbered Europeans by approximately 40:1, but by the late 1850s the numbers were roughly equal.[92] In March 1855 the Colonial Secretary advised the surgeon at New Plymouth to admit 'any Europeans who may apply for admission provided that by so doing you are not likely to prevent the Hospital being as useful as possible to the Native race'.[93] This balancing act would become ever more difficult to achieve. Two years after this directive, Dr Edward Hulme of the Dunedin Hospital complained that there was no room in the hospital for a mentally-ill Maori woman because the chief constable was occupying the spare room.[94]

The historian Margaret Tennant has noted that it was significant that Grey's hospitals were to provide medical treatment for both Maori and 'indigent settlers'.[95] However, while the right of admission had been originally restricted to destitute Europeans, by the mid 1850s there was a growing tendency to admit paying patients. As George Rees of Wanganui explained in 1853, the comparatively high number of European outpatients was a direct consequence of there being no other doctor in town; 'until medical men are more numerous, if applications of this kind continue, it will be just to apply to them the rule by which the admissions into the hospital are governed, viz., a payment according to the means of the applicant'.[96]

In response, the Colonial Secretary informed Rees that European patients must guarantee a daily payment of 2s for maintenance.[97] Fifteen months later, in response to a plea from Rees, the charge was increased to

Return of Patients treated in the Colonial Hospital at Whanganui during the half year ending 30th June 1855.

Name	Sex	Age	Residence	Race	Disease	Admitted	Discharged	Remarks
William Knight	M	43	Whanganui	European	Subluxatio	Decr 19	Jany 6	Cured
Watarowi	M	11	Whanganui	Native	Fractura	Jany 7	" 14	Discharged to attend as out patient.
Jeremiah Harrington	M	40	Whanganui	European	Orchitis traumaticus	" 12	" 20	Cured
Tetaihu	M	40	Whanganui	Native	Ulcus	" 26	" 30	To attend as out patient, doing well
James Williams	M	31	Whanganui	European	Abscessus	Feby 1	Mar 30	Discharged doing well to attend as out patient.
Thomas Murray	M	34	Whanganui	European	Febris rheumaticus	Mar 10	Apl 26	Discharged convalescent
Tepatu	M	10	Whanganui	Native	Enteritis	" 21	" 18	Cured
Pete	F	35	Whanganui	Native	Venenum	" 25	" 27	(Doing well (From Mercury)
Richard Smith	M	32	Whanganui	European	Orchitis	June 10	June 25	Cured
Edmund Tipler	M	23	Whanganui	European	Enteritis	" 19	" 25	Recovery.

[illegible]
Colonial Surgeon

Wanganui Hospital's return of patients for January–June 1855 included six Europeans and four 'Natives'. *NA, IA 1, 1855/2887*

3s per day.[98] Many defaulted on this payment, according to FitzGerald's successor in Wellington, Dr Alexander Johnson.[99]

It is almost impossible to provide reliable data on the number of Maori patients admitted to hospital from the mid 1850s. Even FitzGerald, regarded as a champion of the Maori, ceased to indicate the number of Maori patients in his annual returns, and his 1853 report on the new hospital at Thorndon gave no indication as to who would use the facilities.[100] In 1859 Arthur Thomson analysed 2,580 Maori admissions to hospitals in the Bay of Islands, Auckland, Wellington, Wanganui, and New Plymouth, but gave no dates.[101] Later hospital historians have rarely attempted to quantify usage and most published histories of New Zealand hospitals contain little or no reference to Maori.

One of Grey's dispatches to the Colonial Office boasted that the maintenance of hospitals was a 'matter of paramount importance to the native race'.[102] Many of his contemporaries held a different opinion. F.D. Bell, a New Zealand Company official who was to become a politician, had in 1848 informed his distant second cousin, Edward Gibbon Wakefield, that New Plymouth's 'Maori hospital' was no better than an 'absurd waste of money'. It was ridiculous, he claimed, to spend £1,000 on such a 'toy' when roads and bridges were in a state of disrepair.[103] Bell's view would never entirely prevail, but neither would the 'Maori hospital' reach its intended potential.

'All our ailments': subsidised doctors

Government-sponsored medical care for Maori began in the early 1840s. Most of this work was undertaken by the colonial surgeons based in the major European settlements. John FitzGerald of Wellington, whose medical attendance on Maori soon became the main focus of his work, was the exemplar.[104] Financial constraints and the reluctance of the government to accept responsibility for such expenditure hampered these efforts. In May 1843 Bishop Selwyn complained he had no funds to pay a forage allowance to FitzGerald in his role as Native Medical Officer (NMO).[105] FitzGerald appealed to the Colonial Secretary, pointing to the fatigue and labour involved in attending to Maori, and their ever-increasing willingness to seek medical treatment.[106] His pleas went largely unheeded. The Colonial Secretary advised that he could pay only half the doctor's bill for February and March 1844. FitzGerald stressed that his efforts would continue unabated but that he would have to dispose of his horse, which he kept solely for his 'native' work. The repercussions might be serious, he warned, citing the recent example of a chief's son at Petone who would probably have died without his intervention.[107]

Ten days later FitzGerald furnished the Colonial Secretary with a duplicate copy of his account for treating Maori in January 1844, since he had received no response to the original. This document stated that he had made more than 600 visits and was often obliged to travel up to eighteen miles in inclement weather. Although his invoice was for £20 12s, he calculated the true cost of his services at £60, a figure he submitted for future consideration by the Governor. Uncertain as to which department would pay his bill, FitzGerald left this section blank.[108]

Similar problems beset the other doctors who undertook such work. Prior to 1844 the accounts rendered by James Evans, Colonial Surgeon for New Plymouth, and his partner, George St George, had been handed to the Governor by the Bishop of New Zealand. In August 1844, on the instructions of the agent to the Trustees of the Native Reserves, the Resident Magistrate sent the account covering the period from February 1843 to August 1844 to the Colonial Secretary.[109] The existence of such administrative hurdles could have done little to inspire confidence among either doctors or patients.

In the mid 1840s Samuel Martin suggested the appointment of district medical officers who would be responsible for Maori welfare. This concept found favour in principle with George Clarke, the Chief Protector of Aborigines, who wished to establish educational, medical and advisory services but realised these were currently impractical because of the expense. They would also, he recognised, require 'many trained men', still something of a rarity in New Zealand.[110]

Responsibility for administering expenditure on Maori health appears to have been devolved to the resident magistrates, the first of whom were appointed in 1846. In 1847 Donald Sinclair reported from Nelson that he had accepted a tender of £6 5s per month from Alexander MacShane to provide medical attendance, medicines and surgical operations for 'all sick Natives' resorting to Nelson. Under the contract MacShane was obliged to seek written authorisation for each patient and to submit weekly returns,

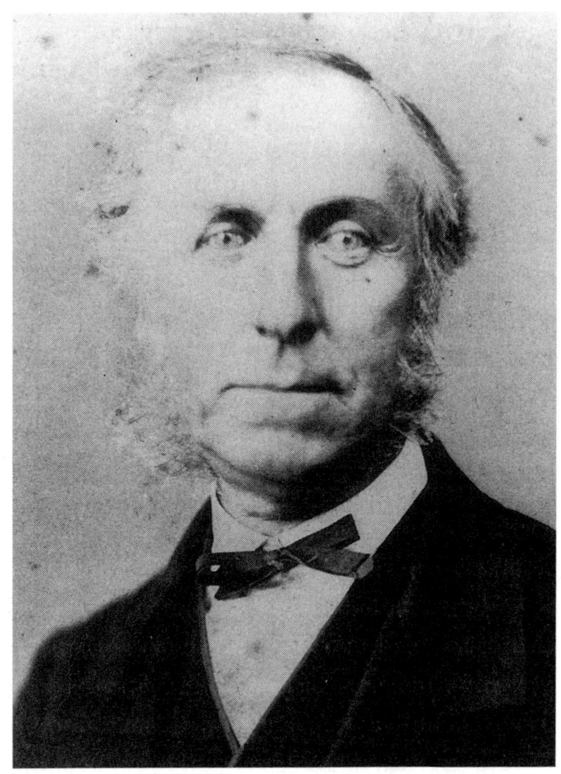

Dr John Patrick FitzGerald (1815–97) resigned from Wellington Hospital and left the colony in 1854 after a prolonged dispute with Dr John Dorset and his allies in the Provincial Government. *ATL, F41832 1/2*

while the government retained the right to end the contract on ten days' notice. MacShane's offer undercut George Bush's rival tender of £6 10s. The latter, wrote Sinclair, would retain his gaol appointment until March 1848, after which he hoped to combine the two appointments.[111]

MacShane and Bush had arrived at Nelson some six years earlier as surgeon superintendents aboard two of the early ships. Their rivalry was comparable to the cut-throat competition under the poor law systems in both England and Scotland, where practitioners would vie for modestly paid appointments which made the difference between financial survival and failure. Although this practice could mean savings for the funding body, the disadvantages sometimes outweighed the benefits.

Just days after settling this particular contract, Sinclair again wrote to the Colonial Secretary, enclosing correspondence from John Greenwood of Motueka. Having learned that other local doctors were recompensed for providing medical and surgical care to Maori, Greenwood wished to file a claim against his efforts at Motueka, Massacre (Tasman) Bay and

Queen Charlotte Sound since his arrival in 1843. This work had cost him dear in time and drugs, he stated, with many travelling from the outlying settlements especially to see him. He was now tending an increased number of patients, who were 'no longer congregating together in their Pahs, but separating and spreading themselves over their cultivations'. In addition, he claimed to act as a de facto magistrate in resolving disputes between Maori and settlers.[112] Within three months Greenwood had been appointed registrar of births, marriages and deaths for Motueka, perhaps as a means of compensating him for these other responsibilities.

In one case health care was provided by the New Zealand Company, which in 1849 sent Dr William Donald to Lyttelton to attend to the labourers, many of them Maori, who were constructing the Sumner Road.[113]

At an official level, Governor Grey informed the Secretary of State for the Colonies in April 1848 of his attempts 'to introduce a tolerably efficient system of medical attendance into those portions of this colony which are most densely inhabited by natives'.[114] It is hard to avoid the conclusion that this 'system' developed in an ad hoc fashion. In 1848, for example, Henry King, New Plymouth's Resident Magistrate, authorised treatment for a Maori injured by a local European, on the grounds that the victim did not wish to bring charges. The bill for £11 10s 6d subsequently presented by Dr Peter Wilson led to a flurry of correspondence.[115]

The following year the Colonial Secretary instructed the Resident Magistrate at Russell, in the Bay of Islands, to issue 'medical comforts' to local Maori whenever Richard Bannatine, a staff surgeon with the 58th Regiment, decreed this to be necessary.[116] Some years later a second regimental surgeon, Alexander Montgomery, assumed this role. His experience perhaps typified the gap between supply and demand at a time when governments were constantly short of cash. In January 1855 Russell's Resident Magistrate, concerned at over-spending, asked Montgomery to suspend the issuing of medicines other than in cases of absolute necessity. On 24 April Montgomery offered an explanation for a budget blowout which had seen him spending £21 per month instead of the £6 per quarter targeted by the Auditor-General. There was, he explained, a high incidence of sickness in the district, and he frequently received more than 50 requests for assistance in a single day.[117]

Other parts of the country fared no better in the quest for funds. In

June 1854 Colonial Surgeon George Rees asked for an addition to his budget to enable him to visit sick Maori along a 60-mile stretch of the Wanganui River. His intention was to hospitalise where appropriate, and to persuade the healthy to look after the sick. The Colonial Secretary sanctioned a meagre £16 per annum for the purpose.[118]

In 1854 William FitzHerbert, Wellington's Provincial Secretary, attempted to place health care for Maori on a systematic colony-wide footing. FitzHerbert, a London-trained doctor who had opted for a business and political career upon his arrival in New Zealand in 1841, contacted the Colonial Secretary to foster the 'claims of humanity'. He recommended dividing the colony into several medical districts, in each of which a resident doctor would receive a modest salary for Maori work as a supplement to private practice. 'Medical destitution becomes painfully apparent', he wrote; there was no qualified doctor with any Native commission on the east coast between Wellington and Ahuriri (Napier), a distance of 200 miles, while the vulnerability of the Maori to introduced disease had increased. FitzHerbert suggested that the costs could be met from 'the £7,000'—the Civil List allocation set aside for Maori purposes under the 1852 Constitution Act.[119]

FitzHerbert's ambitious proposal was not acted upon in the short term. When Parliament discussed 'Medical Assistance to Natives' in September 1855 it did so on the basis of special pleading rather than overall need. Joseph Greenwood (Pensioner Settlements) moved that £100 be added to the supplementary estimates to provide medical assistance for Bay of Islands Maori, explaining that the local military doctor currently supplied aid at considerable personal cost. The plea was backed by Hugh Carleton (Bay of Islands): this was 'one of those sums the necessity for which was so obvious that he apprehended the House could not refuse it'. Not everyone agreed. Henry Sewell (Christchurch) sounded a cautionary note about the dangers of ad hoc solutions: 'If such a practice were tolerated there would be no end to it.' A second dissenting voice was that of Thomas Forsaith, who argued that the £100 would be better spent on supplying medicines through the mission network, which would benefit inland Maori as well as those around Russell. Their warnings went unheeded and the motion was carried.[120]

The late 1850s brought a modest expansion of the subsidised system. Thomas Hitchings became NMO at Ahuriri in August 1857. He doubled as Coroner for Napier from January 1858 and was a member of the Provincial Council from 1859 to 1867. A number of other doctors became NMOs in the late 1850s, some serving for extended periods. Henry Thomas Spratt, for example, was appointed to the Wairarapa in May 1859 and remained in the post until 1883.[121] The rationale behind such appointments is unclear.

The essence of FitzHerbert's 1854 proposals was revived in Grey's 'Plan of Native Government' of October 1861. This followed hard on the heels of a complaint by William Colenso, the former CMS missionary who was now MHR for Napier: 'With reference to medical attendance, proper medical men had not been appointed to look after the Natives. They must have men who would not wait till the Natives came to them, but would travel about amongst them and interest themselves in their welfare.'[122] Grey proposed that 'The Native portions of the Northern Island . . . be divided into, say, twenty Districts, each under a Civil Commissioner, with a Clerk and Interpreter, and a Medical man as district surgeon attached to his District'. The estimated annual cost of £49,000 included £6,000 to cover annual payments of £150 to the surgeons and clerk/interpreters.[123]

Grey's proposals were widely disseminated. Hepata Turingenge stated at a meeting at Rua Kotare on Aotea Harbour in April 1862 that 'Governor Grey said he would send doctors to every place. . . . We saw it in the *Karere Maori*'.[124] Discussions at a series of runanga in early 1862 reveal both the attitudes of Maori and the deficiencies in the existing provision. Unlike Hitchings and Spratt, not all the 1850s appointees were properly qualified. George Topp had become NMO at Waiuku in July 1858 despite having no formal medical qualification; three years later the runanga of Ngatitipa discussed whether a doctor should be located at Waiuku or Taupiri. One speaker wished to send a letter to the Governor asking him to 'station a doctor here, an elderly man, not given to women'. His concerns were shared by a number of others, who cited examples of doctors at unnamed locations who misbehaved with women or drank rum. Despite these failings the speakers were convinced that a doctor would 'cure all our ailments'.[125] The complaints seem to have borne fruit; Topp was replaced by Dr Joseph Giles in March 1862.

Similar disquiet was voiced at a gathering at Whaingaroa (Raglan): 'Several complained of the doctor not visiting them when sick, and objected to him as a doctor for that reason.' 'Mr Wallace' was praised for his attention during sickness and the efficacy of his medicine, while opinion was divided on the merits of Captain Johnstone as a doctor. (Neither man appears on any list of qualified medical men in New Zealand.) At another meeting at Whaingaroa, the runanga asked James Armitage, Resident Magistrate, to appoint 'Mr Bishop, a quondam medical student'. Armitage could not endorse this suggestion but reported favourably on the medical work of James Wallis, Methodist missionary at Raglan (probably the 'Wallace' mentioned earlier), who 'has the confidence of the natives for his skill therein. If you did not think it worth while to station a doctor here, I should recommend that he be supplied with drugs, and receive a small salary for his services if he would accept it.'[126]

No attention was paid to the wishes of local residents; instead, an incumbent official was relocated. Dr Walter Harsant had been Resident Magistrate from 1854 to 1857 in the upper Waikato, where he had 'scarcely attempted to act as magistrate'.[127] Transferred to Whaingaroa as Resident Magistrate and NMO, he subsequently became Coroner (1858) and Registrar (1865). He was still acting as NMO in 1875.[128]

It is difficult to be certain about the number of subsidised doctors at any given time. The official returns contain errors in the spelling of names and on occasion the stated dates differ from those printed in other sources.[129] Some were very short-lived engagements. Thomas Kenderdine became Coroner for Whangarei in December 1856 and NMO in November 1858. He resigned the former post the following January and later lived in Auckland, though the date of his transfer is not known. William Perston, a Glasgow medical graduate who had settled in Whangarei around 1859, filled the position of NMO from February 1861. Still there in October 1863, his name was omitted from the list drawn up four months later. Three years later 'R. Perston' of 'Kaipara' appeared in the return of medical attendants whose services had been dispensed with some time after 30 June 1865. Two other 'Kaipara' doctors—James Bell and John Nicholson—suffered the same fate as Perston in 1865.[130] Whangarei/Kaipara does not seem to have been granted a replacement.

In 1862 five NMOs were appointed at the same time; all were added to the establishment before the runanga discussions had been completed. Three were classed as new appointments and the others described as

NATIVE INSTITUTIONS.

Resident Magistrates, &c., Native Districts.

Jan. 14	J. E. Gorst, R.M., Upper Waikato	New	350 0 0
" "	J. Armitage, R.M., Lower Waikato	New	350 0 0
" 16	J. Speedy, R.M., Waiuku	New	350 0 0
" "	G. Clarke, Civil Commissioner, Bay of Islands	New	550 0 0
" "	H. Clarke, Interpreter, Bay of Islands	New	150 0 0
" "	M. Clarke, Clerk and Interpreter, Upper Waikato	New	150 0 0
" "	W. B. Baker, R.M., Waiapu	Substitute	350 0 0
" "	R. Parsons, Clerk and Schoolmaster, Waiapu	New	150 0 0
Feb. 1	H. Taylor, Inspector Native Schools	New	500 0 0
" "	C. O. Davis, Editor Maori Messenger	Substitute	300 0 0
" 14	W. L. Buller, R.M., Manawatu	New	350 0 0
" "	P. King, Interpreter, Waiuku	New	150 0 0
" 7	Dr. Watling, Medical Attendant, Waimate	Substitute	100 0 0
" 21	Dr. Catling do. do. Akaroa	New	50 0 0
" "	Dr. Beswick do. do. Kaiapoi	New	50 0 0
Mar. 1	Dr. Giles do. do. Waiuku	Substitute	150 0 0
" 6	Col. A. H. Russell, R.M., Hawke's Bay, and Civil Commissioner	New	550 0 0
" "	G. Law, R.M., Taupo	New	350 0 0
" 7	T. H. Smith, Civil Commissioner, Bay of Plenty	New	550 0 0
" "	G. S. Cooper, R.M., Waipukarau	New	350 0 0
" "	C. P. Baker, R.M., Tokomaru	New	350 0 0
April 1	J. Shepherd, Interpreter, Taupo	New	150 0 0
" 2	E. M. Williams, R.M., Waimate	New	350 0 0
" 5	Dr. Curl, Medical Attendant, Wanganui	New	150 0 0
May 1	C. Vickers, Road Surveyor, Maketu	New	250 0 0
" 12	J. H. Greenway, Interpreter, Russell	New	150 0 0
" "	W. Webster, do. Hokianga	Substitute	150 0 0
June 1	E. Maunsell, do. Lower Waikato	New	150 0 0
" 20	R. H. McGregor, R.M., Raglan	Substitute	365 0 0
" 28	G. Falwasser, Clerk, Raglan	New	150 0 0
July 1	R. Todd, Surveyor, Raglan	New	250 0 0
" "	W. Farmer, Messenger to Inspector of Native Schools	New	60 0 0

In 1861/2 just £500 was spent on medical attendants in a total expenditure of £8,375 on 'Native Institutions'. *AJHR, 1862, D-17, p.4*

substitutes. Although Grey's 1861 plan contained no reference to South Island needs, two of these appointees were located at Akaroa and Kaiapoi. They received salaries of £50 per annum while their North Island counterparts, stationed at Wanganui, Waimate [North] and Waiuku, were paid £150, £100 and £50 respectively.[131] It is hard to discern any pattern or consistency in these appointments, or in those which followed.

Two years later an official return of NMOs listed seventeen doctors. Two of the five recruited in 1862 had disappeared. Joseph Giles of Waiuku had joined the Auckland Militia and served in the Waikato campaign, while George Catling of Akaroa had been convicted of habitual drunkenness and opium abuse in August 1863; he died three months later of 'intemperance'.[132] Samuel Beswick of Kaiapoi was now listed as serving 'Canterbury' while Samuel Curl, formerly shown at Wanganui, was now at 'Rangitikei'. These two changes were perhaps more terminological than geographical. Only the listing for Henry Watling of Waimate remained unaltered.

The seventeen NMOs covered an area from Mangonui in the north to Canterbury in the south. Only Beswick served in the South Island. Some held dual or even multiple appointments, as NMOs, coroners, registrars and, in the cases of Walter Harsant and William Nesbitt of Maketu, as resident magistrates. Workloads varied enormously, as did salaries, though there seems to have been little correlation between the two.

Most of these returns gave no indication of the number of Maori within each catchment area. Where figures were given, they have to be viewed with suspicion. In July 1862 Hunter Brown, Resident Magistrate for Wairoa in northern Hawke's Bay, reported on an official visit to the Urewera tribes and cautioned that Maori habitually over-stated their numbers in order to support claims for medical aid.[133] It is well-nigh impossible to assess how far these figures, inflated or otherwise, influenced the location of subsidised medical men. Nevertheless, they do give some indication of apparent inconsistencies of approach.

In particular there appears to have been no direct correlation between payment received and catchment area or number of patients. Thomas Trimnell, Mangonui's NMO for more than 40 years from 1859, received £100 in 1864 to look after the 1,500 Maori of the district. Robert Hooper of Taupo, who covered eight settlements with a total population of 460, received £150, while William Nesbitt, who was Resident Magistrate for Rotorua as well as NMO for both there and Tauranga from July 1863, earned a combined salary of £400. His medical duties alone involved the care of some 5,000 Maori.[134]

Nesbitt presumably was the 'competent medical man' appointed following instructions from the Attorney-General, Henry Sewell, to the Civil Commissioner in March 1863.[135] Nesbitt's contribution demonstrated both the hazards and benefits of sending doctors as part of the advance guard of the European presence. In 1870 he was dismissed from his post at Maketu after getting into financial difficulties and borrowing from the local runanga against his salary.[136] He then became Resident Magistrate and Coroner at Gisborne. One contemporary observer concluded that the presence of a doctor, albeit one largely occupied with magisterial work, was a boon to the small community of the time. There was no mention of how he was regarded by Maori.[137]

The ranks of NMOs swelled from seventeen to 29 between 1864 and 1866, a period during which there was a partial lull in the fighting between Maori and Europeans which had begun in the early 1860s.[138] Turnover in the initial cohort was high, with more than a third of those listed in 1864 (six out of seventeen) omitted two years later. Much of the increase was accounted for by appointments in the South Island, where there had been no hostilities. Five new posts were created in Nelson and Marlborough in mid 1864, with each doctor receiving a stipend of £50 from the rents paid on Native Reserves. Significantly, a third of the 1866 cohort, including four of the five Nelson/Marlborough men, held medical posts in the militia or regular army before, during or after their NMO service.[139] This trend was equally marked among the doctors whose services were dispensed with between 1865 and 1868, a number of whom had been temporary appointees. The 1867 return, for example, described Edward O'Connell and Thomas Best, attached to Maketu and Tauranga respectively, as 'returned to England surg. H.M. 68th Regt.'[140] There is no record of the impact such military links had upon their standing among Maori.

When subsidised doctors were introduced in New Zealand in the 1840s there seems to have been no expectation that Maori would contribute directly to the cost of the service by paying fees. By the mid 1860s parliamentarians and others had begun to question this aspect of the existing scheme. On 8 August 1866 Colonel Ponsonby Peacocke of Auckland raised the matter in the Legislative Council. He asked 'Whether, having reference to the small salaries paid to certain medical gentlemen for professional attendance in Native districts, it has ever been distinctly explained to the Natives of such districts that these salaries are to be regarded merely in the light of contributions, and that the Government does not intend thereby, nor otherwise profess, to furnish gratuitous medical attendance in Native districts?' The Native Minister, Colonel Andrew Russell of Hawke's Bay, seized the opportunity to clarify the government's philosophy. It had been intended from the outset, he replied, that Maori 'should contribute to the income of their medical men', and he personally 'objected to the system of pauperizing the Natives by giving them so much gratuitously.' His sentiments echoed the growing concern about the influx to the colony of

European paupers. It probably reflected also a belief that Maori income from land sales should be utilised to meet their needs. There was no simple solution to this problem; the question of which Maori were eligible for free health care would exercise the minds of legislators and officials for another three-quarters of a century.

Russell also suggested that subsidised doctors in most 'Native districts' would experience no trouble in deriving a more than adequate income. It was never envisaged that they would be able to survive on the subsidy alone. Most had 'rather a large white population, from whom a considerable addition to the medical man's salary was obtained'. In his own rather remote district, he stated, the local doctor had a practice of at least £500 per annum.[141] The example quoted, however, has to be regarded as atypical; most rural practitioners survived on much more modest incomes. Michael Belgrave has identified three broad categories of medical immigrants before 1880: successful practitioners with access to some wealthy clients, marginal doctors who relied on other work to boost their income, and those who abandoned medicine in favour of land-holding, mercantile pursuits or government service. According to Belgrave, it was not until the later 1880s that medicine could provide a 'full-time career occupation'.[142]

Alan Ward states that Russell dismissed several NMOs on the grounds that they did little work and that Maori, who allegedly had plenty of money to spend on liquor, ought to have emulated settlers by paying their own doctors' bills. Russell's successor, according to Ward, continued this policy of retrenchment, with Native Department expenditure slashed from £60,000 in 1864/5 to £34,000 in 1866/7. Ward does not, however, provide a separate breakdown for medical services.[143]

One outcome of this negative attitude in government towards the NMOs seems to have been a reluctance to use their expertise and knowledge in planning future services for Maori. In February 1868 the Under-Secretary of the Native Department instructed his officers to supply full details about the social and political conditions affecting Maori in recent years. The results were to form briefing papers for the incoming Governor, Sir George Bowen.[144] The topics covered were to include population data (with the causes of increases or decreases), attitudes towards Europeans, physical and moral conditions, and 'Hauhauism'. Only one respondent sought evidence from a local NMO in complying with this request. Samuel

Deighton, Resident Magistrate at Wairoa, forwarded in its entirety a report by Dr Matthew Scott. This report described diseases prevailing since pre-European times, commented on the prevalence of scrofulous ailments as a result of lifestyle and habits, noted the existence of pre-European phthisis (tuberculosis), gave an account of the incidence of typhoid from 1863, and mentioned the recent increase in sexually transmitted diseases. Such professional assessments could have been invaluable in planning Maori health services, but officialdom paid them little heed.[145]

The first generation of NMOs have been castigated for intemperate habits or other moral lapses.[146] It is true that some fitted the profile of the frontier doctor escaping or driven from the confines of a conventional career, but many were eminently respectable and respected members of society. This conclusion is supported by analysis of the 29 NMOs in 1866. Only three had no formal qualifications, having entered the profession long before 1858 when medical registration became compulsory in Britain. Most would have been apprenticed to a surgeon, as was William Williams of the CMS mission. Of the remainder, sixteen held membership of the Royal College of Surgeons of England; half of this number were also licentiates of the Worshipful Society of Apothecaries. This combination of surgical and medical qualifications was the hallmark of the general practitioner, who had come into his own in the first half of the nineteenth century.[147] The other thirteen appointees had been educated at Edinburgh or Glasgow, with the exception of the Irish-trained William Jackson of Hokianga. Only six individuals boasted university degrees, reflecting the fact that many of the medical graduates who emigrated to New Zealand at this time sought alternative careers, for example in politics.[148]

The first national Register of Medical Practitioners in New Zealand was published in January 1870. It contained 181 names.[149] Had the exercise been conducted three years earlier the number would have been smaller. It is reasonable to assume, therefore, that in 1866 approximately 20 per cent of the colony's doctors held paid appointments to provide care for Maori. These figures indicate a higher level of commitment to alleviating Maori health conditions than has generally been acknowledged. The reality of the subsidised medical scheme was a far cry from claims that medical services for Maori were virtually non-existent in the nineteenth century.[150]

REGISTER OF MEDICAL PRACTITIONERS FOR 1869.

LIST of MEDICAL PRACTITIONERS who are registered under the provisions of the Act of Parliament of New Zealand, 31 Vict., No. 30.

Date of Registration.	Name.	Residence.	Qualification.
1868, Nov. 19	Agassiz, Alfred	Mercury Bay, Auckland	Mem. R. Coll. Surg. Eng. 1863.
„ April 11	Aickin, Thomas	Auckland	Lic. 1839, Lic. Midwif. 1839, Fell. 1844, R. Coll. Surg. Irel. M.D. Univ. Berlin, 1842.
„ July 31	Alexander, Edward William...	Dunedin, Otago	Mem. R. Coll. Surg. Eng. 1853. Lic. R. Coll. Phys. Lond. 1861.
1869, May 14	Armitage, Frederick William	Tauranga	Mem. R. Coll. Surg. Eng. 1865.
„ Sept. 23	Barker, Alfred Charles ...	Christchurch, Canterbury	Registered under New Munster Ordinance.
1868, Mar. 7	Bayntun, Francis Thomas ...	Auckland	Mem. R. Coll. Surg. Eng. 1858.
„ April 29	Beale, Bernard Charles ...	Hamilton, Waikato ...	Mem. R. Coll. Surg. Eng. 1852. Lic. Soc. Apoth. Lond. 1854.
1869, May 14	Beaver, Henry Bibergiel ...	Dunedin, Otago	M.D. Berlin, 1835. Lic. Fac. Phys. Surg. Glasg. 1860. M.D. Wilna.
1868, June 27	Bell, James	Kaipara, Auckland ...	Lic. R. Coll. Surg. Edin. 1857. Lic. R. Coll. Phys. Edin. 1860.
„ April 11	Beswick, Samuel	Hokitika	Registered under New Munster Ordinance.
„ „ 11	Bond, Joseph Francis ...	Motueka, Nelson ...	Lic. Apoth. Hall, Dubl. 1858.
„ Jan. 9	Boor, Leonard	Wellington	Mem. R. Coll. Surg. Eng. 1852. Lic. Soc. Apoth. Lond. 1851.
1869, May 14	Borrows, Robert	Tokomairiro, Otago ...	Lic. Fac. Phys. Surg. Glasg. 1853. M.D. Univ. St. And. 1861. Lic. R. Coll. Phys. Lond. 1865.
„ „ 14	Bruen, Patrick Joseph ...	Westport, Nelson ...	Lic. R. Coll. Surg. Irel. 1863.
„ Sept. 23	Buchanan, Andrew	Chingford, Dunedin ...	Registered under Otago Act.
1868, Nov. 19	Burns, Robert	Dunedin	Registered under Otago Act.
„ Dec. 9	Burrows, William Adcock ...	Wellington	Lic. Soc. Apoth. Lond. 1852. Mem. R. Coll. Surg. Eng. 1859.
„ April 29	Butler, Edward	Timaru, Canterbury ...	Registered under New Munster Ordinance.

Entries in the first Medical Register can be misleading. All five of those listed here as registered under previous ordinances possessed acknowledged British qualifications (four MRCS and one LRCPEd). *New Zealand Gazette, 1870, p.36*

'Incalculable advantage': vaccinating Maori

Western medicine in the 1840s was of limited value. Physicians were dependent on a restricted range of medicines, many of dubious utility. Anaesthesia was introduced in 1846, but the antiseptic surgical revolution would not occur until the mid 1860s. Preventive medicine was still in its infancy. Vaccination against smallpox was one of the few proven and accepted preventive measures available to the medical profession. Its use among Maori is assessed in this section as an indicator of European willingness to combat the supposedly 'fatal impact' of introduced disease. The commitment to the vaccination of Maori also challenges any suggestion that the settler community from the 1850s onwards was resigned to the notion that the Maori race was doomed to extinction.

The effect of introduced Western diseases on Maori has been a recurring motif for both contemporary observers and historians since before 1840.[151] The nineteenth century concept of Maori as a dying race was depicted most famously in 1856 by Isaac Featherston, another medical graduate turned politician: 'The Maoris are dying out, and nothing can save them. Our plain duty as good, compassionate colonists is to *smooth down their dying pillow*. Then history will have nothing to reproach us with.'[152] Featherston's words have been described by one modern commentator as a succinct expression of a central tenet of settler legislation.[153] However, the predicted extinction of the Maori people did not prevent doctors and others from urging positive action to ameliorate or repel infectious disease.

The responses to epidemics in Britain and Australia are relevant to health strategies designed for Maori in this period. The first confirmed case of Asiatic cholera in Britain was verified in October 1831, and the disease quickly spread. Its presence sparked intense moral and medical debate, fuelled by the failure to identify any cure or effective treatment.[154] (The parallels with AIDS in the early 1980s are striking.) Concern soon extended to New Zealand. Henry Williams, the leader of the CMS mission, noted in his diary for 15 July 1832 that 'In the afternoon Mr Brown and I went over to Kororarika, mostly women, a few lads, their attention surprising, some of them wishing to go with us to the settlement, much enquiry concerning the Cholera'.[155] The initial fear soon passed, and cholera was never again perceived as a major threat in New Zealand.

Prior to large-scale European settlement there appear to have been only sporadic outbreaks of infectious disease among Maori. Surgeon John Watkins told the 1837 United Kingdom parliamentary select committee that he was not aware of the existence in New Zealand of either smallpox or measles.[156] He was presumably ignorant of the country's first outbreak of measles at Port Molyneux in 1835, when the former whaling station was home to a dwindling band of Maori who were 'wretched, ill-fed and ill-clothed'. Within months a second outbreak occurred at Preservation Bay, 160 miles from Port Molyneux. The epidemic had apparently travelled from Sydney after arriving there from South Africa.[157] Neither outbreak occasioned any great alarm.

Harrison Wright listed a number of diseases that Maori had never come into contact with in 1840: 'Small pox was one. Yellow fever, cholera, and typhus were others.'[158] It is debatable whether the last three ever reached these shores, and only a handful of smallpox deaths were recorded during the entire nineteenth century.[159] Unlike the other diseases cited by Wright,

INSTRUCTIONS TO THE SURGEON-SUPERINTENDENT ON BOARD THE EMIGRANT SHIPS OF THE NEW ZEALAND COMPANY

II. You are to keep up such a succession of vaccinated cases as may enable you to convey fresh virus to the Colony, if any occasion should occur on the ship; fresh virus must always be procured for the use of the Colony; and it is to be obtained by you previous to sailing, from the London Vaccine Institution, in the name of the Directors.

W.H. Skinner, Pioneer Medical Men of Taranaki, 1834 to 1880, p.44 preventive measures had been devised to combat smallpox. Their application to the Maori population is instructive.

The extent of the smallpox problem in Britain can be gauged from contemporary statistics. From 1830 to 1837 London alone averaged 560 deaths each year; the 1837–40 smallpox epidemic in England and Wales claimed 41,644 lives. The fight against smallpox saw the distribution of 800,000 doses of Edward Jenner's calf lymph in the years 1837–9.[160] It is against this background that we must view the measures adopted in New Zealand.

Jenner's successful use of cowpox vaccine to protect humans against smallpox was announced in 1796. It was widely adopted in Britain and overseas. In the late 1830s New Zealand Company surgeons were instructed to offer passengers vaccination on board ship, and to convey fresh vaccine to New Zealand.[161] The magnitude of this task should not be underestimated. There were difficulties in transporting vaccine before the advent of refrigeration, particularly over long distances. Japan, the last major country to receive smallpox vaccine, did not do so until 1849, half a century after Jenner's announcement.[162]

Surgeon Watkins suggested in 1837 that the absence of smallpox in New Zealand might be explained by the length of the journey from Europe, but confessed that he was 'not quite clear upon that subject'.[163] This uncertainty, and the prospect of large-scale emigration to New Zealand at a time when smallpox was in the ascendant in Britain, help to explain concerns about the potential threat to the indigenous population.

Vaccination was traditionally conducted in Britain by clergymen as well as by health professionals. It is no surprise that missionaries were vigorous advocates of the practice in New Zealand. In 1845 William Williams confided to his diary that 'There is an alarm among some natives about an eruptive disease with which a man is affected at this place [Patutahi, near Gisborne], fearing it may be the small pox. I am glad to find it is groundless, but I propose to take the present occasion for vaccinating the whole population in this quarter.' Four weeks later Williams vaccinated another 24 Maori children and adults at Taruheru.[164]

Such instances are representative of a more extensive campaign. Williams' colleagues, including those without medical training, were equally keen to promote vaccination. In August 1851, for example, following reports of smallpox at the East Cape, William Colenso wrote to Donald McLean, then a government land purchase agent, begging for vaccine so 'that I may do all I can for the infants and others here who are not vaccinated. I have at different times vaccinated a large number, but there are still hundreds who have not been done'.[165]

The extent of co-operation by Maori is difficult to assess. As with the European population, their attitudes covered a wide spectrum. In November 1848 Edmund Halswell, New Zealand Company Protector of Aborigines and Commissioner for the Management of Native Reserves, reported to the company secretary on his attempts to promote vaccination. An emigrant ship, the *Martha Ridgway*, had arrived at Wellington with smallpox on board. Initially reluctant to submit to vaccination, even after seeing the ravages of the disease at first hand, many Maori soon relented; others remained suspicious. It required Halswell's personal intervention to break the impasse: 'and when it was proposed to vaccinate some of the younger people at Pah Te Aro, the principal elders (for there are no chiefs there) made it a condition that, if I would submit to the operation first, they would allow the children to be treated as I wished. To this I consented'. Other nearby communities only 'partially submitted'.[166] Halswell probably cannot claim the entire credit for this breakthrough. In the same year Dr John FitzGerald of Wellington published a short pamphlet in Maori on the importance of smallpox vaccination.[167] To some extent this move backfired. Peter Wilson, Colonial Surgeon at New Plymouth, lamented the tone of this 'indiscreetly alarming account', which had created a 'singularly urgent anxiety to be vaccinated'. Panic had resulted in Maori self-vaccination, imperfectly administered. Wilson despaired of rectifying the 'prevalent conceit that they are duly qualified to vaccinate themselves'.[168]

Wilson's warning brought no immediate government response. Five years later, events in Britain prompted a revival in official interest. In 1853, England and Wales replaced the voluntary Vaccination Act of 1840 with legislation which required all infants to be vaccinated during the first three months of life. South Australia, Victoria, Tasmania and Western Australia introduced mandatory vaccination between 1853 and 1860, while the Queensland and New South Wales legislatures rejected such a move.[169]

New Zealand was slower to act, and did not introduce a general

Classes of Diseases.	Number of Cases presenting themselves for Treatment in an English Infirmary.	Number of Cases presenting themselves for Treatment in the New Zealand Hospitals.	Proportion among each Race; out of a Thousand Cases of Disease there were among the	
			English	New Zealanders
Fevers	390	190	20	74
Diseases of the lungs	2165	435	109	169
„ liver	228	—	12	—
„ stomach and bowels	1418	304	71	119
„ brain	1031	15	52	5
Dropsies	451	2	23	—
Rheumatic affections	2365	495	119	191
Venereal	86	99	4	38
Abscesses and ulcers	2195	278	111	108
Wounds and injuries	1952	89	92	34
Diseases of the eyes	703	91	35	35
„ skin	801	181	45	70
Scrofula	1173	210	59	82
Eruptive fevers	—	—	—	—
All other diseases	4908	191	248	75
Total	19,866	2580	1000	1000

A.S. Thomson's 1859 comparison of New Zealand data with that obtained from Sheffield Infirmary inpatients was the first attempt to quantify the state of Maori health. A higher incidence of categories such as fevers, lung disease (i.e. tuberculosis), digestive disorders and 'rheumatic affections' also featured in later assessments. *A.S. Thomson, The Story of New Zealand, p.323*

Vaccination Act until 1863.[170] A greater sense of urgency was evident in relation to Maori, however. In June 1854 Loughlin O'Brien (City of Auckland) proposed that Parliament appoint a 'Committee for Consideration of the Introduction of Vaccination amongst the Natives'. Just three weeks later the committee's report was ordered to be printed,[171] and before the end of the year the government acted on it by setting up a 'Central Board of Vaccination for the Aborigines of New Zealand'. The select committee's view that missionaries and colonial surgeons were best placed to undertake such work was reflected in the composition of the board. While neither the Roman Catholic nor Anglican Bishops of New Zealand accepted nomination, Jean Pompallier stressed that he was very keen on the 'preservation of the interesting and dear race of the Natives'. George Selwyn was more practical in his reponse, nominating George Kissling, who had conducted the 1852 Auckland Hospital inquiry, in his stead. Informing the Colonial Secretary of this, Kissling stated that he himself had already vaccinated hundreds and distributed lymph in pursuit of this goal. One of the most interesting communications came from Isaac Featherston, the Superintendent of Wellington Province. Keen to take advantage of Maori co-operation after a recent epidemic, he asked what proportion of the £500 set aside for this work would be allocated to Wellington.[172]

Little evidence as to the vaccination board's effectiveness is available. The medical members, who appear to have been largely Auckland-based, included coroners and those who held appointments at the hospital and gaol.[173] Arthur Thomson, one of the original members, suggested in 1859 that Maori were 'strongly predisposed' to smallpox, and considered it fortunate that around two-thirds of them had been vaccinated. He did not reveal how this figure had been arrived at, nor did he indicate how compliant Maori had been.[174]

In 1863 J.B. Tuke considered that smallpox and cholera posed a real danger to Maori, who 'not infrequently aggravate the disease, and often tacitly refuse to make themselves amenable to treatment'.[175] Despite this warning, smallpox vaccination was apparently shed by the Native Department in 1865 as part of a cost-cutting exercise; there is no evidence that it was assumed by any other agency.[176] With no obvious sign of smallpox in the colony during the 1860s, the reluctance of the authorities to continue vaccinating against it is understandable. Retrenchment also affected New Zealand as a whole. The Vaccination Act of 1863 empowered provincial superintendents to appoint medical officers as vaccinators for each district but made no provision for their payment. Although the government promised to change this in 1866, payments were not sanctioned until the

1871 Vaccination Act. This legislation also permitted the appointment as public vaccinators of suitable persons other than doctors, if this was approved by a medically qualified certifying officer.[177]

Individual doctors seem to have continued vaccinating, with or without official assistance. Matthew Scott's 1868 report on the physical condition of Wairoa Maori concluded: 'I might state that I consider the process of vaccination has been of incalculable advantage to the present generation of Maori children.' While not prepared to argue that vaccination was prophylactic or afforded protection against diseases other than smallpox, Scott did claim that it seemed 'to impart a vigour and stimulus to the [Maori] constitution which it did not naturally possess'.[178]

A threatened smallpox epidemic in 1872 revealed the absence of any administrative structure to facilitate the vaccination of Maori. The deficiency was highlighted by John Nicholson, one of the Kaipara NMOs whose services had been dispensed with in the mid 1860s. By the end of the decade Nicholson had been elected to the Auckland Provincial Council, acting as Provincial Secretary and Treasurer in 1869–70. In June 1872 he became principal vaccinator for the province. Anticipating the spread of smallpox to Maori, Nicholson decided to contact his professional brethren in districts 'contiguous to or occupied by Maoris'. He was heartened by their positive response, despite the lack of funds for vaccinating Maori, but was concerned at the lack of organisation. Tauranga provided an example. The Civil Commissioner in Auckland asked Nicholson to send supplies to one gentleman; Dr Daniel Pollen, Agent to the General Government, asked him to do likewise to another; the local authorities wished vaccine to be sent to a third; then Frederick Armitage, Surgeon to the Armed Constabulary stationed at Tauranga, whose name had not been mentioned by any of the others, wrote asking for a supply of lymph. As Nicholson wrote: 'This may possibly be regarded by you as showing the necessity for some controlling head for vaccination in the Province.'[179]

Whatever the bureaucratic defects, Nicholson's evidence bears testimony to widespread individual goodwill. More importantly, central government had taken steps to meet the smallpox threat even before Nicholson penned his report. On 18 July 1872 Alexander Mackay, Commissioner of Native Reserves for Nelson, wrote to the Native Minister enclosing a return of

820 cases treated by the Nelson and Marlborough NMOs in 1869–71, and acknowledging receipt of a circular urging vaccination due to the presence of smallpox in the colony.[180]

This vaccination programme was supervised by the resident magistrates. In at least one instance, that of Walter Harsant of Raglan, the magistrate acted in person while wearing his other hat as local medical officer.[181] Around the same time Herbert Brabant, the Resident Magistrate at Opotiki, reported that local Maori 'generally show a great desire for the services of European doctors in their illnesses'. They were also willing to submit to vaccination, provided he travelled to them. As a result Brabant had undertaken more than a thousand vaccinations. In addition, a considerable number of Maori had vaccinated one another. The quality of lymph was often a cause of concern at this time. Inadequate storage conditions and the poor technique of some public vaccinators could render the lymph unusable. This was probably the reason for Brabant advising the Native Department in 1873 that Urewera Maori had missed out on the vaccination campaign because his supply had failed.[182]

There are no reliable figures on the coverage or effectiveness of the early vaccination campaigns aimed at Maori. (The same, of course, is true of the European statistics for the period.) Nor do we have accurate estimates of the incidence of the disease. This was almost certainly negligible as smallpox was easily identifiable and any occurrence would have been reported. Of greater significance than any numerical record, however, is the record of government's reaction to the perceived danger, and the contrast with earlier events in Australia.

During the late 1820s and early 1830s smallpox broke out in the Aboriginal population of Australia. Modern accounts of this outbreak emphasise the complacency of colonists, who rarely came into contact with Aboriginals. Little was done to help the sufferers.[183] Official responses in New Zealand were far more proactive. Some of this can be explained by the very different circumstances of the two communities. Smallpox vaccine was more readily available from the 1840s than it had been in the 1820s. Another important factor was the belief in medical institutions and knowledge as tools of racial amalgamation.[184] Settler links with Maori were much closer than those between whites and Aboriginals. There is little evidence, however, that the vaccination campaign was driven by fear of cross-infection from Maori to European, a factor which helped fuel later concerns about Maori sanitation and susceptibility to infection.

Finally, the commitment to vaccinating Maori is one strand of evidence which suggests a need to review the 'dying pillow' forecast of future Maori extinction. The episode highlights some of the difficulties of interpreting comments on nineteenth century Maori health. It is probable that men such as Featherston could calmly discuss the demise of the race in the abstract while participating in practical measures to combat disease. The vaccination programme, though limited in scope, was indicative of a continuing concern for the health of the indigenous population.

2
'Open to Natives Equally' 1870–1900

This chapter begins with a summary of the funding and administrative changes which shaped the evolution of Maori health care in the last three decades of the nineteenth century. The hospital sector became increasingly directed towards European needs, with provision for Maori varying greatly between localities. The extent to which Maori made use of hospitals is difficult to quantify. The period also saw some consolidation and expansion of subsidised medical attendance, although this was far from uniform. The allocation of both services and personnel changed considerably over time, with an increasing emphasis on South Island communities. The final section examines initiatives relating to infectious diseases and environmental health.

Between 1858 and 1874 the Pakeha population of New Zealand increased from 59,000 to nearly 300,000. During the same period Maori were officially estimated to have declined in number from 56,000 to 47,000. By 1901 the respective figures were approximately 770,000 and 45,000.[1] Maori health was to some extent impaired by this influx of Europeans and the changes in lifestyle which followed. Pakeha responses to the resulting problems were more committed than has sometimes been recognised. Considerable effort was expended in the related fields of infectious disease, hospitals, medical services and health education, although constraints on medical knowledge and lack of funding limited the effectiveness of health personnel and bureaucrats.

'Existing machinery': administration and funding

No clear policy considerations seem to have guided the application of money from the annual £7,000 Civil List allocation and from Native Reserve trust funds to Maori health in this period. Political expediency appears to have been the most important factor, and the level of funding fluctuated accordingly. In 1871 the Civil List disbursement was £6,145, of which just £882 was expended on medical officers.[2] In most years until the late 1890s, spending on medical officers was less than £1,000.[3] This resulted in part from the many competing claims on the Civil List. In 1875, for instance, more than half of the £6,074 set aside for this purpose was used to pay the salaries of Native Department officials and the Taranaki Civil Commissioner, who received £650.[4] From the late 1870s Native Ministers were increasingly keen to ensure that their expenditure did not exceed the £7,000 allocated a quarter of a century previously. John Bryce took office in 1879 committed to a reduction to this level. Spending on contingencies over and above this sum, including medical care, was severely curtailed.[5] In 1879/80 total expenditure fell to £3,683 and the outlay on medical attendance and medicines to £552.[6] Such reductions may have been partly offset by the decline in the Maori population from around 47,000 in 1874 to just over 42,000 in 1896.

Most of Bryce's successors as Native Minister were equally keen to limit the sums devoted to health, by creative accounting or by other means. In 1887, for example, Edwin Mitchelson introduced fresh measures to keep spending below the designated £7,000. One was a circular issued to hospital and charitable aid boards in 1888, announcing that 'free medical attendance to indigent persons of the native race must in future be borne by the local bodies receiving subsidies from the Government'.[7] This directive urging local charitable bodies to regard destitute Maori in the same light as their European counterparts seems to have had only limited impact.[8] While the Otago Hospital Board minutes noted receipt of the circular without comment, it 'got short shrift from the Hawke's Bay Board'.[9]

When the Native Department was disbanded in 1893, responsibility for the areas covered by the Civil List passed to the Justice Department.[10] The transition led to a vigorous debate between government and opposition members about the administration of funds. Native Department head office salaries had been paid from the Civil List £7,000 for some two decades.[11] The Justice Department's intention to pay some of its head office staff from this source was challenged in September 1893 by the Western Maori MHR H.P.R. Taipua and his Northern Maori colleague, E.M. Kapa.[12] In addition to misusing these funds, Kapa complained, the government consistently refused to subsidise a doctor for a Far North Maori community whose nearest doctor lived two days' journey away.

The two Maori members were supported by a number of Pakeha colleagues. Robert Houston (Bay of Islands) confirmed that the Mangonui doctor, who received a subsidy, could offer little assistance to Kapa's constituents since the roads were impassable in bad weather, while the Kaitaia chemist, who was paid to supply medicines to Maori, lived 70 miles from Kapa's home. Taipua's allegations were endorsed by William Rolleston, who had been Native Minister briefly in 1881, while Robert Stout, who had been Premier from 1884 to 1887, accused the government of abusing trust funds.

Richard Seddon, the new Premier and Minister of Native Affairs, promised to look into the matter. The death of Premier John Ballance in April 1893 had left the Liberal government in a state of disarray. During the ensuing five months there were no fewer than four Native Ministers. Seddon, Ballance's successor, held the portfolio briefly in May and retrieved it in September. Having made their protest, Taipua and his colleagues apparently allowed the matter to lapse. Concerns over the allocation of the Civil List funds, however, would be revived in the following decades in a series of undignified squabbles between the Health Department and a reconstituted Native Department.

The transfer of Maori matters to the Justice Department in 1893 made little difference to overall funding, which continued to follow no clear pattern. While the Civil List outlay remained close to the theoretical figure of £7,000, a greater proportion was spent on medical provision. Over the next five years this figure was almost three times the £538 of 1892/3. It was never again to drop below £1,500, and from 1905 always exceeded £3,000 per annum.

The second source of funding for medical assistance to Maori in specific locations, most notably in Nelson and Marlborough, was Native Reserve trust funds. Setting aside Native Reserves to provide Maori with a guaranteed income was originally conceived by the New Zealand Company as a protection against the 'want of foresight' believed to be a common failing of aboriginal peoples.[13] Income from this source was commonly referred to as 'tenths'. Implementation of the scheme during the 1850s was haphazard, for Governor Grey was allegedly 'capricious' in allocating Crown land as Maori reserves.[14] Matters were not helped by poor record keeping and the fact that Grey later 'declined to remember' what he had ordered concerning the Otago tenths. Low population density also contributed to the logistical problems of implementing any social welfare structures. In 1865 the Native Minister noted the impossibility of providing clergy, schools and hospitals for every community of a dozen inhabitants and urged Maori to congregate in one place, where these could be supplied.[15]

Alexander Mackay, Native Commissioner in Nelson, did his best in the 1860s and 1870s to use income from these sources to provide education and medicine.[16] Fluctuations in the annual expenditure from both the Civil List and the Native Reserves make it impossible to be precise about the relative importance of the two funds. In the early 1880s, however, when annual returns were published, the outlay from reserve funds on doctors and medicines was equivalent to somewhere between 10 and 20 per cent of the Civil List total—a significant sum considering the small populations involved. In the main, the money was used to fund subsidised doctors at a number of upper South Island locations.[17] The uneven distribution of funding for Maori health care would later cause headaches for Health Department officials charged with administering medical subsidies.

'Practically shut out'?: Maori and hospitals

New Zealand's hospital system underwent both a major expansion and significant change between 1860 and 1900. From 1852 to 1876 hospitals were controlled by the provincial governments, and from 1877 to 1885 they were overseen by central government under what Julius Vogel described as 'the present hybrid system'.[18] The Hospitals and Charitable Institutions Act 1885 established a system of hospital administration based on local hospital boards.[19]

One of the major changes in this period related to the ethnic composition of the patient base. The rapid increase in the European population from the 1860s brought the earlier relative equality of treatment to an end and changed the ethos and function of New Zealand's hospital system. It has been claimed that 'The early spatial pattern of health care provision was characterized by private hospital development near the goldmines and largest settlements of the South Island, and public hospital establishment in North Island settlements with a large Maori population'.[20] The perception of a two-tier structure is mistaken, although it is true that henceforth health care for Maori was no longer their primary focus. All hospitals became funded by a mixture of government subsidies, local or hospital authority rates, voluntary contributions and patient payments.[21] Maori might or might not be involved in this funding process.

The utility of hospital services for Maori had been clearly established during the 1850s. At the end of the decade consideration was given to expanding the network beyond the five existing hospitals at Auckland, Wellington, New Plymouth, Wanganui and Dunedin. In April 1859 the new Hawke's Bay Province asked the Colonial Secretary to assist in the establishment of a general hospital at Napier 'for the reception of Native as well as European patients.' Nothing came of the proposal.[22]

Total Public Hospital Income 1886–1910

(in £ sterling, percentages in brackets)

	A	B	C	D	Total
1886–1890	119,294 (39.22)	108,212 (35.58)	27,221 (8.95)	27,177 (8.93)	304,167
1890–1895	160,132 (40.61)	122,148 (30.98)	36,530 (9.26)	49,625 (12.59)	394,289
1895–1900	205,526 (40.21)	160,816 (31.46)	52,949 (10.36)	65,844 (12.89)	511,159
1900–1905	276,389 (38.96)	215,746 (30.41)	64,335 (9.07)	96,676 (13.63)	709,355
1905–1910	414,560 (38.94)	326,734 (30.69)	86,303 (8.11)	144,197 (13.55)	1,064,509

The four categories, adapted from tables printed in the *AJHR*, are: A: government; B: local and hospital authorities; C: voluntary contributions; D: patient payments. The balance of the total consisted of rents and unspecified other income.

The eruption of hostilities between the government and Taranaki Maori in 1860 encouraged the kind of backlash exemplified by Dillon Bell's dismissal in 1848 of Maori hospital services as an absurd waste of money. In May 1862 William Fox, Premier for the previous ten months, instructed James Armitage, Civil Commissioner for the Waikato, that such matters as 'your own place of residence, the erection of a gaol, Court-houses, Hospital, and other objects in which the whole district may have a common interest, had better be postponed till the meeting of the general District Runanga.'[23] Fox's decision was primarily dictated by settler antagonism, and within three months he had resigned, disheartened by a perceived lack of support for his Maori policy.[24]

Racial tension adversely influenced events in some parts of the colony. Waikato Maori gave land at Te Awamutu in 1862 for a long promised 'Native' hospital, only to see the proposal abandoned when the town was evacuated in April 1863.[25] Attorney-General Henry Sewell attempted to implement the returned Governor Grey's 'Plan of Native Government' in the Bay of Plenty, specifically to provide funds for 'some kind of hospital [for Maori] at Rotorua'. His rationale was both clinical and political. The Rotorua waters were believed to possess special medicinal properties; and the 'earnestness and sincerity of the Government would be well shown by giving the natives the benefit of medical aid in so populous a locality'.[26]

Grey's gesture was not entirely philanthropic. As Civil Commissioner T.H. Smith reminded Sewell in January 1862, following a runanga at Te Rotoiti which united the hapu of Ngati Pikiao and Ngati Tarawhai, local Maori had ceded land to the government in 1850 as an endowment for a hospital. Participants in the runanga expressed the hope that the hospital would be built on this land, 'and a medical man appointed'.[27] Their expectations were not fulfilled; Rotorua did not obtain a hospital until the government sanatorium opened in 1886, and its King George V Hospital was not erected until 1916.[28]

Grey's promise of seed-funding for a Rotorua hospital was in line with his intention that Maori self-government, under the intended runanga system, would be largely self-funded. Henry Halse, the acting Native Secretary, explained this approach in a letter of 26 March 1862 to Taupo's Resident Magistrate: 'the Natives must be made to understand that in establishing Schools, and like Institutions, the Government is not prepared to do more than commence the work.' Maori would be expected to sustain operations.[29] While this goal might have been feasible in relation to Maori schools, it was impractical in terms of a hospital system which from the outset was designed to meet both Maori and European needs. The concept of a Maori-only hospital was never implemented (a point discussed further in chapter 3).

The importance of hospital care was stressed in 1863 by Dr J.B. Tuke. He described the impossibility of issuing more than a single dose of medicine to Maori patients, as they usually either swallowed it all or distributed it among family and friends. Tuke believed that only a hospital, where remedies were dispensed in proper doses and at regular intervals, could be effective. Institutional cleanliness and regular habits offered the best hope for apparently hopeless cases.[30] Other contemporary observations throw doubt on the feasibility of this suggestion. In 1864 Nelson's Provincial Surgeon, Foord Wilson, drew attention to the small number of tuberculosis patients admitted to Nelson Hospital and speculated that the incidence of the disease must be much higher among Maori, 'who are not very willing to avail themselves of hospital treatment'.[31]

As has already been noted, it is difficult to obtain accurate data on Maori use of hospitals from the 1850s. Nevertheless, there is evidence of a decline in the proportion of care devoted to Maori. In the mid 1850s Europeans had made extensive use of outpatient facilities at the 'Natives' Hospital' in Wanganui because of a lack of local general practitioners. During the 1860s, however, Europeans came to dominate inpatient treatment. Though Maori outpatients outnumbered Pakeha in 1865 by 51 to 18, there were only 31 Maori inpatients compared with 54 Pakeha.[32] Between March and December 1867 Wanganui admitted 58 inpatients, only four of whom were Maori. The remainder comprised 38 Pakeha paupers, thirteen paying patients and three military personnel.[33]

The changing balance between Maori and European in the early 1860s can to some extent be accounted for by the fighting which disrupted both communications and normal hospital services. The severity of war injuries among hospitalised Maori probably discouraged others from seeking admission. After the battle of Te Ranga in 1864, for instance, fourteen wounded Maori prisoners died in the military hospital at Te Papa, near Tauranga.[34] Even when the fighting was over, occasional deaths in custody perhaps heightened antipathy to hospitals. In 1871/2, for instance, Dunedin Hospital's high death rate was attributed to the inclusion of thirteen Chinese with beriberi, several 'moribund' accident cases, and seven Maori prisoners who had been transferred from the local gaol.[35] Incidents of this kind have led to the conclusion that 'Hospitals had a bad name among Maori: they were thought of as places where one went to die.'[36]

Other factors originating within the Maori community had a bearing on Maori willingness to enter hospital and the success or otherwise of the outcome. The most important of these was the role of tohunga. In 1872 William Mair, then a Native Department 'official correspondent' at Alexandra (now Pirongia) in the Waikato, informed his Under-Secretary that arrangements were in place to erect a hospital 'whenever they choose to bring their sick'. Mair had obtained the services of a medical officer but was not sanguine of success, since 'as a rule it is only when a case is hopelessly given up by their own "tohunga" that they will place a patient in proper hands'.[37] The following year Mair wrote to the Native Minister about the difficulty of persuading Maori to make the best use of the services on offer: 'They do not object to medical attendance at their own homes, but, like their brethren elsewhere, will not take the trouble to bring their sick to hospital.'[38] Mair's comment ignored the very real difficulties facing prospective patients. The Alexandra hospital proposal, like the earlier Te Awamutu venture, was never implemented. No hospital was erected in the Waikato until 1887; the nearest hospitals in 1872 were at Auckland, Thames and New Plymouth.[39]

Mair's concerns were echoed by other Native Department officials. Hopkins Clarke, Native Officer in Tauranga, complained in 1875 that Maori often delayed bringing patients to hospital until the 'Maori doctor' had exhausted his repertoire, by which time the patient was 'past all hope'.[40] Another who spoke out on more than one occasion was R.S. Bush, Resident Magistrate at Opotiki. Bush's ire at the 'foolish conduct' of the Whakatohea people during a typhoid epidemic in 1883 spilled over in his report to the Under-Secretary. He argued that hospitalisation, with a sufficient complement of attendants, was the only way to ensure compliance with the doctor's instructions.[41] Three years later Bush made the point even more forcefully. A chief suffering from pleurisy had discharged himself into the care of a tohunga and returned to the Pakeha doctor only when

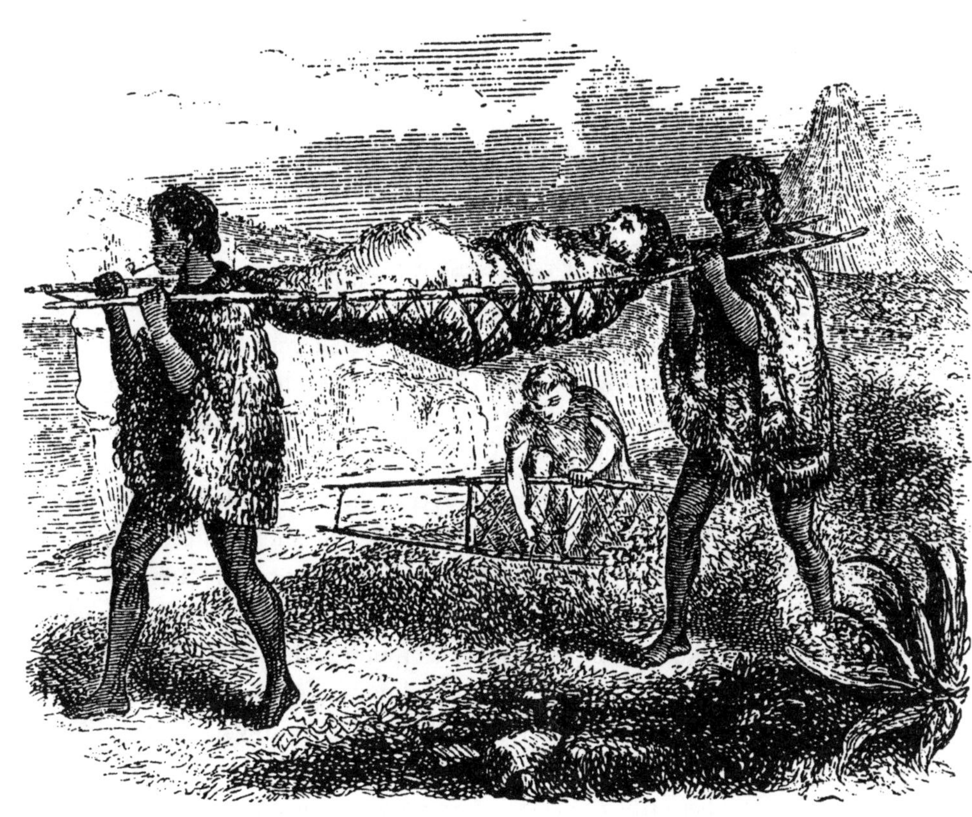

This 1859 engraving of a 'Native litter for the conveyance of the sick and wounded' demonstrates how Maori were transported over considerable distances to seek medical help. *A.S. Thomson, The Story of New Zealand, p.129*

on the verge of death. He had, claimed Bush, 'really killed himself'. It is questionable whether Western medicine would have made any difference in this instance, but Bush's solution was the same as that proposed by Tuke and others over the years: 'It appears to me that little or nothing can be done for Natives in this way unless they can be placed in a hospital and thus compelled to obey the doctor; otherwise it is labour in vain.'[42]

Such a policy was simple to formulate but impossible to implement. Patients could not be compelled to undergo treatment. On the other side of the equation, the government had no power to force hospitals to admit patients, and with the expanding settler population the majority of hospitals were increasingly geared towards treating Pakeha. In the end, Maori presence in hospitals depended upon a multiplicity of local factors. The claim that most hospitals in the 1880s were too small or too far from centres of Maori population to accommodate Maori patients offers only a partial explanation for their absence.[43]

Almost half of the hospitals opened between 1861 and 1900 were established to serve the needs of the goldfields. Their size, and in some cases their relatively rapid decline, was determined by the transient mining population. But lack of size does not appear to have been a factor in determining use by Maori; smaller hospitals within reach of Maori seem to have been more rather than less willing to accept Maori patients.

Evidence for the last quarter of the nineteenth century is, like that for the previous two decades, patchy and in many ways contradictory. In 1877 H.T. Kemp, then Civil Commissioner for Auckland, commented that Maori desired to become inmates of the colonial hospital only 'in extreme cases'.[44] He defined neither the number of such instances nor what constituted an extreme case. In New Plymouth two years later, the medical officer and his medicines were popular but 'in no case will they go into hospital, looking upon it as almost certain death, and preferring to die at their own places'.[45] Herbert Brabant, Tauranga's Resident Magistrate, was just as vague as Kemp in his report for 1879/80, stating baldly that 'hospital comforts' were accorded Maori when necessary.[46]

Under the terms of an 1872 Crown grant, Wanganui's public hospital was to treat 'all races'.[47] Yet the admission of a Maori patient in July 1876 prompted the *Wanganui Chronicle* to note that it had been 'some considerable time since any of the aboriginal race have received treatment at this institution'.[48] Some months later, Wanganui's Resident Magistrate R.W. Woon revealed the reason for this situation. Thanking the Under-Secretary of the Native Department for supplying Native School teachers with medicines, Woon stressed the importance of this 'liberal response', since Maori were 'practically shut out of the Wanganui Hospital, an institution originally endowed and set apart for their special benefit'.[49] The development typifies the kind of impasse that could exist between central and local health administration.

Relations were more co-operative in some parts of the country. An 1877 newspaper appeal to raise funds for a 'Hawke's Bay hospital' specifically invited Maori to contribute on the basis this would create a friendlier feeling between the two races. It was hoped they would provide land rather than money. Local Maori undertook to contribute to the hospital Sunday Fund, a common means of community fundraising. Napier Hospital opened its doors in mid 1880, but the extent to which Maori were involved in its establishment is unclear. In 1885, however, the hospital's visiting committee drew attention to the urgent need to construct 'the Maori ward and fever ward, as we consider delay in this matter is likely to lead to very serious results'.[50]

The concept of a hospital facility exclusively for Maori was carried a stage further when John Ballance, Native Minister in the Stout–Vogel government, undertook an extensive tour of the North Island to hear Maori grievances on the eve of the passage of the Hospitals and Charitable Institutions Act 1885. At Mokoia Island on Lake Rotorua he told his audience what medical assistance they might expect from the state. In return for ceding the township lands of Ohinemutu to permit the extension of Rotorua, local Maori would be provided with a hospital free of charge. The offer, however, was not unconditional. Ballance emphasised the facility would be reserved for 'dangerous and serious' cases only. He added a further condition during a meeting the next day with Tuhourangi Maori, stating that they themselves must provide transport to and from hospital: 'We think they should do that, considering that the Government has gone to great expense in providing treatment for people who are dangerously ill.'[51]

No evidence confirming the existence of this proposed hospital has been found. Instead, Maori were to share in the development of Rotorua's thermal resources. On 5 March 1885, within weeks of Ballance's visit, the Inspector-General of Hospitals announced plans 'to erect two additional "Priest's" baths on the shore of the lake, where a good deal of hot water now runs to waste. One of these will be set aside for the Maoris, in accordance with the terms of their agreement.'[52] Eight years later his successor commented on the relatively high salary paid to the Rotorua Sanatorium medical officer. This was due to 'the difficulty of inducing a good man to remain in such an isolated place all the year round, whose services should be available for the general public and for the Natives'.[53] Decades later, Te Arawa people received free medical care in the King George V Hospital. The concept of a 'Maori hospital' would be revived, though not implemented, in the early twentieth century.

Such local arrangements in return for co-operation on land issues echoed earlier events in the South Island. In May 1887 Alexander Mackay told the Native Minister that during the 1860s Ngai Tahu had been offered schools and hospitals to compensate in some measure for the unfulfilled pledges given when their lands were ceded in the 1840s and 1850s, with the promise that such institutions would not have to wait until 'the requirements of the European community rendered them necessary'.[54] A committee investigating Middle Island Native Claims in 1889 concluded that separate hospitals had never been provided for Ngai Tahu 'but that the public hospitals are open to Natives equally with Europeans'.[55] This conclusion was based, it appears, on the flimsiest of evidence.

The committee's principal informant was T.W. Lewis, Under-Secretary of the Native Department from 1879 to 1891. Although he had been associated with the Department for some twenty years, Lewis was either remarkably ill-informed or reticent almost to the point of silence. Questioned about the existence of any 'Native hospitals' in the South Island, he replied that he had asked the Inspector-General whether Natives availed themselves of hospitals. When pressed for a more specific answer he could not say if this usage was large or limited. He then tried to deflect questions to 'some hospital authority' on the grounds that officially he knew nothing about the hospitals. All attempts by the committee to obtain hard information were met by similar stonewalling tactics. Asked if Maori were so prejudiced against European hospitals that 'hospital accommodation [was] comparatively useless to them', he responded: 'I have heard so; but the Natives do use the hospitals occasionally.' Unable to quantify this, Lewis could only add that he had found 'at least four Natives in hospitals in the Middle Island; he thought there were more'.[56] The most charitable view of Lewis's performance is that it reflected the quality of contemporary information about Maori use of hospitals.

From 1882 the Inspector-General of Hospitals was required to make at least one visit per year to each of the colony's hospitals and report his findings. His occasional comments on Maori use of hospital facilities, coupled with the meagre details in annual patient returns, provide some clues about Maori admissions.[57] From 1883 these returns provided a breakdown by sex, religion and 'country'. The last category was never consistently defined. Some hospitals identified Maori or 'New Zealand Maori'; others included classifications for 'natives' or 'aboriginals' or 'aboriginal natives', and 'half castes'. Few hospitals reported more than a handful of Maori patients each year. In most, if the returns are to be believed, fewer than 5 per cent of patients were Maori. Some of the largest hospitals, such as Auckland and Christchurch, did not submit returns. At Wellington, the colony's biggest hospital, the figure for Maori was consistently under 1 per cent.[58] Dunedin rarely furnished details of Maori patients, but occasional comments in the hospital board minutes indicate their existence. On 14 May 1902, for instance, it was noted that 'An ex-patient named J Miller (a Maori) sent a donation of fish &c for use of the hospital'.[59]

Published figures suggest that some hospitals, particularly smaller ones, manipulated Maori patient numbers to justify the protection, consolidation or expansion of facilities. On the one hand, hospital administrators repeatedly expressed concern about chronic or incurable cases who occupied beds for an extended period, linking this to the spectre of pauperisation.[60] Some smaller hospitals, however, were willing to admit Maori patients to help ensure their viability. For example, in 1882 the Inspector-General, Dr George Grabham, reported that the eight-bed Greytown Hospital's 'other cottage can be utilized as a fever-hospital, but has been occupied for ten months by a Maori boy, who has a severe gunshot wound of the knee. His whole family appear to have taken up their residence here.'[61] Four years later Grabham still adhered to his previously-expressed view that the hospital, however well conducted, 'could well be dispensed with'.[62]

The rate of Maori admissions to such small hospitals far exceeded the average. At Coromandel only two out of 30 patients were Maori in 1888; by the time new buildings were erected in 1898 ten of the 78 patients came into this category, and in 1903 'aboriginals' comprised 21 of the 94 admissions.[63] Two years later, the Inspector-General revealed that 'The township is going downhill, and altogether the Hospital is in a bad way financially'.[64] There was no indication that the high proportion of Maori patients had contributed to these financial woes. The extent to which the hospital had survived and expanded because it attracted Maori patients is unclear.

At Wairoa on the East Coast a hospital was opened about 1897 as an offshoot of Napier Hospital. The geographical isolation of this institution was graphically illustrated by the Inspector-General's explanation in 1900 that he had not visited Wairoa 'because of the danger of too long a detention,

Foundation Dates of New Zealand Hospitals 1847–1909

name	date	name	date
Auckland	1847	Patea	1876
Wellington	1847	Akaroa	1877?
New Plymouth	1848	Riverton (Wallace & Fiord)	1877
Wanganui	1851	Blenheim (Wairau)	1878
Dunedin	1852	Waipawa	1878
Nelson	1853	Arrowtown	1879?
Invercargill (Southland)	1861	Masterton	1879
Christchurch	1862	Ashburton	1880
Lawrence (Tuapeka)	1862	Napier	1880
Dunstan	1863	Waikato	1887
Queenstown (Wakatipu)	1863	Palmerston North	1893
Timaru	1864	Hawera	1894
Hokitika (Westland)	1865	Wairoa	1897?
Picton	1865	Mercury Bay	1898
Ross	1865?	Otaki	1899
Greymouth (Grey River)	1866	Whangarei	1901
Charleston	1867	Pahiatua	1902
Westport (Buller)	1868	Northern Wairoa (Te Kopuru)	1903
Thames	1869	Waihi	1903
Naseby	1872	Rawene	1905
Oamaru	1872	Dannevirke	1906
Reefton	1872	Havelock	1906?
Coromandel	1873?	Mangonui	1907
Waimate	1874	Stratford	1907
Cromwell	1875	Waiapu (Te Puia Springs)	1907
Greytown (South Wairarapa)	1875	Kaitangata	1909
Gisborne (Cook)	1876	Taumarunui	1909?
Kumara	1876	Gore	1909

Dates derived from official and other sources

owing to the uncertainty of communication and the consequent disproportionate expense'. During the 1897/8 year the new venture admitted eleven 'Natives' and 26 Europeans. For 1898/9 the respective figures were fourteen and 29, and for 1899/1900 ten and 30.[65]

Any firm conclusions on the dynamics of hospital care for Maori await a detailed analysis of admission patterns. These examples, representative of a larger sample, seem to indicate that Maori were often more visible in those marginal hospitals whose continued existence was open to question. These institutions had opened to meet the needs of expanding European communities in the more distant rural reaches rather than to provide care for Maori, but it appears that settlers and Maori discovered a greater degree of interdependence than did their counterparts in the less remote corners of the colony.

Margaret Tennant has claimed that the increasingly localised funding and management of social services encouraged settlers to adopt the stance that as Maori paid no local rates they 'had no entitlement to hospital and relief services financed partly, at least, from such sources'.[66] In some instances this attitude was intensified by a rise in the number of Maori seeking admission. At Waikato Hospital, opened in 1887, the board argued that Maori land should be rated to provide it with an income sufficient to treat indigent Maori under the 1888 Native Department instruction.[67] This debate was one which would intensify in the twentieth century.

The interaction between Maori and hospitals in the latter decades of the nineteenth century presents a complex and varied picture. Some Pakeha actively discouraged Maori participation, for a variety of reasons. On the other hand, many Maori became disillusioned with Western medicine, or were discouraged by opposition from Europeans. Hospitals were often thought to be exclusively for the treatment of Pakeha illnesses, and to be run by people who were disdainful of Maori beliefs. However, the claim that Maori regarded hospitals as places to die is an over-simplification. While this was true of many Maori, others actively sought hospital treatment; some were persuaded to do so by doctors or Native Department officials.

Conclusions remain tentative, but there appears to have been no uniformity of view or approach, either geographically or over time. Some Maori in some regions made use of hospitals at least some of the time; others missed out, either deliberately or involuntarily. A number of factors contributed to these outcomes: tensions between Maori and Pakeha during the 1860s resulting in active hostilities; the uncertainties of the political system; the lack of a strong lead from central government. In the light of all these variables it is hardly surprising that modern observers cannot discern any clear government policy towards Maori and hospitals in the second half of the nineteenth century.

'Medical comforts': subsidised doctors

The last three decades of the nineteenth century saw a significant rise in the number of European doctors resident in New Zealand. The 181 names in the first medical register of 1869 were eclipsed by the 504 who appeared in 1900. This rise, however, failed to keep pace with population growth. In 1874 there was one doctor for each 1,391 residents; in 1901 the ratio was 1:1,863. The geographical distribution remained fairly constant. Between 1871 and 1901 36 to 38 per cent of all doctors practised in the four main urban centres, while 33 to 35 per cent were located in small towns and rural areas.[68] The number of rural doctors increased from 66 in 1871 to 172 in 1901. It was these rural practitioners who continued to offer services to Maori through subsidised medical attendance.

Donald McLean, the Native Minister from 1869 to 1876, has been credited with establishing within this portfolio area what was essentially a mini-government. Based on a core of resident magistrates, this operated in the spheres of justice, police and education, and supplied medical and economic assistance to Maori. These magistrates have been praised for their 'significant achievement' in restoring the network of subsidised doctors, which had been cut back by McLean's predecessor, Russell.[69] McLean appointed 'about' 24 Native Medical Officers (NMOs) to Maori districts in the early 1870s, 'and required of them regular circuits and monthly reports'.[70] These reports provide an indication of how doctors operated in what was essentially an ad hoc system.

The most striking feature of the NMO scheme was its uneven coverage. The 'Nominal Roll of the Civil Establishment of New Zealand' named eighteen NMOs in 1875. Seven were located in the South Island; five served in Nelson and Marlborough, and one each in Otago and Canterbury. Another seven were to be found north of Wellington and in the coastal communities between the capital and New Plymouth. Waikato had two doctors, at Raglan and Cambridge; there was one at Wairoa (Hawke's Bay) and only one north of Auckland, at Russell.[71] Yet only some 4 per cent of Maori lived in the South Island in 1874, compared with 15 per cent in Waikato, 13 per cent in Hawke's Bay and 18 per cent in Northland.[72]

There is no comprehensive index of NMOs, and no list of names seems to have been published in the decade after 1875. In April 1885 the Under-Secretary of the Native Department issued a circular to fifteen NMOs calling for a report on the sanitary condition of the Maori population; it is not clear if these were all the NMOs. They were located at Mangonui, Hokianga, Waimate North, Thames, Tauranga, Rotorua, Galatea, Wairoa

(Hawke's Bay), Napier, New Plymouth, Wanganui, Hutt (Wellington), Kaikoura, Kaiapoi and Port Chalmers. Not all possessed medical qualifications. Although designated as medical officers, the three based at Hokianga, Waimate North and Wairoa were unqualified 'native dispensers'.[73]

Probably the most accurate source for the later part of the century is the Audit Office salary registers held at National Archives in Wellington.[74] Unfortunately the quality of information varies from volume to volume. Dispensers were not differentiated from doctors in the nineteen names given for the period 1888–91, and there were few particulars of dates of appointment or resignation. The register detailed annual salaries ranging from £8 for one of the 'native dispensers' to a maximum of £50. Most received either £25 or £30.

The register for 1891–4 contained a reduced number of appointees (thirteen in total), divided almost equally between the North and South Islands. The volume for 1894–7 revealed a major expansion, following the transfer of responsibility from the Native Department to the Justice Department. Most of these new appointments dated from 1895–6. By this time there were 27 NMOs, thirteen in the South Island. The enlarged South Island complement during the early 1890s included Kaiapoi, Little River, Temuka, Moeraki, and Riverton. These were supplemented between 1894 and 1897 by additional posts at Kaikoura, Rapaki and Port Levy, Waimate, Oamaru, Palmerston South, Henley, Balclutha and Bluff.

In 1901 South Island iwi still constituted only 6 per cent of the Maori population. The repercussions from this uneven distribution of medical provision between the North and South Islands lasted well into the new century. The imbalance was accentuated by the appointments made by the Nelson Native Reserve Fund, which administered revenue from the rents of Native Reserves in Nelson and Marlborough. The first five doctors recruited under this scheme had taken up office at Takaka, Motueka, Nelson, Wairau and Queen Charlotte Sound in July 1864.[75] Their positions continued to be funded from the Reserve Fund throughout the nineteenth and into the twentieth century. A smaller sum from the Greymouth Native Reserve Fund paid for a medical presence in that region.[76] In his evidence to the Middle Island Native Claims Commission of 1889, T.W. Lewis denied any Native Department knowledge of these activities, stating they fell within the domain of the Public Trustee, not his Department. Lewis was able, nevertheless, to supply names and dates of tenure for sixteen medical officers who had held appointments in Canterbury, Otago and Southland between 1848 and 1889.[77]

Native Department records help explain some of the discrepancies between regions. The complexity of the issues revealed in this official correspondence makes it difficult to ascertain how the Native Department set its priorities. Some of the considerations which determined the operation of the system are outlined below.

The first of these factors was the role of the Resident Magistrate or Native Agent, the mainstay of the departmental infrastructure in the 1870s and 1880s. The attitudes of individual staff could prove crucial in determining whether a particular locality received the benefit of a subsidised doctor. Resident magistrates furnished annual reports on Maori social and economic conditions in their localities from the early 1870s until 1893, when the institution was abolished. These reports were tabled in Parliament and many were published in the *Appendix to the Journals of the Houses of Representatives*. Criticisms and suggestions were thus subject to parliamentary and public scrutiny. On occasion these accounts were surprisingly frank, though more contentious issues were generally restricted to the magistrates' unpublished correspondence with head office.

In 1871 Herbert Brabant, Clerk to the Bench in Raglan, described the health of Maori in his district and commented on the Raglan NMO's contribution during an epidemic some three years previously.[78] By 1873 Brabant had been promoted to Resident Magistrate for the Bay of Plenty. One of his first reports noted: 'The Natives generally show a great desire for the services of European doctors in their illnesses, and I doubt not derive benefit from the medical attendance and drugs provided for them by the Government'.[79] The following year Brabant claimed that such attendance had saved many lives.[80] Senior officials did not always agree with this viewpoint. Under-Secretary Lewis was especially sceptical in 1886 about the value of medical attention: 'A sort of craze has taken Maories of late to have an unlimited supply of doctors and medicine—to, I am sure, the great detriment of their health.'[81]

Maori requests for medical attendance were a second factor in deciding the location of subsidised doctors. Officials generally attempted to assess requests objectively and to deal with the problems of over-servicing and of areas with changing needs. In February 1885 Native Minister John Ballance met a deputation of Hauraki Maori to discuss their application for a government medical officer at Coromandel. Ballance declined to act, on the grounds that the combination of good climate and strong constitutions meant the services of the previous incumbent had been rarely needed, and the government felt it 'not worth while to pay him £25 a year for doing next to nothing'.[82]

In the following year the Maori of Rapaki near Lyttelton applied for a government doctor since all three local practitioners had recently died.[83] The ensuing Native Department correspondence illustrates the complexity of the issues that had to be worked through. T.W. Lewis initially informed Native Commissioner Alexander Mackay that it was impossible to provide every small settlement with a doctor. Mackay then explained that the region contained two settlements which had received medical attendance for a good many years. He believed the combined population of 118, according to the 1881 census, justified an appointment. Asked to verify Mackay's statement, another of Lewis's officials calculated that 129 Maori resided in the district. He could find no trace of any central government payment to a medical man at Rapaki, although William Donald (one of the three deceased doctors) might have received something from the provincial government.[84] After reviewing other South Island districts which already employed subsidised doctors and discovering that their services were rarely called upon, Lewis and the Minister vetoed the Rapaki proposal. The claimants persisted, backed by the Member for Southern Maori, T.H. Parata. The campaign finally bore fruit in June 1897 with the appointment of Dr Thomas Pairman as NMO for Rapaki and Port Levy.[85]

Successful applications were sometimes determined by ad hoc reactions to specific incidents, with outcomes that were not always satisfactory. In 1879 an outbreak of fever at Little River on Banks Peninsula brought an 'urgent request' from Maori residents that government engage a medical man to attend them. 'Loud in their praises' of his treatment, they nevertheless disregarded his instructions when he departed.[86] Partly as a result of this attitude, there were 23 deaths during the epidemic.[87] The doctor in charge was John Guthrie, a former Christchurch Hospital Medical Superintendent, who had moved to Akaroa in 1877. In order to settle

Guthrie's large claim for attendance, the Native Department made him NMO for the district. This strategy was misguided: 'After his appointment the health of the natives so much improved that his duties became very small almost nil.' In the long term the cost of the retainer paid to Guthrie outweighed any savings made by appointing him as NMO in lieu of payment on a fee for service basis for his efforts during the epidemic. As a result, Under-Secretary Lewis recommended that no replacement be appointed when Guthrie moved back to Christchurch in 1882. He later commented ruefully on the considerable expense that had been incurred because of the decision to appoint Guthrie.[88]

Once committed to a particular location, officials often found it hard to resist calls for a continued presence. By 1890 Little River Maori were so well integrated with their European neighbours that the Education Department decided to close the local Native School.[89] Despite this, the Native Department considered appointing a new NMO for Wairewa. Initial discussions with Dr William Fisher of Akaroa foundered when he rejected the proposed subsidy as totally inadequate.[90] The proposal then lay dormant for more than three years until Parata raised the matter in the House.[91] Within months Fisher accepted a salary of £50, twice the original offer. He retained the position for only a year, after which there was a hiatus until he was succeeded in April 1896 by Wilhelm Morris, a young German-trained doctor.

The third consideration in the appointment of subsidised medical staff was the availability of doctors to undertake this work. William Bertram White, who had been Resident Magistrate for Mangonui since the late 1840s, approached the Native Minister in 1872 with a request from Maori that the government subsidise a medical man: 'Mr Trimnell, it is true, is farming at Pukepoto, but he will not attend to medical practice except he receives a very high fee, and is very inattentive; consequently, he is beyond the reach of the inhabitants.'[92] Thomas Trimnell, though reluctant, was at least accessible; many communities did not even have this option. In June 1874 the Waiapu Resident Magistrate highlighted the need for a resident medical man, 'there being none between Turanga and Opotiki, a distance of 200 miles'.[93] Special circumstances sometimes facilitated such appointments. In 1879 Herbert Brabant sought a government subsidy to attract a 'man of ability' to Ohinemutu, where the Maori were 'very desirous' of obtaining a resident doctor. On this occasion the wish was granted, with the appointment of Thomas Lewis under the Thermal Springs Act.[94] The decision may have owed more to the cession of Ohinemutu township and to the commercial opportunities offered by the local spas than it did to Brabant's appeal.[95]

The problem of attracting affordable doctors was eased or removed in many remote areas by the expansion of European settlement. At Thames, for example, Native Department officials enjoyed a buyer's market in the 1870s and 1880s due to the presence of a substantial medical community attracted by the new goldfields. Martin Payne, whose appointment as NMO dated from 1874, found himself subject in 1882 to the threat of competitive tendering by another local practitioner. While Under-Secretary Lewis claimed to be unhappy about this development, he used it as a lever to reduce the salary on offer before appointing Payne's rival. The gain was short-lived, for the new appointee left Thames in disgrace shortly afterwards. Payne was restored to his former position, but at the reduced salary.

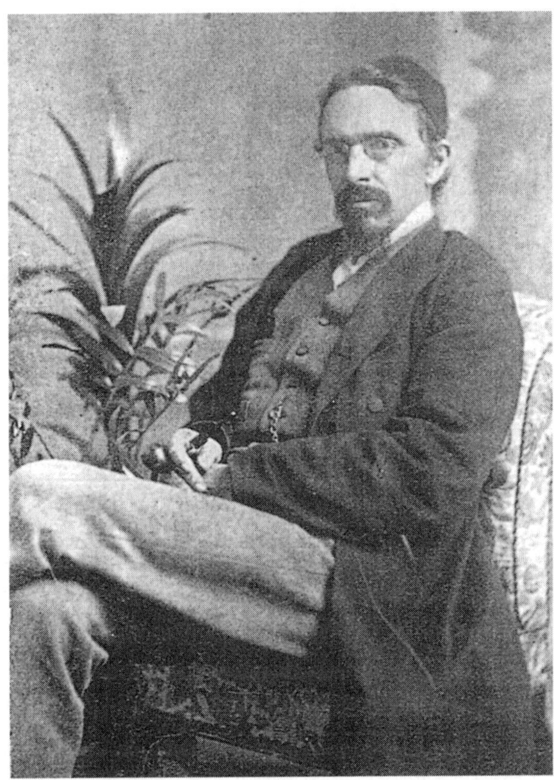

Martin Henry Payne LRCPEd LSA MRCS. The 1889 Maori petitioners claimed that 'Peina' had been 'most attentive to his Maori patients when he was our own doctor'. *J.E. Macdonald, Thames Reminiscences, p.25*

Eventually this policy of erosion forced his resignation, with Payne complaining bitterly that a proposed further reduction in his salary would barely cover the cost of medicines, let alone medical attendance. Despite a petition from local Maori for his reinstatement, the vacancy remained unfilled, which seems to have been the real aim of the exercise.[96]

Whatever the potential drawbacks of dealing with the Native Department bureaucracy, some doctors were eager to obtain the title of NMO. Alfred Perkins, surgeon to Patea Hospital since 1887, reported to the Native Minister in March 1889 that he had been unanimously chosen by local Maori as their medical adviser. He therefore wished the Minister to consult the community before proceeding with the rumoured appointment of a government medical officer.[97] His expectations were dashed. The only appointment made in the region between New Plymouth and Wanganui during the following decade was the replacement in 1895 of Robert Earle as NMO for Wanganui by George Saunders.

The fourth element to be taken into account before appointing an NMO was the question of cost. Depression in the early 1880s caused both officials and politicians to look for ways to service Maori health needs for a minimal outlay. Captain Porter of Gisborne suggested to Lewis in 1881 that it should be feasible to establish a network of 'proper medical officers' without imposing on the colonial revenue. He proposed that Maori be obliged to set aside a percentage of rents on leased lands as an incentive for doctors who currently had 'no inducement whatever to practice in Native districts'.[98] Given the scattered and limited revenues from this source, a more realistic approach would have been to promote medical services as part of the infrastructure of settlement and to link Maori subsidies with the requirements of an expanding Pakeha presence. In 1882, for instance, Mr Morpeth of the Native Department stated that provision of the 'usual Native Office subsidy' would be an inducement if the Europeans of Hokianga were seeking a doctor, 'but no steps of the kind are being taken that I am aware of'.[99] Again, the East Coast MHR Samuel Locke asked the government in 1885 to help locate a medical man between Tolaga Bay and East Cape, a district with a large but scattered Maori and European population. Native Minister John Ballance replied that Matthew Scott of Wairoa had been appointed. Four days later Locke made a second request, for wire and labour to extend the telegraph from Gisborne to Tolaga Bay and thus reduce its isolation. Premier Julius Vogel expressed concern about the expense but promised to look into the matter.[100]

Some applicants for medical assistance believed that subsidised doctors would quickly become self-sufficient and no longer require government funds. This solution appealed to G. Kelly, W.B. White's successor at Mangonui. Kelly was frequently urged by both Maori and Europeans to impress upon the government the value of a district medical officer. In 1879 he claimed that a £100 subsidy for a few years would enable a doctor to establish himself and secure a good income, after which he would no longer need any government help.[101] This sentiment was echoed by Opotiki's Resident Magistrate, Captain Preece, in 1880: 'The Natives residing near Opotiki never ask for medical aid from Government, but go to the doctor in the same manner as Europeans, and I am informed that they pay for attendance cheerfully, and much more speedily than some Europeans.'[102] This was not the experience of other departmental informants. Taupo's Resident Magistrate reported in 1887 that the town's nearest doctors resided at Napier and Rotorua, which meant that their fees for attendance were prohibitively high.[103]

Faced with such conflicting evidence, Under-Secretary Lewis was understandably wary. On 26 November 1886 he warned his Minister that applications for medical assistance were becoming more frequent and expenditure was already considerable.[104] His attitude was coloured by the conviction that many Maori could 'well afford to pay their medical attendant', a belief which led to the rejection of Dr Perkins' attempt to secure a position in 1889. In his evidence to the 1889 Native Claims Commission, however, Lewis admitted that others were not in such a fortunate position and attempted to justify the refusal of applications for medical assistance from communities which had no doctor within a 'reasonable distance': 'If a doctor did not reside within a hundred miles you could not expect him to visit a Native settlement except at a rate of remuneration beyond the means of the department to pay.' When pressed, Lewis recanted slightly, admitting that 100 miles was an exaggeration, though it could be 'a good many miles'.[105]

The dearth of doctors led to a dependence in some cases on the use of unqualified personnel, generally teachers in Native Schools or individuals with some knowledge of pharmacy. These form the fifth factor in the story of late nineteenth century medical care. Writing from Maketu in 1874, the Resident Magistrate, F.E. Hamlin, lamented the absence of the schoolmaster, 'Dr Cowan', who was called out to serious cases. Whatever his background, Cowan was never registered as a doctor in New Zealand.[106] Two years later the district still had no legally qualified practitioner. Hamlin's concern was eased by the presence of a Mr Pinker, the Native School master, who had an intimate knowledge of homoeopathy, had been of 'infinite' service to Maori and was 'invariably successful'. With such a glowing reference the Under-Secretary might have been excused for wondering why a doctor was needed at all.[107]

Such instances were far from unique. In 1886 G.T. Wilkinson, Native Agent at Pirongia, expressed his thanks to the 'Government Medical Officer (Mr Aubin)' for his efforts during an epidemic of low fever among 'King natives' at Whatiwhatihoe. The following year he commented that Aubin, now described simply as a 'local doctor', had dealt with numerous cases of sickness. Fortunately, he added, there had been only one death among people of importance in the community.[108] The New Zealand Medical Register contains no reference to a Dr Aubin in this period.[109]

Aubin may have had a medical education but have chosen not to register in New Zealand. But as he was officially classified as one of three 'native medical dispensers' in 1888, as distinct from the NMOs, this seems unlikely.[110] His colleagues included Robinson Spencer, a Whangarei chemist appointed by the Native Department in 1882 to be 'Dispenser of Medicines' in Hokianga.[111] The local spokesman, R. Hobbs, reluctantly agreed to this if the Native Minister believed that Spencer was up to the task. A departmental memo of 2 June 1882 stressed the desirability of appointing duly qualified practitioners. Under-Secretary Lewis acknowledged in February 1883 that Hokianga was the largest Maori population centre in the colony, but resisted any increased allowance for an unqualified man. Nor did he suggest his replacement by a trained doctor. This decision was not driven by financial considerations, for Spencer's £40 per annum exceeded the payments to all but a handful of NMOs. Even then, Spencer claimed in 1883 that the subsidy did not cover the cost of drugs and sought an additional payment. Matters came to a head the following year as a result of an 'unusual amount of sickness' in Hokianga. While Lewis sympathised with his plight he could not recommend any increase in salary other than as part of a general increase to NMOs. It is unclear if this refusal had any bearing on Spencer's resignation in 1885, when he transferred to an Education Department post. Whatever Lewis's rationale, it was not until November 1896 that medically qualified NMOs were appointed to Hokianga—Valentine Barr to Kaikohe and Clive De Lowe to Rawene.[112]

The sixth and final facet of medical attendance on Maori in this period relates to the nature of the work involved and the impact this had upon the willingness of medical practitioners to continue it. In many cases the duties appear to have been excessive in relation to the remuneration. The scattered nature of Maori settlements was a major obstacle. In Northland, for example, the kainga around Whangarei varied in size from three to 26 individuals; in Hokianga the range was eleven to 220. Wairarapa in the 1870s and 1880s contained just over 700 Maori; the largest settlement had approximately 70 persons, and the average size was around 20 individuals.[113]

Returns submitted by the NMOs to the Native Department give some indication of their commitment to these Maori communities. They also illustrate the difficulty of establishing what was normal or typical. In Nelson and Marlborough the five medical officers treated 820 cases between 1869 and 1871, including 336 for 'diseases of the chest'. This averages out to a caseload for each doctor of approximately one patient per week.[114] In contrast, the quarterly report for July–September 1877 of Henry Spratt, NMO in the Wairarapa since 1859, listed 137 patients, equivalent to 1.5 per day. One-third of these were children. Respiratory ailments, digestive disorders, sexually transmitted diseases and dentistry featured prominently in Spratt's account. More than three-quarters of patients were visited in their own homes, which involved the doctor in return journeys of between four and 35 miles. Where possible, Spratt would visit a number of patients in the same locality during the one trip. At the end of his report he commented: 'This quarter has been unusually heavy. The *express* visits to distant villages have been unusually large in number, although the mortality among the natives has not been very high.'[115] The use of an annual retainer rather than a fee for service produced wild fluctations in the level of remuneration for each treatment. Martin Payne of Thames, for instance, reported his patient numbers for the years 1885–8 as 77, 148, 151, and 111.[116]

The workloads of Spratt and Payne appear modest compared with some other returns. In 1886 Alexander Leslie (a Scottish medical graduate, though

date	name	address	disorder &c	distance in miles	Remarks
Sept 25	Mani huna child	Papawai	feverish &c	4	Visited
	Fanny	do	cough	4	Visited
	Sarah	do	vermin	4	do
	Hori clark's child	Greytown	[illegible]	½	do
28	Mani huna child	Papawai	feverish &c	4	Visited
	Hami	Greytown	constipation sore gums		seen at home
29	Hori child	Papawai	cough	4	Visited
	Sara	do	do	4	do
	Ngatuere	Waihine	cough	2	do
	— wife	do	do	2	do
	Several others	do	sundry trifling ailments	2	do

This quarter has been unusually heavy – the expenses visiting distant villages have been unusually large in number – altho the mortality among the natives has not been high.

[illegible] Thos. Spratt.

An extract from Dr Spratt's report for the quarter ending 30 September 1877. *NA, MA 21/19*

never registered in New Zealand) acted for some time as medical officer for the Taupo district. In the course of three months he attended between 400 and 500 cases. The Resident Magistrate, D. Scannell, noted these were 'happily not of a very fatal nature' and that there had been no dangerous epidemics other than whooping cough during this time.[117]

Such inequities and inconsistencies added to the problems of formulating and administering the NMO scheme. There was no standardised pattern or workload. The Native Department was almost invariably constrained by financial considerations. Although it might bring short-term benefits, the practice of pitting doctor against doctor, as happened at Thames and elsewhere, was fraught with hazards. Not all doctors were interested in serving, though economic necessity obliged many at least to consider taking up the work. Where there was a choice of personnel the wishes of local Maori might have to be taken into account, and their satisfaction frequently depended on more than the technical competence of the doctor. Remote areas brought additional problems, in that they were often unattractive to medical men.

These uncertainties were reflected in a relatively high turnover of subsidised doctors. The Audit Office returns for 1894 to 1897 identified NMOs in 28 locations, of which ten experienced a change of personnel in the period under review. The corresponding figures for 1897 to 1900 were 31 and ten. In some cases, though not all, the retiring doctor nominated his successor; this might be his partner or the purchaser of his practice if he were leaving town. The ability of officials to find replacements, usually within weeks rather than months, indicates an ongoing commitment to the scheme, an interpretation at odds with some previous analyses. This was offset to some extent by the department's failure to provide any assistance to some areas which appear to have been equally in need.

John Moore, who practised medicine in New Zealand throughout the 1880s, subsequently published a book in which he provided guidelines for his fellow professionals. Moore claimed that Maori did not 'trouble the *pakeha* doctor very much',[118] but it is clear Maori could and did utilise the services of a significant minority of European doctors. In 1891 approximately 10 per cent of rural practitioners derived part of their income from acting as NMOs. With the mid 1890s expansion this figure rose to around 16 per cent by 1900.[119] Those paid from the Native Reserves constituted an additional body. Others received ad hoc payments for specific services, especially for the treatment of infectious diseases, although their names do not appear in Audit Office or other NMO lists.[120] A fourth group, like the Opotiki doctor referred to by Captain Preece in 1880, attended Maori on a fee for service footing. For all the reasons outlined above, the coverage was patchy; but subsidised doctors had a more constant presence than has previously been thought.

'To escape extermination': infection and sanitation

The subsidised doctors were not alone in providing health care as a safety net for Maori. Nor did the Native Department carry the entire burden.

Other government agencies such as the Education Department played a part. So too did Maori self-help, which was originally expressed through tohunga but was put on a new footing in the 1890s by the work of the Te Aute College Students' Association, which evolved into the Young Maori Party. This section considers the contributions made by these agencies to official policy on the interconnected themes of environmental health, infectious disease and health education.

In the last decades of the nineteenth century, opinion was divided on the viability of alleviating the deleterious effects of introduced diseases and defective hygiene. At one end of the spectrum were the 'dying pillowers' such as Alfred Newman and Archdeacon Walsh who regarded the demise of the Maori race as inevitable;[121] the opposite pole was occupied by health reformers such as James Pope and members of the Young Maori Party who believed that the situation, though grave, was not irreversible. Many observers and officials were undecided, alternating between optimism and pessimism in their assessment of Maori health status.

As previously noted, the government's first preventive health initiative on behalf of Maori was vaccination against smallpox. These efforts were sporadic rather than constant. The smallpox alarm of 1872 sparked a brief flurry of concern and activity, after which the practice seems to have virtually lapsed. Resident magistrates were charged with ensuring that free vaccination was available to both Maori and European;[122] neither race showed any great inclination to take advantage of this service. As one editorial put it in 1869, New Zealanders awaited the arrival of smallpox with 'a stoical fatalism that would do credit to Mahometans'.[123]

A second smallpox scare in the early 1880s encouraged officials to revive the vaccination question. In 1881 a return showing births, deaths and vaccination rates for European children from 1877 to 1880 was presented to the House of Representatives. It showed a steady rise in the percentage of newborn babies successfully vaccinated, from 63.75 in 1877 to 70.46 in 1880.[124] Two days later the Native Department took 'very earnest steps' to promote vaccination by distributing a circular extolling its advantages.[125] The response was lukewarm. In Wairarapa, about 330 came forward from a Maori population of between 700 and 800, with Dr Spratt reporting 'great difficulty in inducing them to meet or come to him for the purpose'.[126] At Thames the Native Agent enjoyed only 'indifferent success', as the initial enthusiasm turned to apathy and rejection when smallpox failed to make an appearance.[127]

A number of factors contributed to the low uptake of vaccination. Many of these paralleled concerns within the European populace. Some of the more remote communities experienced difficulty in obtaining supplies of lymph.[128] Others were concerned about the quality of the product and deferred action.[129] Such opposition could be intensified by an adverse reaction to the procedure. G.T. Wilkinson of Thames acknowledged that such instances had contributed to apathy and to dislike of the operation, but thought this occurred 'more through the unhealthy state of the children than any fault in the lymph used, or want of care or attention by the medical officer'.[130] At Mataitai, near Clevedon, where only one person had previously been vaccinated, 37 Maori 'fearing the small-pox' came forward to be vaccinated in 1884. Many others refused, 'wishing to see the result in those already vaccinated'. There is no record of any follow-up visit to persuade such defaulters to submit to vaccination.[131]

The scattered nature of Maori communities created dual problems. The first was the difficulty in persuading Maori to congregate in a single location to be vaccinated. Conversely, some vaccinators were unwilling to go to Maori settlements because the travelling allowance was insufficient to cover their costs.[132]

The vaccination issue was aired in Parliament in 1884. H.K. Taiaroa, MHR for Southern Maori, claimed that Maori now recognised the benefits of the procedure, in contrast to their previous ignorance. Taiaroa calculated the cost of vaccinating 45,000 Maori (the entire population) at more than £4,000, although the actual sum would be less since many, especially in the vicinity of towns, had already submitted to the procedure. The Native Minister, John Ballance, replied that only about 7,300 had been vaccinated to date. After further discussion Parliament agreed that medical men should be sent out to vaccinate Maori.[133]

However laudable the intention, it proved impossible to execute this ambitious programme. Matthew Scott, the doctor appointed to the East Coast for this very purpose, met with little success because of 'religious prejudice' on the part of some Maori.[134] Given the anti-vaccination sentiments of many Pakeha,[135] coupled with the absence of smallpox in New Zealand, the failure of the programme was almost inevitable. Not until the appointment of Maui Pomare as Maori Health Officer in 1900 did vaccination again become a live issue.

The first major infectious disease to afflict Maori in the period under review was tuberculosis, variants of which were referred to as scrofula or consumption. The problem was clearly identified but there was no current solution. There was no positive understanding of the etiology of the disease until Robert Koch's identification of the tubercle bacillus in 1882, and no effective preventive measures or treatment until well into the twentieth century. Official comments therefore tended to exhibit a fatalistic attitude; many suggested that Maori sufferers had to some extent brought about their own misfortune.[136]

The tone was set by J.E. Gorst, one of the officers appointed in 1862 to report on Governor Grey's proposed runanga scheme. Describing the 'frightful amount of scrofulous disease in every village', he attributed what he saw as the destruction of the Maori race to defective living conditions, clothing and diet. They were, he added, expending their remaining strength on resisting 'the only help which might save them'.[137] Most observers in the ensuing decades identified a similar catalogue of contributory factors. J.B. Tuke, a near-contemporary of Gorst, expounded at some length on

For many Maori, home was an insanitary whare lacking the most basic amenities. *ATL, F51741 1/2*

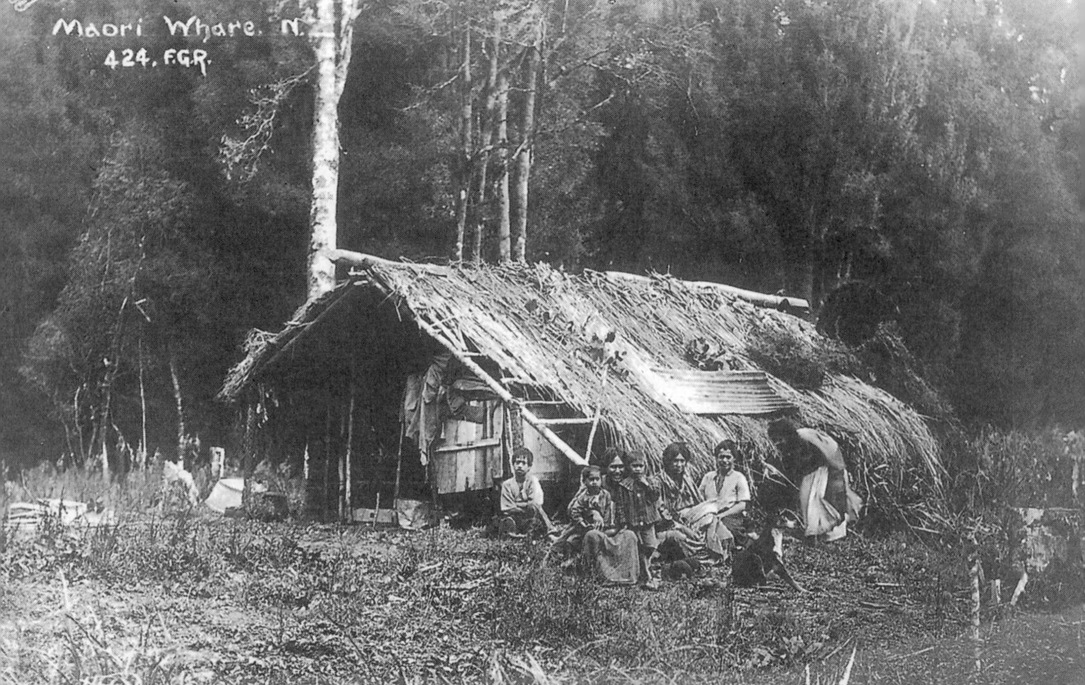

the effects of migration from a warmer to colder climate, and of in-breeding, poor diet, existing habits, and the adoption of European customs.[138] The belief that tuberculosis was largely self-inflicted was expressed time and again in the ensuing decades. This attitude was summed up by H.W. Bishop, Auckland's Resident Magistrate, in 1892. He noted the contribution to 'fatal pulmonary complaints' of low-lying dwellings and inappropriate clothing, and complained: 'Warning is thrown away. They admit the evil, but disregard the consequences.'[139]

Typhoid fever became increasingly prevalent in New Zealand in the second half of the century, although poor record-keeping and an absence of public health officials make it difficult to quantify its prevalence.[140] The problem became more visible as a result of improved systems for reporting on Maori health.[141] Once again, there were allegations that Maori contributed to their own downfall. Opotiki's Resident Magistrate, for example, complained in 1883 that Maori were 'perfectly regardless of the danger of infection, and ridicule the idea of taking any precautionary measures to prevent the spread of the disease'.[142]

Expenditure on public health measures was rarely popular among European ratepayers.[143] As a result, both central and local authorities were generally reluctant to spend money for this purpose. For many Maori the cost of sanitary improvements was prohibitive, and there is little evidence of government spending to meet these needs. Payments from the Civil List for purposes other than medical attendance or medicines were almost derisory and apparently ad hoc. In 1895, for instance, the Civil List Vote for Native Purposes included three payments of 4s 3d for removing nightsoil from 'native cottages, Napier'. Two years later contingencies included £2 for a 'nightsoil contract' at an unspecified location.[144]

Like their European counterparts, Maori were ambivalent about funding for sanitary purposes. Following the transfer of responsibility to the Justice Department in 1893, the Kaiapoi MHR stated that local Maori had raised £25 for sanitary improvements, and asked the government to contribute a further £50. The Minister of Lands, John McKenzie, replied that the original request had been for road improvements, with no mention of sanitation, and that the request had not enjoyed the unanimous support of local Maori.[145]

Budgetary constraints were offered as the justification for government reluctance to meet such costs. In 1898 T.H. Parata, MHR for Southern

Maori, sought funding to erect 22 water tanks at Waikouaiti, a coastal settlement north of Dunedin, at an estimated cost of £102. Richard Seddon, in his joint capacity as Native Minister and Premier, refused because of the 'very large demands on the Native Civil List this year'. Other requests from Otago settlements were turned down on the same grounds.[146]

Ministers also preached the gospel of self-help. Two years after Parata's failed bid, William Field, MHR for Otaki, asked the Native Minister to supply free water tanks at Porirua, where the unwholesome water contributed to high child mortality. Native Minister James Carroll promised to investigate but warned that help would be forthcoming only if the local Maori were found to be destitute.[147] Not until the following decade did the government relax the criteria for meeting such requests.

It has been asserted that Maori schools provided the 'most comprehensive European health work done among Maori' prior to 1900.[148] Native School teachers certainly outnumbered NMOs during the latter part of the nineteenth century, but some weight should be given to the respective skills of the two groups. As James Pope, Organising Inspector for Native Schools, advised in 1884, 'If you cannot get a doctor, the next best thing is to go for advice to a magistrate, or a teacher, or a minister'.[149]

The involvement of teachers in health care had begun with the missionaries before 1840. The Native Schools Act 1867 established a separate network of Maori schools, mostly located in areas with a limited European presence; it would survive until 1969. By 1870 only three schools had been set up with a total of 219 pupils. Five years later there were almost 950 pupils in village schools administered under the act.[150] These institutions were transferred to the Education Department in 1879, and by 1882 the roll had more than doubled to 2,042 pupils.[151] Around 60 teachers were employed by 1880, a figure which increased to 85 by 1900.[152] At least one official regarded the schools as supplementing existing medical provision: 'Everything has been done by a paternal Government to relieve the wants and necessities of the sick by the services of Native medical officers in town, and the gratuitous dispensation of medicines through the Native teacher at Iruharama, the most populous pa on the [Wanganui] river.'[153] Yet many questions remain unanswered about the extent to which Native School and NMO networks co-operated, overlapped or competed.

The 1880 Native Schools Code decreed that teachers were 'expected' to

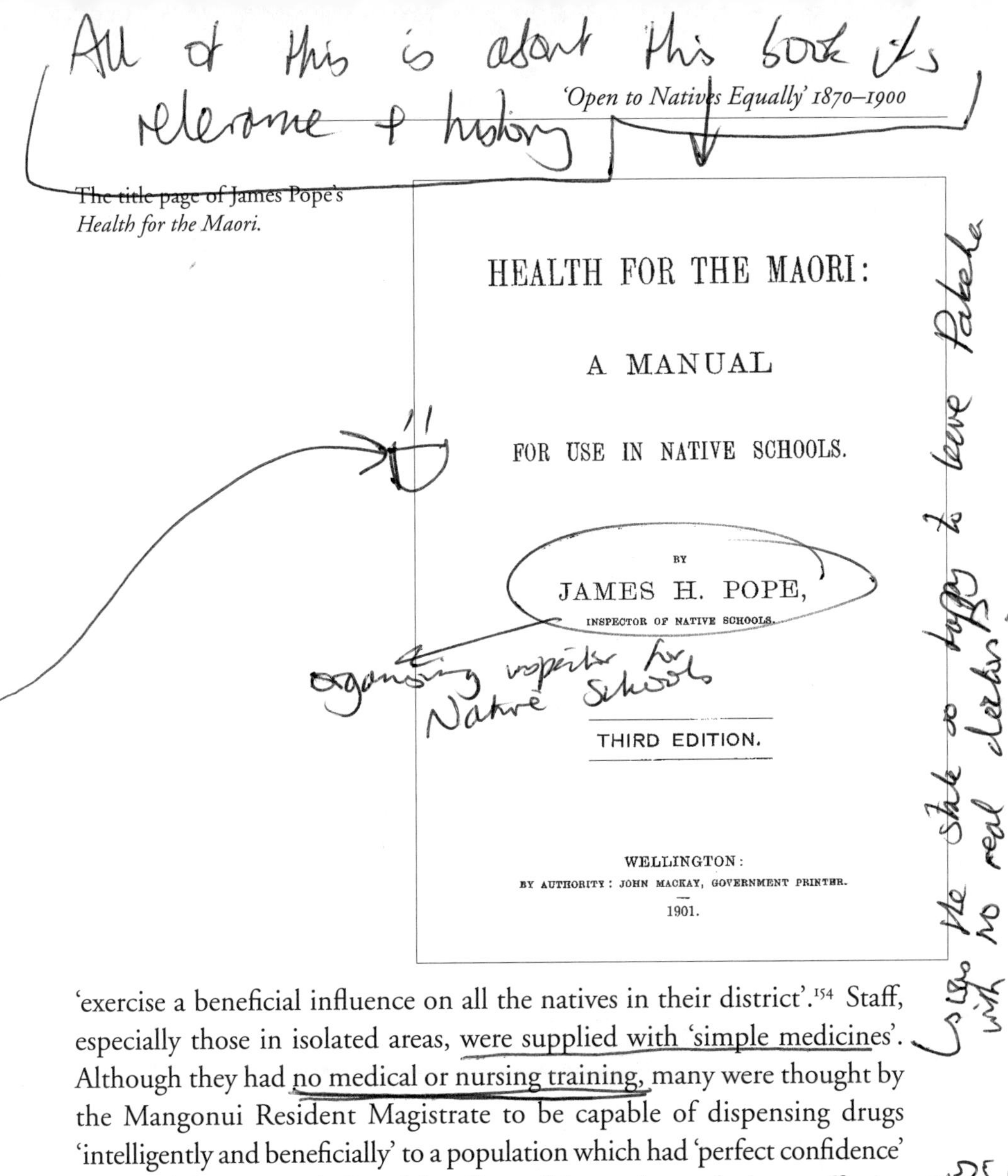
HEALTH FOR THE MAORI:
A MANUAL
FOR USE IN NATIVE SCHOOLS.
BY
JAMES H. POPE,
INSPECTOR OF NATIVE SCHOOLS.
THIRD EDITION.
WELLINGTON:
BY AUTHORITY: JOHN MACKAY, GOVERNMENT PRINTER.
1901.

The title page of James Pope's *Health for the Maori.*

'exercise a beneficial influence on all the natives in their district'.[154] Staff, especially those in isolated areas, were supplied with 'simple medicines'. Although they had no medical or nursing training, many were thought by the Mangonui Resident Magistrate to be capable of dispensing drugs 'intelligently and beneficially' to a population which had 'perfect confidence' in their abilities.[155] He believed the efforts of the teachers to be 'more effective than skilled but irregular medical attendance'.[156] Although it was intended that medicines should be supplied only to pupils, except in cases of 'extreme poverty', such restrictions were rarely enforced.[157] The system was endorsed by the Premier, Richard Seddon, during an extensive tour of North Island Maori communities in 1894, when he travelled almost 1,800 miles and addressed nineteen separate meetings. At Te Whaiti Seddon voiced his conviction that all teachers should be married men with a knowledge of medicine; at a later meeting he referred to the Galatea master as 'also a medicine-man. The Government had supplied him with medicines; he had a slight knowledge thereof, and he was acting as doctor for the district, and had been the means of saving life and alleviating the sufferings of those who were sick.'[158]

Such an approach was closer to providing an ambulance at the foot of the cliff than a fence at the top. James Pope advocated a more preventive agenda.[159] The preface to his *Health for the Maori: A Manual for Use in Native Schools* (1884) described its main purpose as educating the rising generation so that they might 'escape extermination'. The text emphasised prevention as better than cure and gave advice on vaccination, sanitation, burial customs, and exercise. Translated almost immediately into Maori, it was republished at intervals until the final English edition of 1901. It continued to be used in Native Schools for some time thereafter, and provided inspiration for T.W. Ratana in the 1920s.[160]

Pope's book was a direct response to the widely held belief that improvements in Maori health, especially that of children, would depend on 'careful attention to the laws of health'.[161] Its publication coincided with a suggestion from John Grace of Auckland that Maori should receive

Timutimu Tawhai, Reweti Kohere and Maui Pomare, whose 1889 walking tour to promote the gospel of health helped lay the foundations for the Young Maori Party. *J.F. Cody, Man of Two Worlds, facing p.50*

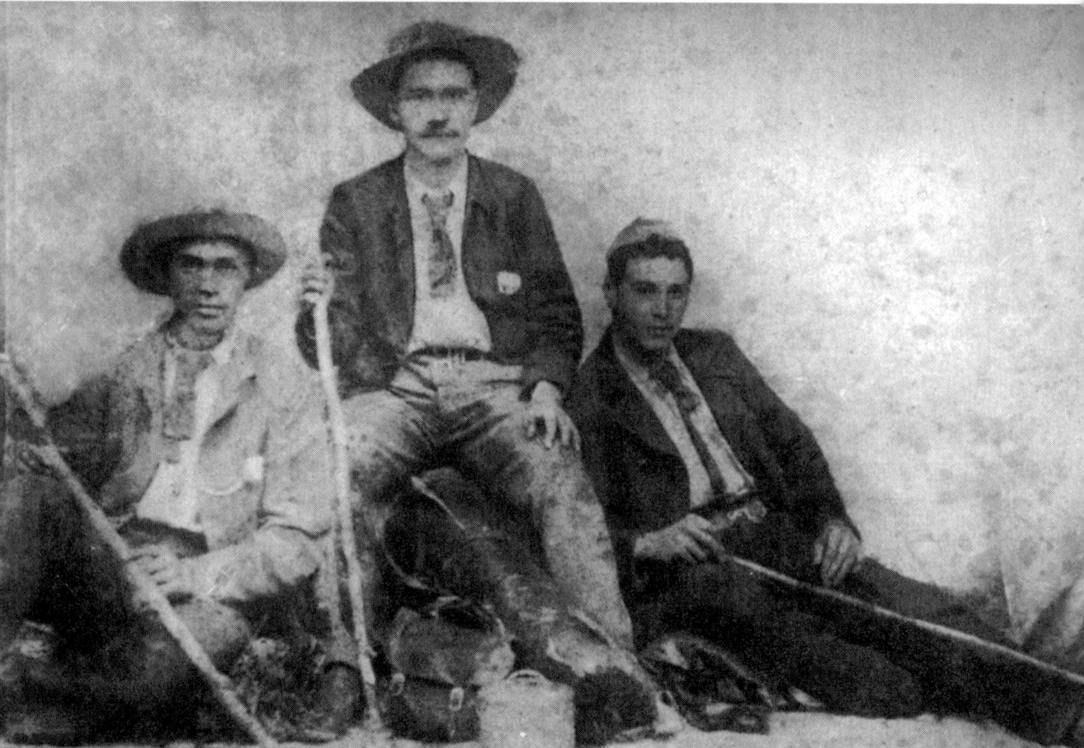

compulsory health education using Mrs Buxton's *Health in the House,* the Revd J. Ridgway's *Rules on Health,* and the Revd D.W. Turner's *Rules for General Health.*[162] Pope's message was quickly endorsed by Native Department officials, many of whom shared his belief that Maori were not necessarily a dying race.[163] Success, however, would require more than the 'little book [on]. . . the laws of health' mentioned in the final paragraph of Pope's report for 1885. In the same report a Native Department official, whose views presumably coincided with those of Pope himself, was cited: 'Mr Bishop concludes by saying that the Maori race is doomed, until sanitary rules are strictly enforced by legislation.'[164]

Enumerators for the 1891 census of the Maori population were invited to comment on the general state of Maori health. Few accepted the invitation. One who did was George Davis, Native Officer in Wellington, who stated that Pope's book contained 'some very valuable and pertinent suggestions'.[165] Others agreed, and strove to promote its message. John Thornton, headmaster of Te Aute College, adopted it as a textbook, hoping his pupils would convey the contents to their families. Some Te Aute students subsequently visited kainga to endorse *Health for the Maori.*[166] One of those involved was Apirana Ngata, who distributed 54 copies during his Christmas holidays, with the promise of a follow-up visit to test the recipients' knowledge.[167]

Pope's involvement extended beyond the written word. During the 1890s he contributed to the deliberations of the Te Aute College Students' Association and the Young Maori Party.[168] Mason Durie has attributed the early twentieth century turnaround in Maori health to the latter organisation, whose 'mission of health reform' had much in common with the old Maori practices of clean water, adequate sanitation, ventilated houses and effective drainage.[169] These were also the central themes of *Health for the Maori,* which in turn was founded on the precepts of mid nineteenth century English sanitary reformers such as Edwin Chadwick.[170] It was a blueprint which offered hope for the future.

3
'All Medical Matters Affecting Natives'
1900–1920

The creation of a Department of Public Health in 1900 completed the formalisation of health initiatives which had begun with the 1872 Public Health Act and continued with the Hospitals and Charitable Institutions Act of 1885. The new Department was regarded by many health professionals and others as long overdue. As the name suggests, it was intended to cover a broad spectrum. The emphasis was on preventive measures rather than treatment and cure, and covered both infectious diseases and environmental health. From the outset, the Department's sphere of responsibility included Maori, though measures to improve their health were hampered by a tortuous chain of command, constant financial restraint, political interference and a substantial degree of bureaucratic bickering. This chapter assesses the Department's influence on Maori health care up to 1920.

'Due proportion': Maori health administration

In the early months of 1900, New Zealand was threatened by an invasion of bubonic plague. Concern focused initially on seaports as points of entry and on the danger to the European population. Dr James Mason and the Chief Veterinarian were appointed as Plague Commissioners for the colony in April 1900. Three weeks later, probably at the instigation of Native Minister James Carroll, Cabinet approved the appointment of a 'Maori chief as Sanitary Commissioner to work with the ordinary Commissioners'.[1]

The feared epidemic never materialised but it did serve as the catalyst for an increased commitment to public health, with implications for both Maori and Pakeha. Mason was appointed in December 1900 as New Zealand's first Chief Health Officer (CHO), a position equivalent to the present-day Director-General of Health. The choice was a favourable omen for Maori. Mason had emigrated to New Zealand in 1895 and settled in Otaki. One of the colony's few doctors with a training in public health, he contacted Premier Richard Seddon soon after his arrival and offered to write simple guidelines for sanitation in Maori kainga. (He was presumably unaware of the existence of Pope's *Health for the Maori*.) Within a short time Mason became NMO for Otaki.[2] The association with Seddon almost certainly played a part in this appointment and in his selection for the demanding position of CHO.

Mason's first report on 'Native Affairs' expressed his belief that the potential exposure of indigenous peoples to plague required special precautions. Displaying a gift for eloquence, he announced the decision to 'continue the work of physical salvation amongst the Natives'. This was to be accomplished by the appointment of Maui Pomare—'an adviser able by reason of his nationality to enter into their thoughts and minds'—as 'Health Commissioner for the Natives throughout the colony'.[3]

The evangelical tone of Mason's words struck a chord with Pomare, who had left Te Aute College in the early 1890s to obtain a medical education at an American Adventist college, with a view to returning as a medical missionary to his people.[4] For almost a decade Mason and Pomare tried to implement their vision, but they were hampered by limited resources.[5] Pomare drew up a fourteen-point blueprint for Maori health in 1904. His aims included training Maori nurses, appointing European women to provide health education and advice on infant welfare and 'sick cookery', better use of medical officers, an increased complement of sanitary inspectors, a separate Maori tuberculosis hospital, the establishment of a leper colony on an unspecified island, the speeding up of the individualisation of Maori lands, and the prohibition of 'the practices of quacks and *tohungas*'.[6] The implementation of these goals met with varied success.

Influential members of the medical profession supported the efforts of Mason and Pomare. The presidential address to the New Zealand Branch of the British Medical Association (NZBMA) was given in 1904 by Dr William Collins, who was to be a member of the Legislative Council from 1907 to 1934. Collins commented on the profession's efforts to halt the 'gradual diminution' of the Maori race, and noted with pleasure that 'one of their own number has been intrusted by the Government with the maintenance and improvement of the health of the Maori people. . . . No doubt Dr Pomare, with the aid of the Natives themselves, will be able to check the death-rate among the Native people.'[7]

Lack of money was a major obstacle to the development of Maori health care. As Pomare ruefully commented to Mason in 1907: 'This year finds me sending you the usual *compte rendu*, the use of which you and I cannot discern, for nearly all the suggestions contained in the previous ones are seldom acted upon.'[8] The Health Department's difficulties were exacerbated by a series of unseemly wrangles about the control and funding of Maori health. The basic problem was the fact that the Native Civil List allowance of £7,000 per annum had remained unchanged since 1852. As James Carroll bluntly put it when challenged to extend services in 1903: 'The Civil List

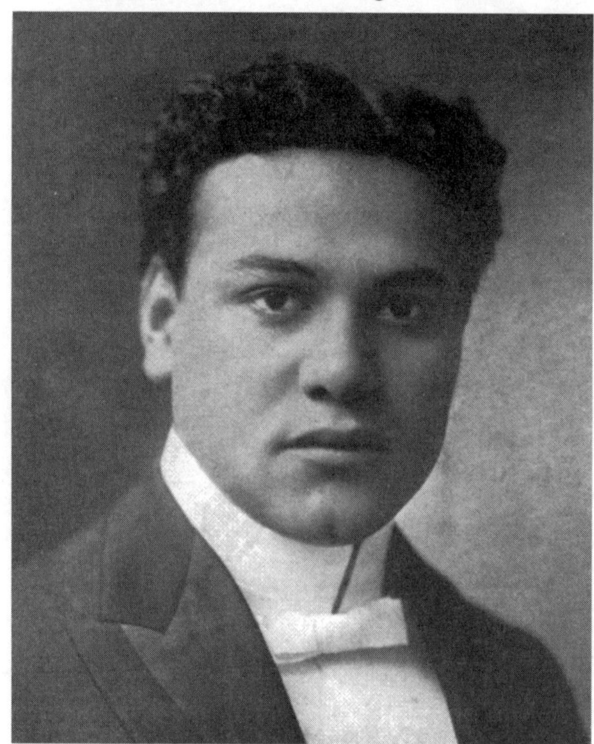

Maui Pomare (1876?–1930) on his graduation with an MD from the American Medical Missionary College, Chicago, in 1899. *J.F. Cody, Man of Two Worlds, facing p.51*

Fund was not a very large one, and the requirements of the Natives of the whole of the colony had to be considered in due proportion to their wants.'[9] At the turn of the century approximately £3,000 was earmarked for health expenditure on Maori.[10]

Responsibility for Maori health was complicated by the involvement of the Justice Department, which had administered Civil List payments since 1893, and the Public Trustee. Pomare's recommendation that the Health Department take control of the Civil List was approved by Carroll and Health Minister Joseph Ward in July 1902, but not implemented. Two years later the question remained enmeshed in the bureaucratic undergrowth despite Pomare's repeated efforts to promote the issue. On 19 October 1904, however, a Health Department memorandum suggested that a recent communication from the Public Trustee 'has brought it forward again, and it now seems that the question ought to be brought to a finality'.[11]

When a second Maori doctor, Peter Buck (Te Rangi Hiroa), was appointed as Pomare's assistant in 1905, he was paid through the Justice Department. The revival of the Native Department in 1906 brought an end to this practice.[12] Mason suggested to Herbert Edgar, the new Under-Secretary of the Native Department, that Pomare and Buck be attached to a 'definite department', with salaries voted in the supplementary estimates rather than paid through the Civil List.[13] On 12 October 1906, during the Health Department Supply debate, Health Minister George Fowlds confessed that no such arrangement was yet in place.[14] On the same day Edgar sent Fowlds details of the responsibilities that were to be handed over to the Health Department. These included complete control of Pomare and Buck and the Maori sanitary inspectors, payments to NMOs, medicines distributed by schoolteachers, the suppression of epidemics, and control of hostelries used as nursing homes.

Edgar calculated the current Civil List expenditure to be £3,950, but recommended that only £2,000 be handed over to the Health Department annually. He argued that additional costs should come from the supplementary estimates, leaving the Native Department with a larger margin to purchase rations for indigent Maori.[15] Five days later the Native Minister proposed to his Health counterpart that 'The health of the people of the colony should be under the care and attention of the Health Department', and that this was a matter of some urgency because of the need to provide medical care for Maori attending the 1906 Christchurch Exhibition.[16] Ignoring Edgar's advice, he agreed that the annual grant from the Civil List should be fixed at £3,000.

Edgar and Mason continued to haggle over the allocation of costs. Alarmed by what he regarded as Edgar's attempted sleight of hand, Mason claimed that the Native Department spent around £900 per annum on the medicines distributed by schoolteachers. He was adamant this should not be deducted from the £3,000 allocated to his Department but ought to be provided for in the Native Department estimates: 'It would be unfair to ask them to take it from the civil list but certainly we ought not, in addition to having to do the work, be out of pocket over it.' Edgar was equally emphatic that the money should come from the Health vote. He claimed that only £233 had been spent on medicines, from a total medical outlay of £573, and since this was 'so much less than is estimated by Dr Mason, perhaps the £3,000 a year will be sufficient to provide the necessary funds'.[17] James Carroll adopted a more conciliatory approach. Replying to a claim by Apirana Ngata (formerly the Organising Inspector of Maori Councils, now MHR for Eastern Maori) during the Tohunga Suppression Bill debate that the Civil List £3,000 could not meet the needs of 46,000 Maori, he conceded this sum was 'insufficient' and stated that he would ask his colleagues to 'rectify' the matter.[18]

A government economy drive resulted in the amalgamation of the chief executive positions of the public health and hospital sectors in 1909.[19] The incoming CHO and Inspector-General of Hospitals, Thomas Valintine, was concerned about the proposed transfer of Maori health back to the Native Department. He opposed any moves to 'disassociate the health of the Maoris from that of the pakeha' or create 'two Government health authorities in the Dominion'.[20] Maui Pomare's dismay was just as great, and more eloquently worded: 'We regret that, owing to stormy weather, the ship of State has to unburden itself by the unloading of our Department . . . [but] the years which we have spent in trying to uplift our fellow-men have not been spent in vain.'[21] Cabinet ignored Valintine's advice. The transfer was authorised on 22 July and Pomare was ordered to report on 2 August to T.W. Fisher, who had succeeded Edgar as Under-Secretary of the Native Department in February 1907.[22]

Fisher's first task was to cut annual expenditure on Maori health, which had risen from £3,000 when the Health Department took over to nearly £5,600 three years later. He identified savings of some £1,300 and suggested fudging the issue until March 1910, since any attempt to make special provision on the departmental estimates would 'no doubt give rise to considerable discussion'. At the same time, Apirana Ngata informed the Acting Prime Minister of his wish to see a more self-reliant policy for Maori health, with Maori contributing one-third of the costs when they were able to do so.[23] Three months later, Carroll admitted that the Civil List £3,000 had been supplemented by an equal amount in the Health Department vote but claimed that the return to the Native Department had seen the limit once more restricted to £3,000.[24]

The transfer from Health to the Native Department created strained relations between the two agencies.[25] Dr Robert Makgill, Auckland's District Health Officer, was particularly scathing about the Native Department's poor understanding of health issues. After a 'somewhat unprofitable and acrimonious' exchange of views with Fisher he warned Valintine that continued confusion over the funding and control of Maori health might erupt into a public scandal. Fisher defended his position by stating the Health Department was responsible for controlling infectious diseases, while his Department's vote was intended to cover medical attendance for 'indigent natives'. Carroll supported this position but also suggested that 'the Native Department might be relieved by the Health Department of duties it at present undertakes'.

Matters came to a head in March 1911, when Dr Joseph Frengley, Makgill's brother-in-law and Valintine's second-in-command, listed the agencies engaged in dealing with three outbreaks of infection in Maori communities. They included Health Department doctors, Native Department-approved nurses, Apirana Ngata, county councils, the police and subsidised NMOs. This multiplicity prevented the Health Department from doing justice to 'either the health of the Natives concerned or the public health generally'. Cabinet considered Frengley's memo on 7 April and resolved that in future the Health Department should deal with 'all medical matters affecting Natives'. During these prolonged discussions Makgill had suggested the formation of a new Department, 'or a special branch of the Health Department', to oversee the notification of infectious diseases among Maori and to promote public health. He pointed out to

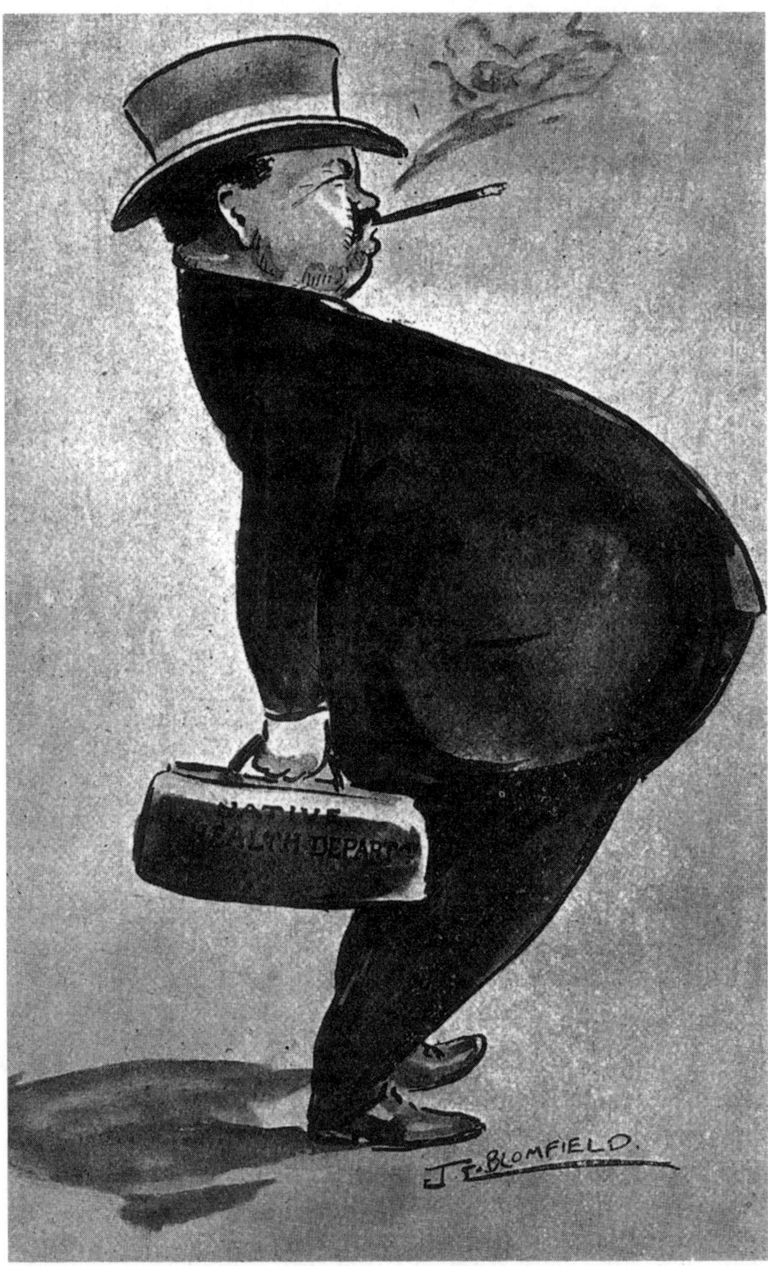

Blomfield's 1910 cartoon of Pomare toting the 'Native Health Department' in his doctor's bag reflects the difficulty in gaining credibility for this work. The sentiment was echoed in 1926 when the *New Zealand Herald* rejoiced in Pomare's removal as Minister of Health, and the return of 'this important portfolio . . . to one who represents a European constituency'. *ATL, N-P 422- (New Zealand Observer, 5 February 1910)*

the Under-Secretary of the Native Department that Maori were not subject to the provisions of the Public Health Act and were thus not required to register either deaths or notifiable diseases. The introduction of birth and death registration in 1913, attributed to Makgill's former Health Department colleague, Maui Pomare, brought some improvement in the monitoring of Maori health. The restructuring of the Department and the creation of a Division of Maori Hygiene, however, did not occur until 1920, when this was one of the consequences of the influenza epidemic which had struck New Zealand two years earlier.

While the two departments bickered about the direction of Maori health, another legislative innovation of 1900 to promote Maori well-being was quietly being consigned to oblivion, at least in the short term. Questioned in Parliament on 3 October 1911 about the ineffectual utilisation of the Civil List, David Buddo claimed that the Health Department had been obliged to take over responsibility for Maori medical care from Maori Councils.[26] This was a misleading inaccuracy from a man who had been Health Minister for nearly three years. In fact, Maori Councils had been given only limited powers to deal with sanitary matters and had never possessed sufficient funds to meet even these obligations.

The Maori Councils Bill of 1900 had its origins in the work of the Te Aute College students and 'did not come unawares on the Maori people'.[27] In moving the Bill's adoption, Native Minister James Carroll described it as an effort on the part of the Maori race to organise themselves for a measure of self-government. He also stated that the councils would redress the lack of statistical information on Maori by collecting data on their general health and causes of death, a task that had been carried out by Native Department officers prior to 1892. Alfred Fraser, who as MHR for Napier showed a keen interest in Maori health, challenged the legisation on the grounds that Maori should be subject to the existing Public Health Act as the only way of raising them to European levels. His claim went unheeded.[28]

The introduction of Maori Councils was greeted in many quarters as a new beginning. At Papawai, near Greytown, the scene of Carroll's announcement in 1899 that the government would establish marae committees to control and improve kainga,[29] the formal constitution of the Rongokaka Maori Council drew approving comments from European observers. The *Evening Times* described the system as 'well fitted to develop self-reliance and the governing faculty in the rank and file of the Maoris'. Praising the improvements brought about by Henare Parata, the Maori Sanitary Commissioner during the plague scare of 1900, the *Evening Post* claimed that his influence on Papawai was 'clearly apparent as the party drove along the road'.[30] By 1902 24 councils had been set up, but there were some serious omissions. Waikato Maori consistently declined to take part because of the threat to the mana of the Maori King.[31] Rua Kenana, the Tuhoe leader, also rejected the council structure.[32]

Maui Pomare, the Health Department's 'chief of the Native Section',[33] considered that the councils had made 'vast improvements' to Maori sanitation and would be instrumental in averting the extinction of the race. His colleague Peter Buck took a more cautious view, complaining in his first report of 1906 about the 'ceremonial verbose style' of many meetings but conceding that Maori were becoming more aware of the tool they now possessed to help improve their condition. His frustration at the delay in achieving these goals became apparent in his second report, which alleged that Maori Councils were as slow as their European equivalents to realise the importance of public health laws.[34]

Gilbert Mair, who was appointed Superintendent of Maori Councils in 1903 at the age of 60 after a lifetime of involvement with Maori, was another whose initial enthusiasm was tempered by subsequent experience: 'I entered upon this duty full of zeal, and with high aspirations, for not only do I personally know almost every Maori in the North Island, but I have the very strongest affection for the Race.' After three years, however, he was increasingly concerned about the lack of office accommodation, loss of and damage to council records, and the failure of tribes to meet their financial obligations to the councils.[35]

Mair resigned in 1906, prompting a suggestion from Under-Secretary Edgar that Pomare be asked to handle the required reorganisation. Echoing the mission of Pope and others down the years, it was anticipated that he would also expand the educational function, 'especially in the matter of sanitary arrangements and the observance of the laws of health'.[36] Asked some weeks later about the failure to replace Mair, Carroll revealed that he was contemplating placing the work under the Health Department, 'if he could get Dr Pomare to take charge'.[37] This scheme never came to fruition and Mair's role devolved to a Native Department records clerk, J.B. Hackworth, who remained in the post until 1919.[38]

With hindsight, the misgivings expressed by Alfred Fraser in 1900 can be seen to have had some merit, for the Maori Councils failed to achieve many of their objectives.[39] Some of their defects, such as those pointed out by Mair, were beyond the control of the councils. Almost from the outset they were hamstrung by chronic under-funding. During the Supply debate in 1908 Ngata observed that 'Subsidies to Maori Councils' had been disbursed only in 1902 and 1903. Carroll deflected the criticism by attacking the poor accounting procedures of Maori Councils, and the matter went no further.[40]

The economy drive which saw the removal of James Mason from the position of CHO in 1909 further affected the councils' activities. Peter Buck, who had recently entered Parliament as successor to Northern Maori MHR Hone Heke, spoke with the authority of an insider during that year's Supply debate. The Maori Councils vote was £659, down from the previous year's £840, a sum rendered even more inadequate since councils had now to undertake some functions previously discharged by the Health Department. The salaries of Pomare and the Maori sanitary inspectors had also been cut. Buck's conclusion was harsh: 'Unless the Government were willing to spend a reasonable amount in attending to the health of the Maoris, they might as well let them die out.'[41]

The work of the councils was seriously handicapped by these cutbacks. Despite this, in 1911 a number of Maori census enumerators lauded the councils' contribution to improved Maori health standards.[42] Buck, despite his earlier impatience, attributed much of the population increase recorded in the census to the work of the councils and the Native Department.[43] Two years later, when the councils' work was again debated in Parliament, Tame Parata (the Southern Maori MHR) commented favourably on the improved sanitation of South Island settlements. Others were less complimentary. Gordon Coates (Kaipara), a future Native Minister, claimed that 'Some years ago Maori Councils did good work, and the Maoris themselves were keen but they had gone back.' Instead of increasing resources to reverse this trend the House voted only £350 for the following year's work.[44]

Any remaining impetus for change, a pattern which had characterised the early years of the century, was abruptly halted by the advent of World

War I in 1914. Many Maori already felt that European medicine discriminated against them, in the paucity of services offered or in the rejection of traditional health practices. Some became disillusioned by a perceived failure to meet binding commitments to improve their health status. Peter Buck summed up their sense of frustration and anger when addressing the 1914 Australasian Medical Congress: 'We Maori people have had much legislation passed in the interests of our health and welfare, but too often the dispensers of that legislation seem to have been more concerned about the mote in their neighbour's eye than the beam in their own.'[45] It would be the role of a new Division of Maori Hygiene, under Buck's leadership, to attempt to reverse this disillusionment after 1920.

'Willing to contribute': Maori and hospitals

Relations between Maori and hospitals continued to exhibit a confused and sometimes contradictory picture in this period. Access to services and Maori attitudes towards institutional care remained problematical, and there is little accurate data about Maori use of hospitals. This section considers the principal factors which determined the attitudes of hospital boards as providers and Maori as consumers, comments on the Health Department's role as a mediator, and outlines various unsuccessful attempts to create a 'Maori' hospital.

The demographic and other factors which affected admissions to hospital in the late nineteenth century continued to complicate this aspect of Maori health care in the first half of the twentieth. As with the earlier period, there are substantial difficulties in obtaining accurate data about admission patterns and trends. Much of the evidence is impressionistic rather than quantitative. Only from the early 1920s did boards, especially those which felt over-burdened with Maori patients, begin to supply patient numbers.

Peter Buck, according to his biographer, was able in 1907 'on the basis of rudimentary hospital statistics to tabulate the causes of Maori illness'.[46] In fact, Buck acknowledged that his figures were derived from returns made by subsidised doctors and dispensers in the Auckland district.[47] Pomare used the same sources for his computation of Maori disease statistics between 1901 and 1908. He admitted that these could not be regarded as the complete picture 'but served in a general way to indicate the diseases most prevalent in the Native race'.[48] Both seem tacitly to have accepted either that hospital admissions were a minor component in Maori health care, or that this information was simply not available.

Between 1897 and 1909 the number of public hospitals in New Zealand rose from 41 to 56.[49] The majority of new units were located in the more remote rural areas. Given the population distribution, it is not surprising that Maori continued to be more visible in the rural hospitals after 1900. It was also no coincidence that these were often the hospitals with the lowest bed occupancy rates.

Some of these smaller hospitals made fairly generous provision for Maori. At Wairoa in northern Hawke's Bay the local hospital contained 'two six-bedded wards for male and female patients, and a four-bedded ward for Maoris' in 1908, yet the annual return claimed that only one of the 53 patients had been Maori.[50] Others, working to a tight budget, improvised. Northern Wairoa Hospital (later renamed Te Kopuru) opened in 1903 to serve the Dargaville district. In 1909 eight of its 110 patients were Maori. One of these was a lad suffering from tuberculosis. On visiting the hospital Inspector-General Valintine suggested that 'a corner of the verandah enclosed with canvas might be used for him' since he disturbed the other

INCIDENCE OF DISEASE.

From the returns supplied by medical officers and two dispensers in the Auckland District for the year 1907 I have compiled the following, which will serve as a beginning in this district to the statistical study of the ailments which afflict the Maori :—

	Males.	Females.	Total.
CLASS I.—Specific febrile or zymotic diseases,—			
Order 1. Miasmatic diseases	91	78	169
,, 2. Diarrhœal diseases	70	61	131
,, 3. Venereal diseases	8	2	10
CLASS II.—Parasitic diseases	18	25	43
CLASS III.—Constitutional diseases	45	29	74
CLASS IV.—Local diseases,—			
Order 1. Diseases of nervous system ...	18	16	34
,, 2. ,, organs of special senses	42	33	75
,, 3. ,, circulatory system ...	13	1	14
,, 4. ,, respiratory system ...	165	114	279
,, 5. ,, digestive system ...	86	76	162
,, 6. ,, lymphatic system ...	7	3	10
,, 7. ,, urinary system ...	6.	6	12
,, 8. ,, reproductive system ...	2	39	41
,, 9. ,, locomotive system ...	1	1	2
,, 10. ,, integumentary system	50	36	86
CLASS V.—Violence	78	23	101
CLASS VI. Ill-defined and not-specified cases ...	22	10	32
	722	553	1,275

The incidence of disease recorded amongst the Maori of the Auckland Native Health District in 1907 mirrored some of the findings of Dr Henry Spratt 30 years earlier. Infectious diseases topped the list, followed by respiratory ailments and digestive disorders. *AJHR, 1908, H-31, p.130* patients. There was apparently no suggestion that he be removed from the hospital.[51]

In 1907 Hone Heke drew attention to the fact that Marsden district Maori lived in the only electorate north of Auckland which had no subsidised NMO. His claim was supported by the local European MHR, Francis Mander, who added that 'every facility' was given to Maori seeking admission to Whangarei Hospital'.[52] Such claims are almost impossible to verify or refute. In the year to 31 March 1907 Whangarei, later the base hospital for Northland, admitted 115 patients, 58 of whom were classified as 'New Zealand'. The return made no distinction between Maori and Pakeha.[53]

The hospital at Rawene in Hokianga offers a microcosm of the dilemmas faced by smaller hospitals. When it opened in 1905 the Inspector-General of Hospitals defended his inability to inspect the facilities: 'It was found that to visit this Hospital would be very difficult, owing to the uncertainty of the boats and the disproportionate expense.'[54] In the following year twelve of the 30 patients were Maori; the 1907 figure was 26 out of 60. Rawene Hospital was a vital provider of health care for Maori in this remote Northland area. Peter Buck, anxious that there should be no reduction in service, queried the withdrawal in 1911 of a £100 Native Department subsidy for Hokianga Maori. This sum had raised the Rawene Hospital subsidy to £250; without it, Buck claimed, there would be no incentive for a medical officer to remain in the district.[55] The situation was resolved in 1914 with the arrival of Dr G.M. Smith, who was to be an eccentric but much loved doctor to Hokianga Maori for more than 30 years.[56] Soon after his arrival Smith faced the difficult problem of balancing individual patient care against wider community needs. On 26 January 1915 he recorded in his diary: 'Went to Kohu Kohu in the afternoon and saw several patients. I interviewed Reid, MP, about the hospital on my return. He is going to try and prevent them forcing us to admit Maori typhoids into our wards.'[57] Smith was not unsympathetic to typhoid sufferers or to Maori, but was concerned at the risk of them spreading the infection to other vulnerable individuals.

Few Maori lived in the large urban centres at this time, but the hospitals there were not exempt from treating Maori patients. However, a number of factors mitigated against their admission, notably territoriality and funding.

Such concerns appear to have been most pressing in the Auckland region. Until 1901 there was no hospital north of Auckland. Thereafter Whangarei (1901) was followed in rapid succession by Northern Wairoa (1903), Rawene (1905), and Mangonui (1907). Patients from these and other regions still went to the metropolitan centre for treatment, especially for more complex procedures. The reaction of the Auckland Hospital Board to this influx, and to its likely increase, was understandable yet has sometimes been misrepresented.

During the first decade of the century the board engaged in a number of disputes with neighbouring authorities over financial responsibility for Maori patients. In 1900, for example, it insisted on payment from the Bay of Plenty Hospital Board, which had advised it to seek recompense from the Native Department. The dispute was not about Maori per se, but about the wider issue of catchment areas and territorial obligations. Two years later, a little belatedly, the board asked its legal advisers about the eligibility for admission of non-ratepayers. Their interpretation, based on section 74 of the Hospitals and Charitable Institutions Act, was that 'any person', including anyone suffering from an infectious disease, was entitled to admission, although the board did have an obligation to prevent injury to other patients. Although the word Maori was never mentioned they were implicitly included in this definition.[58]

In 1905 the Auckland board agreed to admit a Maori patient for ophthalmic treatment only on condition that Bay of Plenty guaranteed payment.[59] Just months later the board refused admission to an Opotiki man on the grounds that it had no spare beds and his complaint, a chronic condition of the knee joint, was not urgent. He was offered accommodation in the adjacent Costley Block (intended primarily for children and convalescent patients) until a room became available in the hospital, but his brother declined and sent him back to Opotiki.[60]

The examples cited above are at odds with the common perception that hospitals simply did not wish to admit Maori. In support of this contention some historians have seized upon a letter of 14 July 1906 from Herbert Edgar to Miss Stewart, Matron of Thames Hospital, written shortly after Edgar became Under-Secretary of the Native Department: 'The hospitals, notably Auckland, are very unsympathetic regarding the admission of Maoris for treatment, their principal argument being that the Maoris pay but little towards the upkeep of the hospital [through rates]'.[61] Edgar's words, however, have been taken out of context.

On 5 July Edgar had alerted the Native Minister to a potential problem arising from the hospital treatment of Maori: 'There are several claims on hand by hospital authorities for treatment of Maori patients. I have consulted Dr Mason on the subject; whose opinion is, that hospitals are as much bound to treat Maoris as Europeans. But some hospitals, Auckland in particular, do not seem to think so.' Concerned at the implications for Native Department finances if such claims could be upheld, Edgar sought a legal opinion from the Solicitor-General. The latter's reply of 12 July stated that he was unaware of any distinctions but would need fuller facts to give a definite opinion, and the submission of a specific case. There is nothing in the Native Department files to indicate the matter was ever tested in this way.

Two days later Edgar sought further advice from Miss Stewart, a family friend.[62] Having outlined the problem, he voiced his conviction that 'if equal or favourable treatment is meted out to Maoris at any hospital, it is at the Thames.' Stewart's reply of 19 July contended the answer was simple: 'Maoris have the same privileges here in every way as Europeans.' She added that the hospital often wished to admit Maori who preferred to stay at home. The hospital currently housed two Maori inpatients, 'and I need not tell you that we are as good to them as to the white men—in fact I believe better. . . . As with Europeans some pay their own fees—some do not.' The issue was clearly never as cut and dried as the selective quotation from Edgar's letter to Stewart might imply.[63]

This comparison with Europeans on the matter of payment was a crucial concern. By the late nineteenth century hospital administrators in both Australia and New Zealand were conducting a vociferous campaign against 'hospital abuse' by those who could afford to pay for treatment but did not do so. Attempts were made to ensure that free treatment was restricted to the indigent, a difficult group to define, let alone identify. This campaign had very limited success in New Zealand. Between 1882 and 1910 patient payments never accounted for more than 15 per cent of hospital income, though there were wide variations between individual hospitals.[64]

The fact that many Maori did not pay rates rather than non-payment of hospital fees by individual patients appears to have been central to what

James Mason described as a 'disinclination on the part of some Hospital Boards to accept Maori patients'. This comment was based in part on Maui Pomare's statement that the Maori 'is so willing to go to some hospitals now, the difficulty is to gain admission'. Mason believed the problem stemmed purely from monetary considerations, not racial dislike, and suggested that the Maori should 'do as his white brother does' and pay rates on all his property holdings.[65] During the Health Supply debate later in 1907 James Allen, the MHR for Bruce, attacked hospital boards which discriminated against Maori. Health Minister George Fowlds dismissed Pomare's annual report as largely 'hyperbolical in character' and claimed he had taken firm action with any board which attempted to prevent Maori access.[66]

The question of Maori admissions was conspicuous only by its absence when hospital board representatives met in June 1908 for what Inspector-General Valintine described as New Zealand's most important conference on hospitals and charitable aid.[67] Two years later the Waikato Hospital Board complained to the Prime Minister about the heavy burden on European ratepayers in areas with a high percentage of Maori land, on which no hospital rates were paid.[68] Valintine showed some sympathy with this view, informing the Native Department Under-Secretary that 'special machinery' might be required in such regions. He was equally concerned, however, about the lack of suitable hospital accommodation in some areas, citing Bay of Plenty and Waikato.[69]

Hospital care for Maori was debated, arguably with more heat than light, at a second hospitals conference in June 1911. This followed the 1909 amalgamation of the Hospitals and Health Departments, which Valintine described as having surmounted the 'overlapping and waste of effort which was vexatious alike to the local authorities and the Departments concerned'.[70] The new system drew contradictory responses from hospital board delegates during a discussion on the 'health of the Native Race'.[71] Charles Horrell, chairman of the North Canterbury Hospital Board, argued that boards were not responsible for helping to control infectious diseases among Maori because they 'paid no rates towards the upkeep of the hospitals, or if they did, it was only a very small proportion as compared with the rates collected from the Europeans.' Horrell's complaint was backed by a South Canterbury delegate, R. Moore, and by James Young, chairman of the Waikato Hospital Board. Young estimated that his hospital district contained approximately a quarter of all Maori, yet they 'could get nothing out of those Native owners in the way of rates'.

Representatives from other areas balanced these negative portrayals. F.C.J. Bellringer of Taranaki claimed that Maori were amongst the 'best payers' in his district and supported the hospitals both directly and indirectly. They also conformed to hospital rules and in many instances proved better patients than their European neighbours. Bellringer was backed by H.C. Blundell of the Bay of Islands Hospital Board, who noted that Maori were 'willing to contribute . . . towards hospital expenses' according to their means, and by E.G. Eton (Wairarapa), whose board had always found them to be 'very good payers'.

Some months later Peter Buck commented in Parliament on the Health Minister's suggestion that boards play a greater role in Maori health. He was not optimistic; his own experience was that boards were 'most unsympathetic' because Maori paid no hospital rates.[72] The range of opinion described in the preceding paragraphs, however, suggests that the situation was more complex and less intolerant than Buck had implied. At the same time, Health Department officials recognised that they faced an uphill struggle in persuading some boards to accept any responsibility. As Valintine wrote in his 1913 annual report, when the dust had settled, 'for the indigent Native there is no doubt as to our obligations, and it is to be hoped that Hospital Boards, who sometimes resent the admission of these patients to their hospitals, will bear this in mind'.[73] As with so many areas of health policy, the advent of World War I meant that further discussion was deferred until the 1920s.

Reluctance to admit Maori was matched in some instances by Maori reluctance to be admitted. In 1902 Pomare inspected 124 'pas' and examined 356 indigent Maori, but sent only nine to hospital.[74] Buck offered an explanation for this pattern in 1906, shortly after he became Pomare's assistant: 'The Natives have a strong prejudice against European hospitals. Behind the barriers of the hospital-wards and behind the barrier of speech they know not what is going on. Therefore they imagine. The result is that the majority refuse to go to the hospital. Many lives are lost which might have been saved.'[75] Buck's fellow medical student, Dr Tutere Wi Repa, was more outspoken. In 1911 he wrote to Valintine about the refusal of Te Araroa

Maori to send typhoid cases to hospital and urged the Department to educate Maori out of their 'childish aversion'.[76]

Neither Buck nor Wi Repa mentioned the earlier dream of cottage hospitals staffed by Maori themselves.[77] Native Minister James Carroll tried to convince Maori Councils that they should help fund Maori cottage hospitals in both the North and South Islands.[78] He was not successful. In August 1904 the Kaipara MHR, Alfred Harding, asked when Carroll would honour his promise to erect such a hospital at Dargaville, prompting the reply that no such promise had been given. Carroll explained that the location of any such hospitals would be determined by the ability to 'meet as equally as possible the requirements of the larger centres of Maori population'.[79] Harding repeated his question in September 1905. On this occasion Carroll confirmed the desirability of the proposed scheme but admitted it had not yet been determined how success could be achieved 'both financially and otherwise'.[80] Three years later the local Maori sanitary inspector plaintively repeated the call for a Maori cottage hospital, but to no avail.[81]

Those Maori who were employed by the Health Department heartily supported Carroll's vision. In 1905 Wairarapa Maori were reportedly willing to pay half the cost of a cottage hospital, and provide a half-acre site.[82] Raureti Mokonuiarangi, Sanitary Inspector for Rotorua, emphasised the value that a Maori hospital would have in 'pakeharising' the local population.[83] Peter Buck, before his election to Parliament, advocated turning the Native Hostelry at New Plymouth into a cottage hospital, noting that 'The Maori prejudice against hospitals has considerably weakened, but it still exists'.[84] Maori and Europeans opened a combined cottage hospital fund at Te Araroa in 1907, and raised enough by 1911 to provide a cottage for the new Maori health nurse.[85] This seems to have been the only practical outcome of the agitation for Maori hospitals prior to the 1920s.

Data on Maori use of hospitals in the period 1900–20 are sadly deficient. Much of the evidence is subjective and, in some cases, contradictory. Individual boards were sometimes inconsistent in their practices towards Maori, as the population base altered and pressure on facilities changed over time. The evidence suggests that much depended on the collective or individual goodwill of hospital board members, and on the persuasiveness of Health Department officials. The examples provided in this section are therefore indicative rather than conclusive. For some Maori the hospital was an undesirable and alien threat. For others it was a welcome and vital component of health care. For a third group, subject to geographical or other restrictions, it was an unattainable goal.

'Specially suitable men'?: subsidised doctors

In the first two decades of the twentieth century, subsidised medical attendance continued to be the mainstay of the provisions made for Maori. The period was marked by repeated debates about the usefulness and location of these doctors and, after 1909, their effectiveness in comparison with the emerging district nursing structure. As with many other facets of Maori health care, it is difficult to identify any coherent policy in this area.

The European population of New Zealand increased by more than 50 per cent in this period, from around 770,000 to almost one and a quarter million, while Maori numbers rose from 45,000 to 57,000.[86] The number of registered doctors resident in New Zealand nearly doubled from 504 to 961, with the ratio of doctors to population improving from 1 in 1,863 to 1 in 1,602.[87] The number of Native Medical Officers also increased, at least in the first decade of the new century.

In 1900 there were fewer than 30 NMOs. The service was administered by the Justice Department but the Native Minister retained ultimate responsibility. From 1900 James Carroll and his Cabinet colleagues fielded numerous parliamentary questions seeking additions to the NMO network. In most cases the requests involved special pleading on behalf of a specific location. One of the most vociferous campaigners was Tame Parata, the MHR for Southern Maori. Parata first broached the question of medical assistance for the Maori of Bluff and Stewart Island in 1893.[88] In 1900 he persuaded the Native Minister to provide funding 'other than the allowance at present made to the doctor' for a group of Maori living at Whangarae, in the Nelson district, some 50 miles from the medical attendant. Carroll duly placed a medicine chest in the local schoolhouse.[89]

Success often required considerable persistence. Charles Major (Hawera) battled for over five years to obtain an NMO for his Taranaki constituency. He first asked Carroll to make an appointment in October 1903. The Minister replied that such a large population would involve considerable expense. He also suggested that many local Maori had an interest in reserves administered by the Public Trustee and 'where they are able to afford it they should contribute something towards the cost of medical attendance'.[90] Almost two years later Major resurrected his plea when endemic typhoid struck the kainga around Manaia, ten miles west of Hawera. This time Carroll evaded action by claiming that the government had not been asked to act by Maori themselves, though he did promise to investigate.[91] Major persevered, aided by a fresh outbreak at Waiokura. Carroll then replied that Pomare had telegraphed to say that only one case was being treated by the local public vaccinator, Dr Patrick Noonan, and there was 'No need for alarm'.[92]

In 1907 Major changed tack and asked Carroll to open a Native Hostelry at Hawera to combat the high pneumonia mortality. Carroll responded: 'An addition to the hospital at Hawera for the treatment of Maori sick would perhaps suit better than the present proposal.'[93] (In the previous year only one Maori had been admitted to the hospital, along with 141 Europeans.)[94] Undeterred, Major finally wrung a promise from Health Minister George Fowlds in mid September to subsidise a doctor if necessary.[95] George Brown, an American, was appointed NMO soon afterwards but enjoyed a relatively short tenure; he died of cirrhosis of the liver in June 1911, aged 46.

These incidents indicate an ad hoc approach to Maori health care. They may depict only the tip of the iceberg, with the parliamentary forum being used as a last resort when other approaches failed. They may also represent attempts to short-circuit bureaucracy by going straight to the Minister.

On several occasions MHRs attempted to raise wider concerns about perceived deficiencies in provisions for Maori health. In July 1903 the House approved Parata's motion that a list of all subsidised NMOs be drawn up. This was to include their locations, payments, numbers of Maori and 'half-castes' treated in the year to 31 March, and a classification of diseases.[96] No return was ever published. Parata's initiative, however, elicited others. A month later Hone Heke again referred to the NMOs during the Health Supply debate. He complained that the South Island received a disproportionate share of Civil List funding and suggested that some subsidised NMOs should be brought under the control of the Health Department if an extension of Pomare's work could not be funded from its own vote. Health Minister Joseph Ward replied that he was discussing the entire question of medical attendance on Maori with the Native Minister but refused to be more specific. Carroll made his position clear later that month, when challenged by Parata to provide medical attendance for Maori at Glenavy (near Oamaru); the Minister replied that medical attendance 'throughout the colony would have to be placed on a better footing' without raising costs.[97]

Another year elapsed before the matter was properly debated in Parliament. Alfred Fraser (Napier) used the Supply debate on Maori Councils to promote increased resources for Maori health and welfare, contrasting the solitary figure of Maui Pomare with the 20 veterinarians appointed to look after 'dumb animals'. Robert Houston (Bay of Islands) retorted that there were other subsidised doctors, including four in his own district. Fraser's response, that there was only one *full-time* doctor, prompted a flurry of denials. Arthur Remington (Rangitikei) claimed that Maori in his area were gratified by what was being done, while James Carroll stated there were currently 31 NMOs and four dispensers in the colony, not to mention the caches of medicines in the hands of schoolteachers. Parata then attacked his fellow Maori MHRs for failing to ensure the appointment of NMOs, contrasting this with his own success throughout the South Island. None replied to his criticism and the discussion swung back to the North Island situation.

As the debate raged on Charles Major accused Fraser of exaggeration: there were already 47 doctors, and he was seeking another for southern Taranaki. In retaliation, Fraser dismissed the existing NMOs as men he had never heard of: 'They were just chemists and others who, by political influence perhaps, had obtained a certain amount for so-called attendance on Maoris.' He advocated full-time appointments in Wellington, Taranaki, Hawke's Bay and Auckland. Carroll ignored Major's 47 doctors but sprang to the defence of the 31 he had previously mentioned, accusing Fraser of insulting their 'high profession'. He also revealed that the system was in a state of constant flux. The Wanganui NMO's subsidy had been withdrawn because the majority of local Maori 'were spreading further back, and those who remained were well enough off to pay. Now the back districts would be in want of medical men, more so than the towns, who could attend not only to the Natives, but also to the back-blocks settlers.'[98]

Ability to pay was one of the thorniest issues facing the managers of the NMO scheme. Defining eligibility was no easier in the case of Maori than it was for Pakeha seeking assistance under the charitable aid system.[99] In 1902 Pomare noted the need to supply qualified doctors to advise indigent Maori patients.[100] Five years later Pomare's superior, James Mason, insisted that Maori ought to pay for medical care if they could afford it; many Maori followed the Pakeha inclination to 'lean against the pillar of the State'.[101] In the absence of any clear guidance other officials applied a more liberal interpretation. Chief Health Officer Thomas Valintine, for example, advised William Mercer of Kaeo in January 1913 that if he accepted a subsidy he 'must undertake the treatment of all Maoris in your district, irrespective of the financial position'.[102] Valintine's annual report later that year noted a growing indignation among NMOs: 'The feelings of a medical man can be imagined who, on account of a subsidy of some £50, is called upon to attend a wealthy Maori in possession of broad acres, a well-furnished house, high-class agricultural implements, a motor-car, a billiard-table, and other luxuries of modern life.'[103] The question remained largely unresolved, with one district health officer reporting in 1919 that Temuka's NMO, John Hastings, was quite within his rights in refusing treatment: 'The appointment is for attendance on indigent Maoris, but a Maori can hardly be considered indigent who in preference to going to a public hospital goes to a private hospital in Timaru.'[104]

If nothing else, the 1904 parliamentary debate revealed how ill-informed and partial many members were when it came to Maori health. The first attempt at a comprehensive analysis of the NMOs did not occur until 1906, when the Native Department briefly resumed responsibility for them. A memorandum to Helyar Bishop, Stipendiary Magistrate in Christchurch, from Under-Secretary Edgar expressed doubts about the current structure's effectiveness and suggested that subsidised NMOs might be replaced by a smaller number of full-time doctors. In an addendum Edgar asked, 'Do you know of any specially suitable men?' Bishop concurred with Edgar's assessment, noting that it had always been difficult to obtain 'the best results for a reasonable expenditure'. He favoured fewer appointments and more defined duties, but warned that it would be hard to persuade doctors in settled practices to absent themselves for the time required. Bishop identified fourteen principal Maori centres in the South Island, with

North Island.

District.	Name.	Yearly Subsidy.	Amount of Subsidy actually received.			Additional Fees.			Number of Patients attended.
		£	£	s.	d.	£	s.	d.	
Mangonui	T. J. Trimnell (resigned 31/3/06)	50	50	0	0	...			144
	F. C. S. Forbes (appointed 1/4/06)		...			6	6	0	...
Kaitaia	T. W. P. Smith (dispenser, from 1/4/06 to 30/9/06)	15	7	10	0	...			107
	J. M. Hope (appointed 1/10/06) ...	50	25	0	0	1	10	0	106
Rawene	J. W. Browne (resigned 30/9/05)	100	50	0	0	4	13	0	74
	D. S. Coto (appointed 1/10/05)		50	0	0	5	10	0	22
Ohaeawai ...	A. G. H. Buckby	50	50	0	0	...			198
Kawakawa ...	H. D. Eccles	50	50	0	0	17	12	2	277
Dargaville	F. M. Purchas (resigned 31/5/05)	50	8	6	8	...			8
	W. H. Horton (appointed 1/7/05)		37	10	0	...			32
Huntly	C. Low (resigned 30/6/05)	50	12	10	0	...			29
	H. G. H. Monk (appointed 1/7/05)		37	10	0	...			84
Raglan ...	W. M. Sanders	50	50	0	0	...			179
Kawhia ...	C. C. Jenkins	50	50	0	0	...			206
Otorohanga and Taumarunui	A. Bell and	15	15	0	0	...			60
	C. P. Winkelmann (dispensers, to be discontinued 30/9/06)	25	25	0	0	...			22
	W. Cairns (appointed 1/4/06)	50	...			...			...
Te Kuiti ...	C. H. Holland (dispenser) ...	25	25	0	0	...			20
Taupo ...	R. W. Prinn (dispenser) ...	30	30	0	0	...			115
Te Puke ...	L. Frazer Hurst	100	100	0	0	...			195
Whakatane ...	H. A. Edmonds (resigned 31/12/06)	75	50	0	0	9	10	0	47
Waipiro Bay	C. S. Davis (to 31/12/06)	100	100	0	0	...			591
	W. F. Neil (appointed *pro tem* 1/4/06)		...			...			...
Tolago Bay	J. S. Reekie (resigned 31/12/05)	75	56	5	0	...			145
	H. Weeks (appointed 1/1/06)		18	15	0	...			59
Wairoa ...	J. Somerville	30	30	0	0	15	15	0	164
New Plymouth	H. A. McClelland (subsidy increased from £25 to £75 on 1/11/05)	75	45	16	8	7	10	0	79
Waipawa ...	J. Ross	25	25	0	0	...			21
Pahiatua ...	H. T. Dawson...	50	50	0	0	...			33
Hutt ...	J. R. Purdy	100	100	0	0	...			108
Totals...	...	1,290	1,149	3	4	68	6	2	3,125

populations ranging from 40 to 180, and noted other unnamed scattered communities with fewer than 30 inhabitants. He commented in detail on the discrepancies in the workloads of existing NMOs. William Fleming of Balclutha, for instance, seemed well paid at £25 per annum, since there were only thirteen Maori and nine 'half-castes' in the whole of Clutha County, while 'Dr Hargreaves of Akaroa is not overpaid at £25 if he does his work. The natives at Tikao Bay and Onuku are difficult sometimes of access, and I know, are a little exacting.' Bishop recommended the appointment of two full-time or three subsidised doctors, based in Christchurch, Oamaru and Riverton, to cover the entire island, though he conceded that distance would exclude Kaikoura, Westport and Hokitika from this scheme.[105]

South Island.

District.	Name.	Yearly Subsidy.	Amount of Subsidy actually received.	Additional Fees.	Number of Patients attended.
		£	£ s. d.	£ s. d.	
Kaikoura ...	B. S. Story	40	40 0 0	...	67
Kaiapoi	J. A. J. Murray (resigned 31/12/05)	75	56 5 0	...	321
	H. A. Davies (appointed 1/1/06)		18 15 0	...	83
Akaroa ...	W. H. Hargreaves (appointed 18/10/05)	25	11 8 0	...	14
Little River ...	J. W. D. Cook	50	50 0 0	...	*
Southbridge ...	T. J. Withers	50	50 0 0	...	35
Rapaki ...	J. A. Newall	40	40 0 0	...	56
Temuka ...	J. S. Hayes	50	50 0 0	...	188
Palmerston ...	W. Hislop	100	100 0 0	...	67
Oamaru ...	A. I. Garland	75	75 0 0	...	29
Waimate ...	H. C. Barclay...	50	50 0 0	...	34
Westport ...	M. McKenzie	25	25 0 0	...	38
Port Chalmers	Hodges and Borrie	50	50 0 0	...	61
Taieri ...	J. Sutherland	50	†37 10 0	...	26
Balclutha ...	W. A. Fleming	25	25 0 0	...	12
Riverton ...	C. H. Gordon	50	50 0 0	47 11 1	136
Bluff ...	J. Torrance	50	†37 10 0	...	71
Totals		805	766 8 0	47 11 1	1,238
North Island		1,290	1,149 3 4	68 6 2	3,125
Grand totals		2,095	1,915 11 4	115 17 3	4,363

* No return furnished; attendance when required. † Claim for last quarter not yet received.

The extent of the district intended to be served by each medical officer cannot be stated, nor can any estimate of the Maori population of such district be given. The general terms under which a medical officer receives a subsidy are that he will supply free medicine and advice at all times to all Maoris at his surgery or within a stated distance therefrom if the patient be to ill or infirm to come to the surgery. Attendance on Maoris at a greater distance to be paid for at a mileage rate. Probably Maoris living within a radius of ten to twenty miles will upon occasion visit the medical officer to obtain medicine and advice.

The 1906 'Return of Subsidised Medical Officers for Natives' (opposite and above) did not include 'the extent of the district intended to be served by each, together with an estimate of the Maori population of such district', as ordered by the House of Representatives. *AJHR, 1906, G-4*

Similar concerns were voiced in the North Island. Gilbert Mair, the Superintendent of Maori Councils, complained to Edgar that Dr James Purdy of Lower Hutt was paid £100 to attend about 24 Maori who were able to pay for medical aid and compared this with Elsdon Best's claim that there were several thousand Maori at Whakatane who could obtain assistance only by visiting Opotiki, at £30 a time.[106]

Before the Native Department could act on this information the NMOs became a Health Department responsibility. William Herries (Bay of Plenty) asked for clarification of the procedures to be followed in applying for a subsidy, and expressed his hope that the Health Minister would be more generous than his Native Department counterpart had been. Fowlds' response was encouraging but qualified. Under the old system the Native Department vote had included a whole range of necessities. He now had £3,000 per annum solely for medical and sanitary purposes, and 'would deal with the matter as generously as possible, consistent with regard to economy'.[107]

When the NMO establishment was handed over by the Native Department in October 1906, Under-Secretary Edgar supplied Mason with a tally of 35 NMOs and two dispensers.[108] The rationale behind the employment of the latter was explained by Edgar's successor, R.W. Fisher, in a 1911 memorandum to the Native Minister: 'A number of medical men all over the Dominion are subsidized from the Native Civil List, together with several dispensers in districts where no medical men reside, and who, though not legally qualified to practise medicine, are quite able to dispense simple remedies for minor complaints.'[109]

Mason's annual report for 1907 claimed that efficiency and economy had improved now that doctors were no longer under lay control. He promised adjustments to the allocation of the 38 doctors currently receiving payments of between £25 and £100 for attending indigent Maori, to take account of population movements.[110] Apirana Ngata was one of the first to challenge the current distribution. In July 1907 he reiterated Mair's criticism of the Lower Hutt situation, describing the payment to Purdy as an absurdity when there were up to a hundred doctors available to treat Maori within 30 minutes travelling time: 'But in the Urewera, the Bay of Plenty and up to Cape Runaway, where the Maori population exceeds three thousand five hundred, there is only one man resident at Opotiki, and he is getting a paltry £75.' Ngata blamed this on a lack of enthusiasm by successive governments, but failed to explain how they could compel doctors to practice in particular locations.[111]

Other MHRs were quick to jump on the bandwagon. Shortly after Ngata's statement William Field (Otaki) queried the Porirua NMO subsidy, following complaints by local Maori. Pomare assessed the health of the community's 70 to 80 inhabitants but made no comment on the doctor. Health Minister Fowlds then announced that the community would in future be treated by a doctor 'resident on the other side of the ranges'.

Twelve months later Field reported an improved standard of care since the Hutt subsidy had been rearranged to provide for Porirua, but criticised the lack of services further up the coast.[112]

Some MHRs quite blatantly invoked Maori needs to support European claims for medical assistance. Frederick Lang (Manukau) sympathised in 1907 with the settlers of Clevedon, who could not afford to engage a doctor from the neighbouring community. Instead of making a direct appeal for help, he asked the Health Minister to 'use his influence to have a sum granted in this case for assistance to Maoris, of whom there were a great many round Clevedon'.[113] Lang's subterfuge went unrewarded.

Pomare's annual report for 1903 had emphasised the value of subsidised NMOs in countering the dual threat of exorbitant doctors' fees and recourse to tohunga.[114] Health Department officials struggled to reconcile the conflicting demands of parliamentarians, doctors and Maori. Their efforts were further hampered by local disputes. In 1907 Buck recommended that John Mountaine of Maungaturoto in Northland be appointed NMO to the 407 Maori of Otamatea County in addition to his role as public vaccinator. The advice was disregarded and Edmund Dukes of Paparoa was appointed instead. When Fowlds visited Maungaturoto in January 1909, he found that local Maori would prefer Mountaine because he had a better knowledge of their language. Buck advised the CHO that it would be difficult to appoint both men; but 'if any feeling continues to exist' they might consider a dual appointment at £25 each. He also noted that there had been no charges of negligence against Dukes, who therefore retained his position.[115]

In spite of these local difficulties the NMO scheme expanded by almost one-third beween 1906 and 1909, from 35 to 46 doctors. In public, departmental officials expressed satisfaction with these practitioners. Indeed, Pomare's 1909 report suggested that the major drawback was the behaviour of the patients themselves: 'The forty-six subsidised medical men have also done very good work. No one but a medical man can appreciate the difficulties which these men have to contend against in treating Maori patients; but no doubt as time goes on the Maoris will learn the lessons of a sick-bedside, and so lessen the disadvantages of a medical practitioner for the Maoris.'[116]

Behind the scenes a more critical appraisal was taking place. Valintine, immediately after taking control as Chief Health Officer in June 1909, asked district health officers to report on the efficiency of the medical men who had received subsidies for treating Maori in the previous year.[117] Valintine's own opinion emerged in a letter to John Purdy, District Health Officer for Auckland and the brother of James Purdy of Lower Hutt: 'I absolutely agree with you that the present system of subsidising medical men for the above is not satisfactory. . . . As far as I can see under the present system the doctors do very little to help the Maoris'.[118] Purdy's response to a departmental circular entitled 'Medical Attendance on Natives' was that he could see little merit in the NMO system, and that the time was ripe for a substantial reduction in costs.[119]

This expansion in the middle years of the decade was typical of the public service as a whole. In 1909, however, there was a sudden reversal as falling government revenues forced it to retrench. Some 940 public servants were retired or laid off.[120] The burden of implementing this policy in relation to Maori affairs fell once more on the Native Minister, although the NMOs had been nominally controlled by the Health Department from 1906 to 1909. In December 1909 Carroll assured his parliamentary colleague Tame Parata that government retrenchment should not appreciably inconvenience 'indigent Native patients'.[121]

To assist with the evaluation of Maori health needs a memorandum entitled 'Medical Attendance on Natives and Proposed Changes' had been drawn up in July 1909. This listed more than 60 locations, two-thirds of them in the North Island.[122] Contrary to popular belief Waikato (with twelve) had the most entries among the North Island districts.[123] All except three of those listed appear to have been qualified doctors. Replacements were being sought or considered for several vacancies. Fourteen positions were to be dispensed with, including ten in the South Island.

The memorandum detailed enormous discrepancies in both recompense and workload. Cyril Davis of Waiapu, one of the highest paid at £100, earned his money, for he had seen 720 patients at an average cost of 2s 9d. Close behind came John Somerville of Wairoa, Hawke's Bay, whose £30 for 175 cases averaged out at 3s 5d. At the other end of the scale, Stanley Warneford of Rawene received a salary of £100, which gave him £5 11s 1d for each of his eighteen patients. The most expensive of all was George Wilson of Palmerston North, whose two patients had cost £18 15s each.

Wilson was dismissed, prompting Manawatu Maori to petition for his replacement by John O'Brien.

The government found it difficult to develop a consistent policy in relation to NMOs. The situation was not helped by the continuing use of Maori health as a political weapon. When Sir William Steward asked the Native Minister in 1910 if his government would deliver medical attendance to Maori in accordance with the provisions of the South Island land purchases, the answer was an unequivocal 'Yes'. When he was asked why Morven Maori had been deprived of medical assistance while Waitaki and Oamaru, with a similar population base, still enjoyed the services of a doctor, Carroll fell back on his well-worn response that the whole scheme was receiving attention.[124]

The following year Steward asked what provision would be made for Waitaki now that the NMOs had been transferred back to the Health Department. He noted that the 200 or so Maori and 'half-castes' in the area had been promised medical attendance at the time of the land sales, and that £100 a year had been disbursed in previous years but nothing had been done for the previous eighteen months. Fowlds could only reply once more that the matter was under consideration, along with 'the whole administration of the Native medical health service'.[125]

The transfer back to the Health Department was not entirely smooth. Questions were again asked in Parliament in July 1913 about the alleged withdrawal of North Island subsidies. William Herries, the new Native Minister, explained that some NMOs might have fallen through the cracks when responsibility passed from his Department to Health. If the Health Minister was unwilling to fund the work he would be happy to see this important function return to the Native Department. Herries, as MHR for the Bay of Plenty, had shown a keen interest in Maori health over the previous decade, but there was an element of political grandstanding in his comments.[126]

This renewed debate gave a further opportunity to raise concerns about medical services for European settlers as well as Maori in the more remote reaches of the country. The Health Department quantified its response to such pressures by reporting that it had spent £864 on subsidies to medical men in the backblocks and £4,377 on medical and nursing attendance for Maori in 1913/14. With the advent of World War I the pattern showed a marked change. Spending on European subsidies rose to £1,143 in 1914/15 while the sum allocated to Maori NMOs fell to £3,219. The Maori share of the total had fallen from 84 to 74 per cent.[127] In the latter year Auckland's District Health Officer, Thomas Hughes, recorded the appointment of four new NMOs, at Rawene, Wellsford, Te Puke, and Taupo. His Christchurch counterpart reported in a similarly upbeat fashion: 'Medical attendance on Natives in all the principal pas in the district has now been arranged for.'[128]

The calibre of those available for service during the war years often left something to be desired. The Bay of Islands seems to have been especially unfortunate.[129] Its local hospital board experienced severe difficulties with the practitioner brought into the district by the Whangaroa Medical Club. Alfred Story was apparently addicted to both drink and drugs, but his continued presence deterred other doctors from settling in the area. Not surprisingly, local Maori were reluctant to use his services, although one board member claimed that this was because he had a German wife and Maori feared he would therefore poison them.

The board's proposed solution, that NMOs be paid through the hospital boards and not the Health Department, was firmly opposed by Dr Hughes in August 1915: 'As the work of medical officers is entirely to do with natives, I am of opinion that it would be better for the Department to have full control of them.' Valintine went further in a letter to his Minister on 4 May 1916 concerning an 'unreliable medical officer': the Department should take over the entire Bay of Islands hospital district. 'This would need an amendment in the Act, but I am quite sure that . . . where the population is comparatively sparse, the land poor and the district generally not affording sufficient inducement to reliable medical men such districts should be staffed and controlled by the Department.'[130] The board kept its independence, but the Department retained its hard-won control of the NMOs.

Historians have often questioned the utility of the subsidised NMO. The numerous requests by parliamentarians and others in the early 1900s for an extension of the scheme suggest a rather different contemporary perception. Such demands came from both Maori and Pakeha, the latter sometimes acting as much from self-interest as philanthropic concern. The criteria for obtaining an NMO appear to have included both genuine need and political pressure. The result was a system which exhibited the effects of what Warwick Brunton has termed 'residualism, parochialism and ad hocracy'.[131] There were marked inconsistencies in payments and workloads. Maori in the larger centres were more likely to enjoy the services of conscientious and competent doctors; others were not so fortunate. Geographical isolation and low population density left some communities without medical care. Once again, a multiplicity of factors were at work.

During the debate on the Tohunga Suppression Bill in 1907 James Carroll noted that many Maori lived 70 miles or more from European doctors. Since they could not afford a trip to the doctor, or pay the doctor to come to them, they were obliged to rely upon tohunga. Carroll showed no inclination, however, to supply more doctors.[132] Even much shorter distances sometimes proved insurmountable. John Thomson (Wallace) asked Carroll in 1903 to provide medical aid for the 30 Maori at Scott's Gap. The Riverton NMO lived 26 miles away and was inaccessible, but a doctor had recently set up shop in Otautau, just eight miles from Scott's Gap. Carroll was non-committal because of the numerous demands on the Civil List vote.[133]

Later that year Carroll received a lesson in the economics of general practice from Herbert Barclay, Medical Superintendent of Waimate Hospital from 1890 to 1917 and NMO for the area at various times since 1895. Barclay had quoted £50 per annum to attend Maori at Waitaki North/Glenavy. Using Friendly Society scales as a yardstick, he explained that the 25 inhabitants would attract an annual retainer of £35, plus a three-guinea travelling fee for the 32-mile return trip from his residence. Given the higher sickness levels among Maori, and his frequent attendance on midwifery cases (an additional charge for Friendly Society members), Barclay believed his quote was justified. Because of his 'great interest in the preservation of the native race', however, he was willing to undertake a one-year trial for £35.[134]

Health Department doctors often sympathised with colleagues like Barclay. One of the most outspoken was Robert Makgill. As District Health Officer for Auckland he defended George Craig's bill of 25 guineas for attending Maori typhoid cases in 1910. His aggressive memorandum to the Native Department Under-Secretary claimed that this was perfectly reasonable for a ride of eighteen miles across the dangerous mountain tracks behind Waihi. With seven cases and three deaths, he argued the outbreak would have warranted an outlay of £40 'by whatever branch of the public service the supervision of the physical welfare of the native race is responsible to'. In a separate note to Valintine, he further vented his spleen: 'It seems absurd to treat so well known a practitioner as Dr Craig in this way—as though he were trying to cheat the Native Department. I cannot understand why Mr Fisher considers that there was no need for this expenditure. I don't know what his Department exists for but to attend to matters like this.'[135]

Many practitioners were less accommodating than Barclay and Craig. Edmund Dukes of Otamatea County complained in 1911 that it was 'quite impossible to properly supervise' a kainga fourteen miles from his home.[136] Ebenezer Teichelmann of Hokitika was even more reluctant to assist. He sought compensation in 1914 for treating two Maori when their usual doctor was ill: 'The Maori pah is 4½ to 5 miles from Hokitika and they demand a good deal of attention.'[137]

The high costs incurred by incidents such as the Waihi typhoid outbreak, the gripings of men like Dukes, and the unsatisfactory behaviour of the likes of Story of Whangaroa were contributory factors in the Department's decision to trial a fresh initiative in 1909. Valintine's letter to John Purdy envisaged the partial replacement of subsidised doctors by a network of district nurses, both Maori and European. The introduction of that scheme, which drew mixed reactions from the medical profession and parliamentarians, is addressed in the next section.

'Our own doctors': Maori health professionals

In 1986 Mason Durie complained about the small number of Maori health professionals in contemporary New Zealand.[138] Yet Maori doctors, sanitary inspectors and nurses were a core element in the development of the health system during the first decade of the twentieth century. The failure to build on these initiatives had lasting implications on health care for Maori.

The proposal in 1906 to replace Gilbert Mair, the Superintendent of Maori Councils, with Maui Pomare, a trained Maori physician, had two major implications. It endorsed the Te Aute College Students' Association viewpoint that European health reforms should be introduced by Maori whose education had given them 'pakeha spectacles'.[139] Secondly, it recognised the talent of individual Maori and reinforced Pomare as a role model. In terms of medical education, he had already achieved this standing. Half a century after the event, Peter Buck recalled the effect Pomare had had upon himself and Tutere Wi Repa, a fellow medical student: 'Resplendent in the top hat, frock coat, and striped trousers that characterized the profession in those days, he visited Wirepa and me in Dunedin and cheered us on the way to acquire similar symbols of success.'[140]

The admission of Buck and Wi Repa to the Otago Medical School in 1899 was facilitated by government scholarships. Apirana Ngata urged the two young men to pass their matriculation and medical preliminary exams, for 'it should not then be difficult to make satisfactory arrangements with the Minister of Education to see you through a five years course at Dunedin'. Qualification as a doctor would allow Buck to 'lay the foundations of a healthier more compact, more powerful social opinion among our people'.[141]

Ngata's comments reflected the desire of the Te Aute College Students' Association to establish a training programme for Maori doctors and nurses.[142] In 1903 Pomare's annual report suggested that 'Native doctors' should become local health officers when they qualified. The call was taken up in Parliament by Hone Heke, whom Buck was to succeed in 1909. During the Education Supply debate he appealed on behalf of an unnamed Maori medical student 'who would be equipped better if he was sent Home to complete his studies. Would the Government assist in sending him to London University?' Premier Seddon promised to investigate, admitting that: 'It was essential for the preservation and well-being of the race that more of them should be assisted to become doctors. It would be money well spent.' Nothing came of the proposal.[143]

Buck graduated from Otago in 1904 and joined Pomare as a Native Health Officer in November 1905. Wi Repa was not so fortunate. He struggled to complete his studies and did not gain his degree until 1908, by which time he had already served a term as a house surgeon in Dunedin Hospital.[144] After graduation Wi Repa moved to Gisborne, where Valintine 'offered me the position of house surgeon at the Gisborne Hospital, but when they discovered that I was a Maori they dismissed me.'[145] He was NMO at Te Karaka in Poverty Bay from 1908 to 1913 before returning to practice among the Ngati Porou around Hicks Bay and Te Araroa.[146] Wi Repa's lasting bitterness and a somewhat erratic temperament created numerous headaches for the Health Department over the years. In 1913

Valintine felt it necessary to inform his Minister of the Department's misgivings about him.[147]

In his annual report for 1906 Pomare welcomed the reconstruction of the Native Department, looking forward to the prospect of 'our own doctors to heal the sick'.[148] His view was shared by Judge Edgar, the Department's new Under-Secretary, whose proposal that Pomare become Superintendent of Maori Councils was founded on the assumption that Buck would take over as Pomare's assistant and that another two assistant health officers would be appointed 'so soon as other Maori students have qualified as Doctors'.[149] During the 1907 debate on the Tohunga Suppression Bill Ngata claimed that the 'bastard tohunga'—as distinct from the experts of olden times—would never be driven out until Maori doctors could be supplied through the university system.[150] The system, however, failed to deliver.

By 1910 Otago had produced 119 medical graduates, including eleven women; Buck and Wi Repa remained the only Maori.[151] The scholarships granted to Buck and Wi Repa appear not to have been continued, but it is not known if this was a conscious decision by the government or the consequence of a dearth of candidates. Whatever the cause, it destroyed the Te Aute College Students' Association's vision of a network of Maori doctors. No other Maori was to take up the challenge of medical training until Edward Pohau Ellison, a lawyer's son, graduated from the Otago Medical School in 1919.

Peter Buck's 1910 MD thesis was entitled 'Medicine Amongst the Maoris, in Ancient and Modern Times'. It contained sections on the introduction of civilisation, which covered topics such as epidemic and sexually transmitted diseases, and the present condition of the race, which examined demographic factors, infant feeding, Maori physique and the role of tohunga. Buck acknowledged the lack of Maori doctors and sought to improve doctors' understanding and treatment of their Maori patients.[152] He conveyed the same message to his parliamentary colleagues in 1911, stressing the need for medical men to have an awareness of Maori language and customs. This was accompanied by a complaint about the failure to replace himself and Pomare, both of whom had swapped medicine for politics earlier that year.[153] The two men seem to have been equally disillusioned at the end of a decade which had begun so promisingly. When

Peter Buck/Te Rangi Hiroa (1877?–1951) attired as a graduate of the University of Otago. *ATL, F37931 1/2*

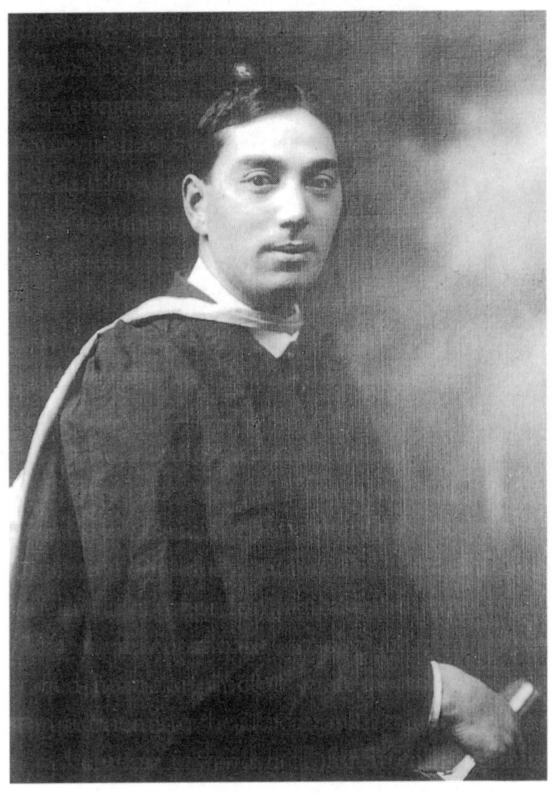

Pomare participated in a conference in 1912 on the control and treatment of tuberculosis as a 'Member of Executive Council representing the Native Race', the report of proceedings made no mention of his clinical background.[154] During the debate on smallpox which followed an outbreak among North Island Maori in 1913, Pomare revealed his distress at the manner in which he had been treated when he left his medical post. It occurred, he said, 'with not even a word of thanks for the services which had been rendered, though humbly perhaps, by myself. That is a matter of taste for those in authority at the time.'[155]

The Maori sanitary officers had equal reason to be dismayed by their treatment. In 1901 the Health Department employed eight Pakeha sanitary inspectors.[156] Pomare used the Rotorua conference of Maori Councils in 1903 to urge the appointment of Maori inspectors.[157] This innovation was welcomed by James Mason, who predicted it would be 'fraught with the greatest good'. Pomare's report to Mason described the venture as fulfilling a 'long-felt want, as it has been almost impossible for one man to do justice to such a large field.' The report also detailed the inspectors' duties.[158]

The appointment of only two inspectors in the first instance was scorned as ridiculous and inadequate by Alfred Fraser, the MHR for Napier.[159] The initial experiment quickly proved its worth, and by 1905 inspectors were located at Kaitaia, Ohaeawai in the Bay of Islands, Dargaville, Ruatoki in the Urewera district, and Masterton. Pomare then recommended extending the system to cover the 'great Native centres' in King Country, East Coast and Waikato.[160] Under-Secretary Edgar concurred. Two years later the death of the prophet Tohu convinced Buck that it was time to appoint a man of tact and influence in Taranaki.[161] By 1908 there were eight inspectors in all, with salaries ranging from £36 to £50 per annum; the one exception was Elsdon Best, the only non-Maori incumbent, who received £150 for his work at Ruatoki.[162] Ngata complained in Parliament about the niggardly payments to those at the bottom of the scale. Health Minister Fowlds reassured him that this would be dealt with through the supplementary estimates,[163] but within a year the salaries had been further reduced and in 1911 the positions were abolished.

Buck castigated this decision as 'unwise' during the 1911 Address in Reply debate. Six days later he sought confirmation that Maori health was back in the hands of the Health Department and asked Fowlds to clarify what was being done. The Minister had to admit that all the Maori inspectors north of Auckland had been dismissed. They were to be superseded in some areas by European inspectors and in others by the new district nurses.[164] On 31 August the General Conference of Maori Councils viewed with regret the decision to 'replace the Maori Sanitary Inspectors by Europeans who through not understanding Maori Customs and sentiment frequently cause unnecessary friction', and invited the Department 'to consider the claims of suitable Maoris for appointment.' The plea fell on deaf ears.[165] At the end of September Buck made a final attempt to have the policy reversed, raising the matter during the Maori Councils Supply debate. Native Minister Carroll expressed surprise at the Health Department's action, considering the amount of work that had been accomplished for such small salaries. Carroll's failure to offer any practical assistance typified the inter-departmental bickering which hindered

Maori health during the first two decades of this century. Thereafter the matter was allowed to lapse.[166]

The first generation of Maori sanitary inspectors had no formal qualifications and little real knowledge of sanitary science when they were appointed.[167] It was only in July 1907 that Pomare managed to arrange a training course which covered a wide range of topics, though not exhaustively.[168] At the Maori Councils conference in 1908 Buck suggested joining forces with the European sanitary inspectors' meeting, which seems to have been held concurrently, but the minutes do not indicate whether this was done.[169] The real strength of the inspectors was their elevated status within Maoridom. When possible, Pomare and Buck were accompanied by inspectors during their visits to Maori Councils, for as Buck noted in 1907: 'They are all chiefs with authority.'[170] By 1909, in Pomare's opinion, they had accomplished in a few years what he had anticipated would take quarter of a century.[171]

The sanitary inspectors were responsible for monitoring environmental health, housing, infectious diseases, vaccination, and the activities of

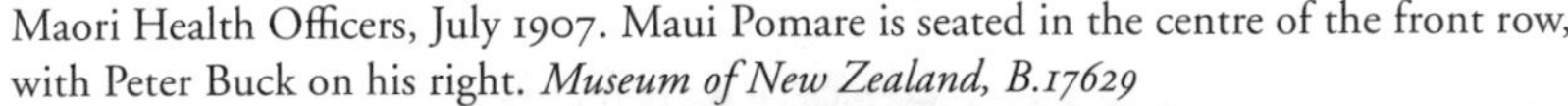

Maori Health Officers, July 1907. Maui Pomare is seated in the centre of the front row, with Peter Buck on his right. *Museum of New Zealand, B.17629*

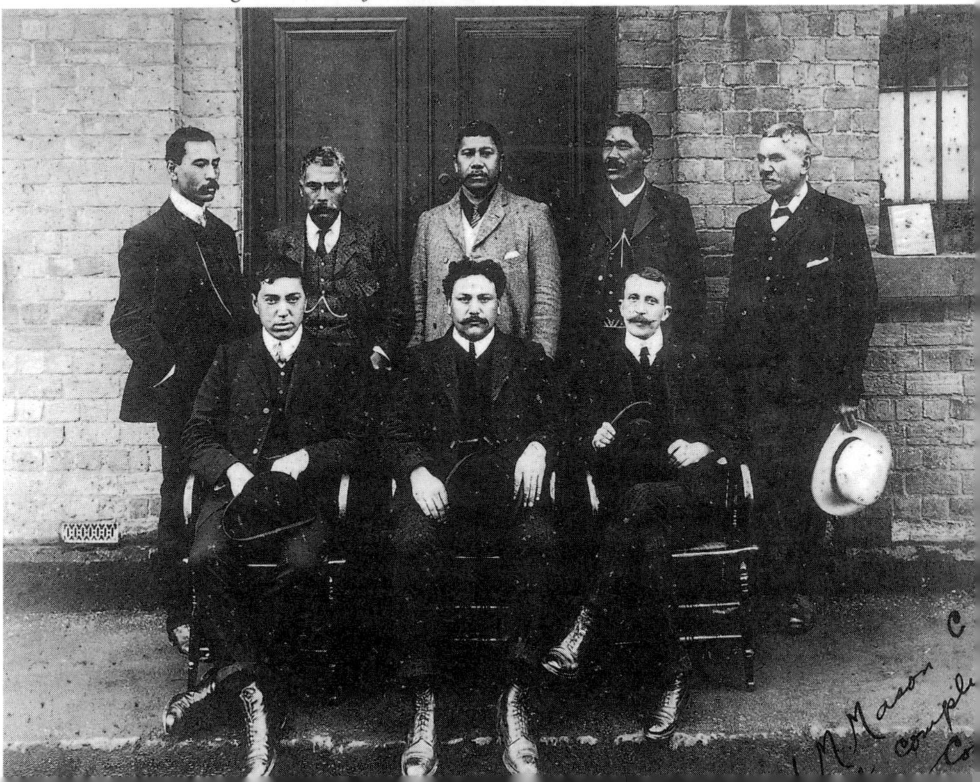

tohunga. Like Ngata, they were opposed to 'bastard tohunga'. Europeans had exhibited varied reactions to tohunga in the nineteenth century. Some, like the CMS missionary William Williams, referred to them as 'native doctors' and noted their skills in administering herbs.[172] Some Native Department officials also accorded them the honorific of 'doctor' and offered qualified approval. G.T. Wilkinson wrote from Otorohanga in the early 1890s that Maori had 'to take their chance between the local Maori *tohunga*, or doctor, and the few proprietary medicines that are on sale at the local stores.' It was unclear which of these he most disliked.[173] Even James Pope acknowledged their competence in treating bruises and wounds, and in curing rheumatism.[174]

By the twentieth century, under the influence of Western-trained Maori

The Tohunga Suppression Act 1907.

New Zealand.

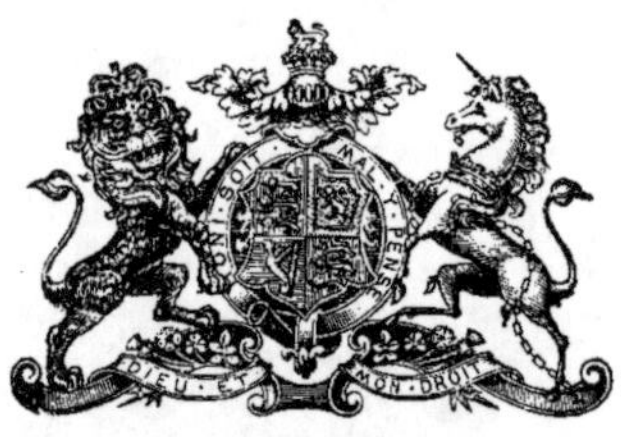

ANALYSIS.

Title.
Preamble.
1. Short Title.
2. Penalty on person practising as a tohunga.
3. Regulations.
4. Repeal.

1907, No. 13.

Title. AN ACT to suppress Tohungas.

[*24th September, 1907.*

Preamble. WHEREAS designing persons, commonly known as tohungas, practise on the superstition and credulity of the Maori people by pretending to possess supernatural powers in the treatment and cure of disease, the foretelling of future events, and otherwise, and thereby induce the Maoris to neglect their proper occupations and gather into meetings where their substance is consumed and their minds are unsettled, to the injury of themselves and to the evil example of the Maori people generally:

BE IT THEREFORE ENACTED by the General Assembly of New Zealand in Parliament assembled, and by the authority of the same, as follows:—

Short Title. 1. This Act may be cited as the Tohunga Suppression Act, 1907.

physicians, tohunga came increasingly under attack. As Charles Hercus rather dramatically put it in 1964, Pomare in particular 'valiantly and successfully contended with apathy and fear, tapu and tohungaism'.[175] Pomare's second report, in 1902, identified 'tohungaism' as a bar to Maori progress and warned that change would take more than one generation. At the same time he acknowledged that high medical fees were a disincentive to Maori, who would 'either do nothing, or sneak off to a tohunga, which is the only alternative'. He proposed a dual strategy to improve Maori health. Compulsory death registration and the notification of infectious diseases would reveal the 'causes of his decay'. This, he claimed, would combat the pernicious influence of tohunga.[176]

During the 1905 Health Supply debate William Herries (Bay of Plenty), a future Native Minister, noted Pomare's views and hoped that the Department would act to curb these practices, since it seemed impossible to mobilise the Native Department.[177] Pomare and Buck took up the challenge, attacking the current generation for adding 'many pernicious things to the ancient mode of treatment' and describing their activities as a caricature of the old-style expert.[178]

At one level, the Tohunga Suppression Act 1907 was an attempt to counter Maori protest movements headed by prophets such as Te Whiti and 'the notorious Rua'.[179] Maori health, however, was a fundamental concern. Herries, for example, used the ammunition supplied by Pomare and Buck to argue that sending qualified doctors to live among the Maori would negate the baneful influence of tohunga. Support for this viewpoint came from influential leaders such as Ngata and Carroll.[180] Health concerns were reflected in the wording of the Act, which outlawed 'attempts to mislead any Maori by professing or pretending to possess supernatural powers in the treatment or cure of any disease'. The Act contained no specific reference to traditional healing per se.[181]

Welcoming the Act's passage, Buck again pilloried the contemporary tohunga as a 'modern quack or sham article'.[182] The choice of phrase was no accident. Hone Heke, the first of the Maori MHRs to speak during the debate on the Tohunga Suppression Bill, had wished the legislation to apply also to Pakeha tohunga, 'who manage to kill their patients in a very similar fashion'.[183] He was to get his wish with the passage of the 1908 Quackery Prevention Act.[184]

Pomare and Buck regarded the Tohunga Suppression Act as a high point in their fight for Maori health. Within four years of its passage both men had effectively quit the health arena, though they were to return briefly during the 1913 smallpox epidemic. Their departure was sorely felt in some quarters. In 1911 Thomas Bevan, a resident of Otaki since 1845, contrasted the 'legitimate' tohunga of former days with the current practitioners. He described Pomare's dismissal as a great mistake, citing his excellent work in 'disabusing their [Maori] minds of these superstitions . . . and teaching and training them as to how they should rule their actions in the interests of their health'.[185]

Buck was to be reappointed to the Health Department in 1919; in a parallel move, the concept of Maori sanitary inspectors was revived in 1920, seven years after Buck had urged their re-introduction. His plea during a debate on the 1913 smallpox epidemic was based on the work undertaken at that time by Maori inspectors. The suggestion brought praise from the new Health Minister Heaton Rhodes for Buck's own contribution, but no commitment to his proposal.[186] A scheme begun with such high hopes in 1900 had ended in apparent defeat a decade later.

A similar fate was to befall attempts to establish a corps of Maori nurses. The Te Aute College Students' Association first suggested such a scheme in 1897. The proposal was embraced by James Pope, Organising Inspector for Native Schools, who asserted that 'The [Education] Department has constantly recognised the importance of directing the attention of the Maori race to the laws of health and to sanitary reform.'[187] The scheme was first trialled in Hawke's Bay, with Emma Mitchell and Mary Jones admitted to Napier Hospital as nurse probationers from Hukarere Girls' School in 1898.[188] Its expansion was hindered by the unwillingness of some hospitals to participate.

Comments by Matron Stewart of Thames Hospital in 1906 typified the ambiguous response of many hospital boards which approved of the scheme in principle but preferred not to participate in it. Stewart and Emil Aubin, the hospital's resident surgeon since 1899, did not wish to disappoint Pakeha girls who were waiting to train by allocating places to Maori, though both agreed that there ought to be a hospital in King Country 'or somewhere' for their training: 'Let them get a Hosp of their own.'[189] Some boards were also worried about the cost of training. Auckland Hospital Board medical staff approved the admission of Maori probationers in 1905 and Martha Nehemia joined the staff in April 1906. Concerns were soon raised about her capabilities compared with those of European entrants. A dispute arose between the hospital, which resolved that board, lodging and uniform were sufficient remuneration for first-year Maori nurses, and the Education Department, which had thought Nehemia would be paid as a first-year probationer. After prolonged discussion with the Inspector of Native Schools, Nehemia was transferred by the Education Department in October 1907 to Rawene Hospital, where the training might be less demanding and, considering the difference in the nature of the two units, less comprehensive.[190] Auckland continued to accept Maori entrants 'as a means of aiding the Maori race', but only as day pupils and on the clear understanding that the Education Department would underwrite the costs.[191]

It was envisaged from the outset that Maori nurses would return to their communities, and relatively few remained within the hospital sector after completing their training. William Collins advocated this step in his 1904 presidential address to the NZBMA. As with the appointment of Pomare some four years earlier, the message was couched in evangelical terms. Collins proposed that female missionaries like those sent to India and China be located in areas of high Maori population as nurses to 'look after the young Maori race under the instruction of Dr Pomare'.[192]

Pomare adopted a similar tone when he announced in 1908 that district nurses were to 'go forth to care for the sick, to lecture, and to uplift humanity'.[193] This was a marked change of tone from the complaint in his 1907 report: 'There ought to be ten girls in training where there is only one at present. We have long advocated the speedy training of Maori girls as nurses.'[194] His new-found optimism probably owed something to the arrival of Valintine as Inspector-General of Hospitals following Dr Duncan Macgregor's death in December 1906. Before joining the Health Department in 1901 Valintine had been a general practitioner at Inglewood in Taranaki, and he had a keen awareness of rural needs. Once again, this was expressed as a religious crusade. He believed backblocks nursing was 'as noble, as unselfish, yes, and as christian-like, as the missionary calls to heathen lands'.[195]

Valintine confided to Auckland's District Health Officer in June 1909 that subsidised NMOs were 'about the best thing that could be done' in the present circumstances, 'but I think we can improve this by a system of district nursing, which I hope to initiate'.[196] Two weeks later he circularised all district health officers, requesting feedback on the existing NMOs and stating his intention to supplement this structure with both Maori and Pakeha nurses.[197] A nursing service for Europeans in the backblocks was inaugurated later that year, but the return of Maori health to the Native Department in July 1909 led to a delay of nearly two years before Valintine could introduce 'Maori health nurses'. The opportunity arose in April 1911, when Amelia Bagley, a Pakeha, was sent to deal with a typhoid outbreak at Ahipara in Northland.[198]

The extension of district nursing to Maori threatened to put Valintine offside with the medical profession and some hospital boards, even though he insisted that nurses had been 'specially directed' to seek medical assistance when necessary and obey the instructions of the doctor.[199] The opening address by the Governor, Lord Islington, to the Hospitals' Conference in June 1911 set out the Health Department's intention to look at the health of Maori settlements in a 'thoroughly effective way' by employing nurses in a preventative role. Discussion was initiated by G.F. Powell of the Waipiro Hospital Board, who supported the employment of Maori girls. Opinion was divided on the wisdom of this policy. James Young of Waikato, a future Health Minister, stated that his board had experimented unsuccessfully with 'Native nurses': 'The discipline, training, and study necessary for their duties seemed to be too much for them.' The session's chairman, James Wilson, MHR for Palmerston North, rebutted this slur, reporting: 'We have a full-blooded Maori who is an excellent nurse.'[200]

The *New Zealand Medical Journal (NZMJ)* criticised Valintine's comment that the need for Maori health nurses arose in part from the poor performance of the subsidised NMOs: 'Until we have had presented the other side of the question we reserve our opinion as to the perfunctory work of the doctors among the native race, but if, for the sake of argument, we admit that the doctors have been unsatisfactory and perfunctory, we cannot describe Dr Valintine's remedy as anything but absurd.' Nurses, stated the editorial, simply could not take the place of doctors.[201]

Even Health Minister David Buddo appeared lukewarm, admitting to Parliament in October 1911 that he was not convinced of the benefits of Maori nurses.[202] Undeterred, Valintine pressed ahead. He reported in 1912 that the scheme, with eight nurses now in post, 'bids fair to be a great success', though he did warn that 'something akin to a "missionary spirit"' was needed to ensure this. This assessment was endorsed by Robert Makgill, arguably the most influential of the Department's policy-makers in the period under review.[203] Conscious of the need to appease his colleagues, Valintine reassured the NZBMA conference in Timaru that the Maori nursing scheme was not intended to supersede the NMOs.[204]

Valintine was only partially successful in defusing criticism. During the 1913 Imprest Supply debate William Macdonald (Bay of Plenty) attacked the government for its alleged withdrawal of subsidies in outlying districts and their replacement by district nurses. He believed that subsidised doctoring was money well spent when diseases such as typhoid broke out in Maori communities, and argued that health care for the 11,000 Maori in his electorate also benefited the European settlers. Apirana Ngata took a slightly different stance. He had previously supported the replacement of NMOs by district nurses as a more effective use of limited resources, but now saw the need for continued subsidies in areas such as the Urewera, Taupo and some parts of North Auckland, East Coast and King Country.[205]

Attempts to integrate the work of Maori and other backblocks nurses met with varied success. In 1915 a suggestion that the Maori health nurse at Opunake might also serve the settler population brought vigorous opposition from the Taranaki Hospital Board, which condemned the proposal as unworkable. At Te Araroa, on the other hand, settlers and Maori combined to erect a cottage for the local nurse.[206] One of Valintine's most loyal supporters was Hester Maclean, the Health Department's Assistant Inspector of Hospitals and proprietor of *Kai Tiaki* (later the *New Zealand Nursing Journal*). *Kai Tiaki* regularly published encouraging accounts of the achievements of district nurses, especially in relation to typhoid cases among Maori.[207] In April 1917 one 'old district nurse' declared: 'There is no doubt a good nurse is better than the average medical practitioner of the back-blocks.'[208]

Despite these confident assessments, the recruitment and retention of Maori nurses proved to be difficult. On several occasions in 1910 and 1911 William Field, MHR for Otaki, challenged the government to reduce the lamentable infant mortality among Maori by appointing district nurses. Field was a close friend of William Collins, who had already advocated the use of district nurses among Maori. His third foray on this issue included a suggestion that European nurses assume this task until Maori had been trained up for it. Buck's riposte about the reluctance of hospitals to accept Maori probationers casts doubts upon the viability of Field's proposal.[209]

Matters were not helped by the fate of the Maori nursing role model, Akenehi Hei. Her brother, Hamiora, had been instrumental in persuading James Pope in 1897 of the merits of Maori nurses.[210] Hei began her training at Napier Hospital in 1901 and qualified seven years later. After some

Maori health nurse Akenehi Hei on duty in her 'tent hospital'. *Canterbury Public Library*

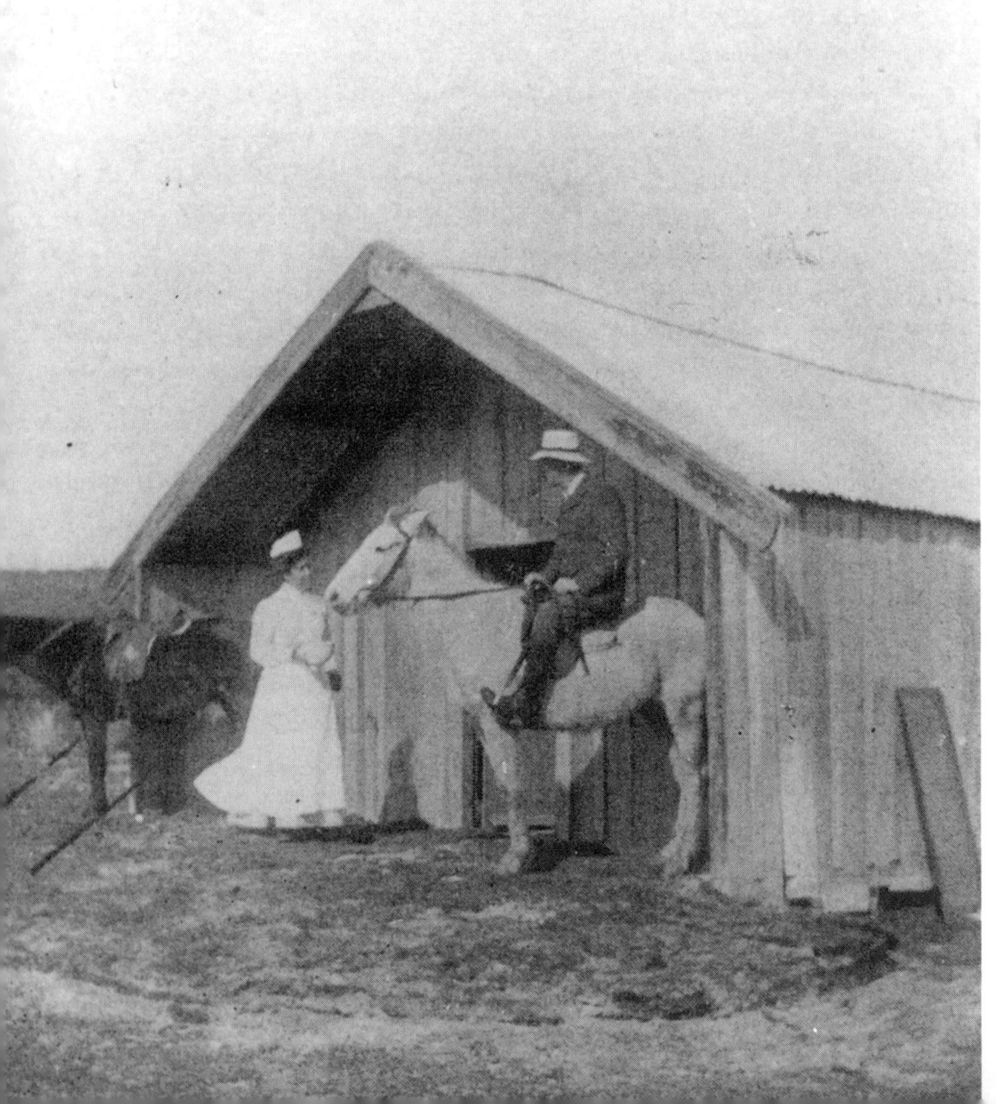

confusion during the transfer of responsibilities between the Native and Health Departments she was appointed to the Taranaki district; two reports on her work there were published in *Kai Tiaki*.[211] Nurse Hei's tragic death from typhoid in November 1910 after successfully nursing family members who had contracted the disease was a body blow. Few other Maori women had the strength of character, education or family connections to take her place.[212]

Valintine's address to the 1911 Hospitals' Conference acknowledged the obstacles faced by Maori nurses. Promising to supply nurses to areas with large Maori populations, he explained: 'In the event of its being necessary to appoint two nurses, one would be European and the other Native. The trouble with the Maori nurse was that she was rather inclined to shirk responsibility. It was found the work was better done when they had a pakeha nurse to stiffen up the Native nurse. Every encouragement would be given to Native girls to receive instruction in the elements of nursing, and so forth.'[213] Whether Valintine's comments are interpreted as supportive or culturally insensitive is largely irrelevant from a policy perspective, since few Maori girls entered the nursing profession. Those who did often found as much difficulty in gaining acceptance from their fellow Maori as from Pakeha.[214]

These various disincentives also led to further resignations from the Health Department by some of the few who actually qualified. Eva Wi Repa (Dr Wi Repa's sister), for instance, resigned shortly after her appointment as a Maori health nurse to undertake private work among wealthy Hawke's Bay Maori.[215] By the mid 1920s the Health Department seems to have become resigned to the dearth of candidates. The 1923 annual report regretted the reluctance of many Maori to heed instruction from members of their own race and contrasted this with their willingness to listen to Pakeha nurses. Noting that Maori nurses were seldom kept on by the hospitals and that there were limited opportunities for them in private nursing, the report hoped they might find future employment among well-to-do Maori.[216] This was hardly the result envisaged by Hamiora Hei in the late 1890s or by Valintine a decade later.

In 1906 Maui Pomare wrote that Maori had longed for the day when 'we could have proper places to take patients to, nurses of our own race to soothe the fevered brow, our own doctors to heal the sick and advise the living how to live'. A lack of suitable candidates and a failure to offer them sufficient financial and other inducements to train had made this a dream whose fulfilment lay much further in the future than Pomare hoped or believed.[217]

'Carriers of infection': preventive medicine

One of the main reasons for the creation of the Department of Public Health in 1900 was to place the control of infectious disease on a more effective footing. James Mason stressed the need for continued vigilance in the wake of the bubonic plague scare of 1900, and his agenda incorporated sanitary improvements, a campaign to combat tuberculosis and vaccination against smallpox.[218]

The vaccination issue was revisited after Maui Pomare's appointment. In 1902 the Health Department published a pamphlet by Pomare, in the Maori language, urging Maori to submit to vaccination. This preceded a similar campaign aimed at the European population in 1904, after minor outbreaks of smallpox in the South Island.[219] In the Department's annual report for 1902/3 Mason commented favourably on Maori eagerness to embrace the sanitary gospel: 'One pleasing feature is that of their own free will an enormous number of Natives have been vaccinated.'[220] Pomare's influence was far-reaching. On a visit to the Chatham Islands he 'found the pamphlet on small-pox had stirred the Natives to the vaccinating-point.' As a result he was able to vaccinate all the children, both Maori and European. Overall, he claimed, his pamphlet had resulted in 2,250 vaccinations colony-wide, 1,827 of them administered by departmental officials.[221]

By the following year this figure had more than doubled to 5,772, about half of them performed by Pomare and his colleagues. In an effort to avoid treading on the toes of the public vaccinators, who were responsible for Europeans as well as Maori, Pomare concentrated his efforts on those who lived outside the vaccinators' catchment areas, and on individuals who had already refused vaccination. It appears that each case was judged on its merits and that he refused to vaccinate those living in unhygienic conditions because of the risk of blood poisoning. His efforts were assisted by the new Maori Councils but the end results were patchy. While more than a thousand vaccinations were recorded in both

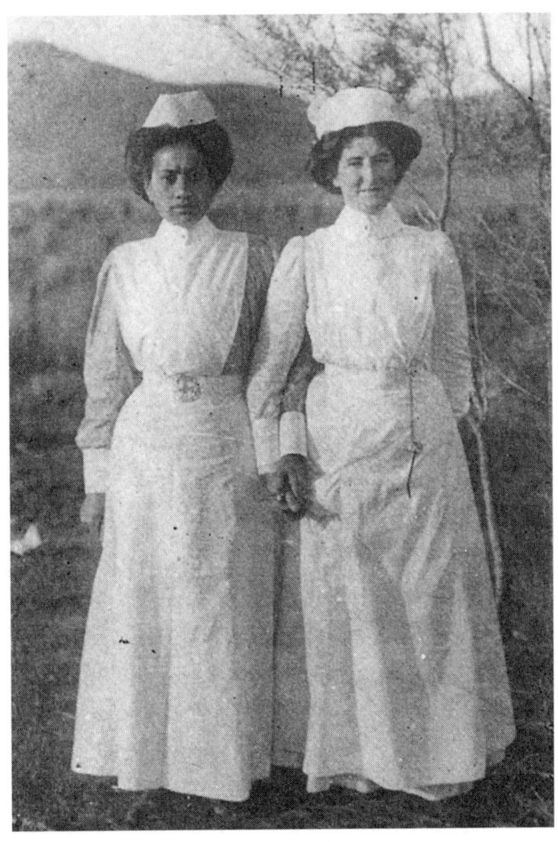

Hand in hand. Maori and European nurses working together at an East Coast fever camp in 1912. *AJHR, 1912, Session II, E-3*

Auckland and Hawke's Bay there were only nine for the whole of Nelson and Westland. Interestingly, in view of its alleged resistance to Western medicine, fourteen villages were visited in the Urewera district, resulting in a total of 630 vaccinations.[222]

The campaign's momentum carried on into 1905. At a dinner in his honour, Health Minister Joseph Ward claimed that the number of vaccinations now stood at 9,846.[223] For a population which according to the 1901 census numbered just 43,143, including 10,120 under ten years old, this was an impressive strike rate.[224] By 1906 the enthusiasm seems to have waned as the imminent danger of smallpox receded. Sanitary Inspector Raureti Mokonuiarangi reported that very few children in the Rotorua and Rotoiti areas had been vaccinated. He attributed this to a mixture of scepticism and reluctance on the part of the public vaccinator to visit the outlying areas. Inspector Rameka Waikerepuru reported only limited success among the Nga Puhi people around Ohaeawai in Northland. He blamed this in part on the schoolmaster's refusal to sanction the practice during school hours.[225] Later annual reports contain few references to vaccination.

These hints of a growing resistance to vaccination mirrored the pattern in the European community. An anti-vaccination lobby had become active in the United Kingdom around the turn of the century. An equivalent group led by Edwin Cox, a septuagenarian dentist, functioned in New Zealand from around 1903 until 1908.[226] In January 1908 the *New Zealand Observer* commented that only a quarter of newborn infants were vaccinated, and that the government did not enforce the law requiring this because it was afraid of Edwin Cox.[227] Nine months later it quoted a *Hawke's Bay Herald* claim that fewer than 8 per cent were now being vaccinated

Another Don Quixote? The *Free Lance* cartoonist focused upon vaccination in his depiction of Peter Buck's efforts to promote Maori health during the 1911 Health Department Supply debate. *ATL, N-P 424- (New Zealand Free Lance, 7 October 1911)*

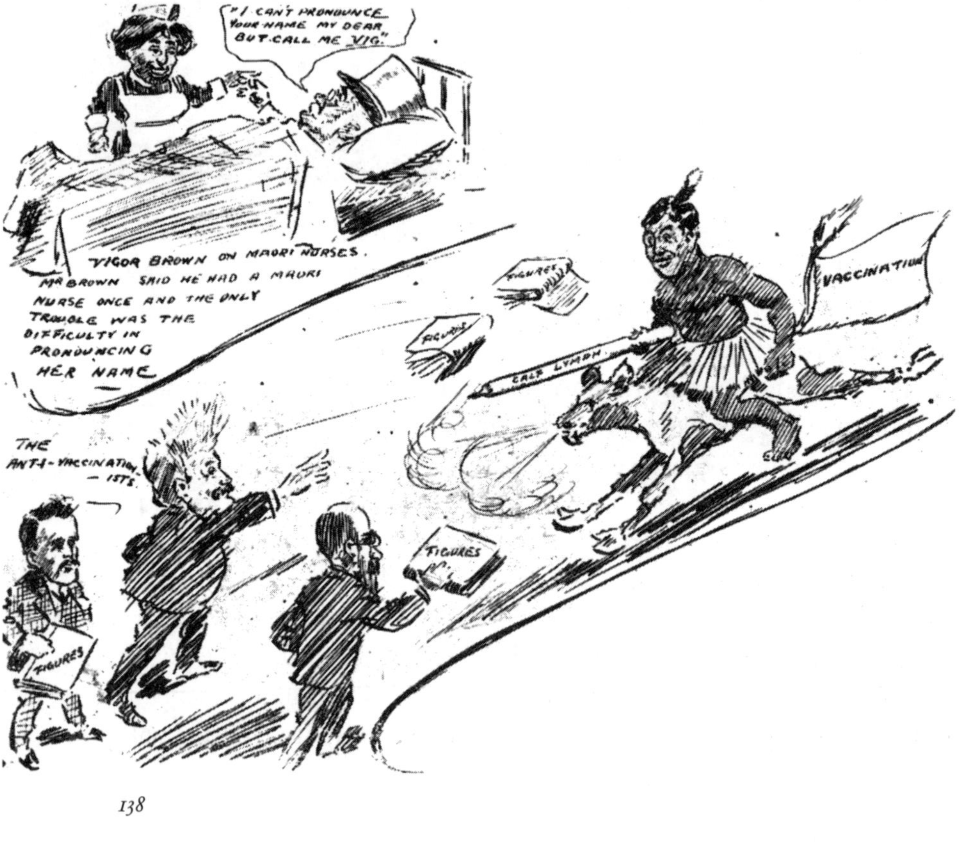

and that within a few years the bulk of the population would be 'unprotected from the ravages of small-pox'.[228]

An outbreak of smallpox among North Island Maori in 1913, following exposure to a Mormon missionary who was a carrier, revived efforts to protect the Maori population.[229] The epidemic broke out near Whangarei at the beginning of May but was not referred to in Parliament until 8 July.[230] Three days later Cabinet decided that precautions must be taken, although medical opinion was still undecided if the disease was smallpox or chickenpox. Discussion centred on the twin issues of quarantine and vaccination.[231] Travel restrictions were imposed on Maori, leading to claims of discrimination both at the time and in the aftermath of the epidemic.[232] This was to be an important precedent for policies adopted to combat typhoid in the 1920s. Of equal importance was the debate on vaccination.

Several anti-vaccinationists made their position clear when the epidemic was discussed in Parliament at the instigation of George Russell (Avon), who served as Health Minister in 1912 and from 1915 to 1919. The consensus approved of vaccination, although some members identified practical difficulties. John Brown (Napier), for example, was concerned by reports of a doctor refusing to vaccinate around twenty Waitoko Maori because it was not a paying proposition. Others queried the purity or availability of lymph, or claimed that Europeans were given preference.[233] Apirana Ngata subsequently alleged that the smallpox epidemic was beyond the resources of the health authorities and called on the Native Department and the government as a whole to become involved. The proposal was not adopted; health remained firmly in the hands of the Health Department.[234] On 29 August Health Minister Heaton Rhodes announced that twelve senior Otago medical students had been recruited to revaccinate North Island Maori.[235]

In the aftermath of the outbreak Peter Buck, who received a government honorarium for his efforts during the epidemic, invited Parliament to make vaccination compulsory for Maori, claiming that he had the support of other Maori MHRs.[236] Buck reiterated this call in 1914 when he reported on the epidemic to the Australasian Medical Congress in Auckland. He insisted that Maori would support such legislation and that smallpox was kept alive in New Zealand by unvaccinated Europeans.[237] The latter allegation was a dubious one. It was true that none of the 116 European victims of smallpox in 1913 had been vaccinated, but it was also estimated that at least 85 per cent of Maori were unvaccinated in May 1913.[238] However, as Robert Makgill, District Health Officer for Auckland, pointed out: 'Their willingness, indeed, eagerness, to undergo vaccination was a pleasant change from the indifference and opposition of the European.'[239]

Smallpox was never again a sufficient threat to prompt action on the lines envisaged by Buck, but the principle of enforced compliance was taken up in relation to another infectious disease. During the Native Schools Supply debate in September 1913 Ngata confirmed Buck's assertion that Maori would raise no objection to mandatory smallpox vaccination. He then advocated compulsory anti-typhoid inoculation provided the medical profession verified its preventive powers. Health Minister Rhodes welcomed this suggestion, and Buck confirmed the doctors' faith in the protective value of inoculation, adding that this would be more cost-effective than the current practice of setting up typhoid camps to isolate victims.[240]

Typhoid, one of the major 'filth' diseases spread by poor housing and sanitation, had been a major public health concern since the 1870s.[241] Because it had a proportionately greater impact on Maori communities by the turn of the century, it remained central to the Health Department's endeavours for several decades. Between 1905 and 1910 Maori sanitary

Health officials acted swiftly to combat the risk of cross-infection during the 1913 smallpox epidemic, burning down Maori whare where deaths were known to have occurred. *Hocken Library (Otago Witness, 24 September 1913)*

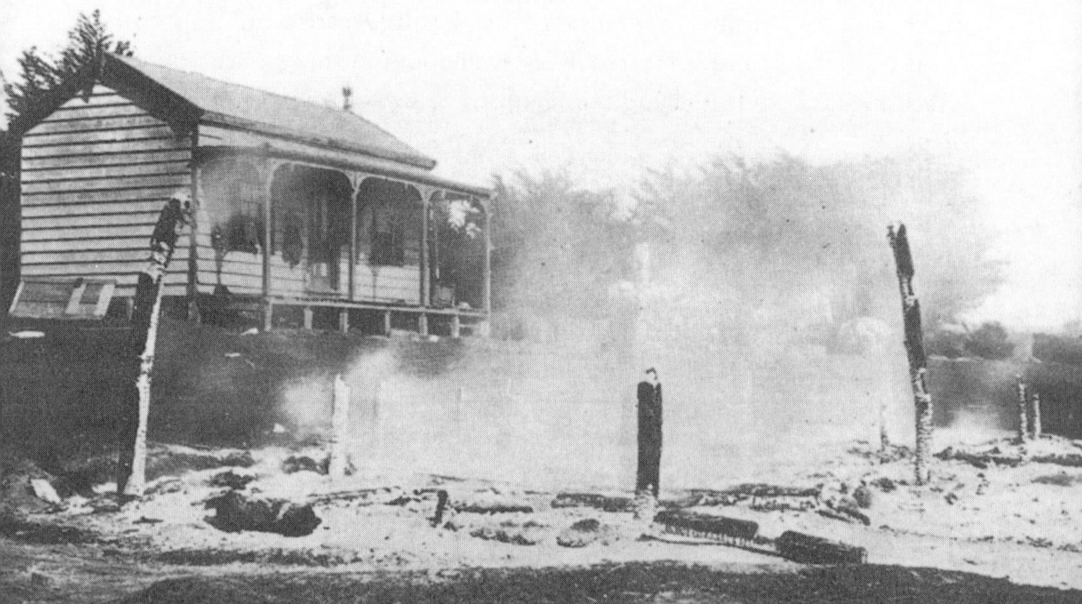

A SEASON (VACCINATION) TICKET.
At least one instance has been reported to the Health Officers of unvaccinated Maoris in the North of Auckland district travelling upon a certificate borrowed from vaccinated friends.
"I GO TO THE RACES YESTERDAY. YOU TAKE IT THE TICKET TO GO THE FOOTBALL TOMORRA"

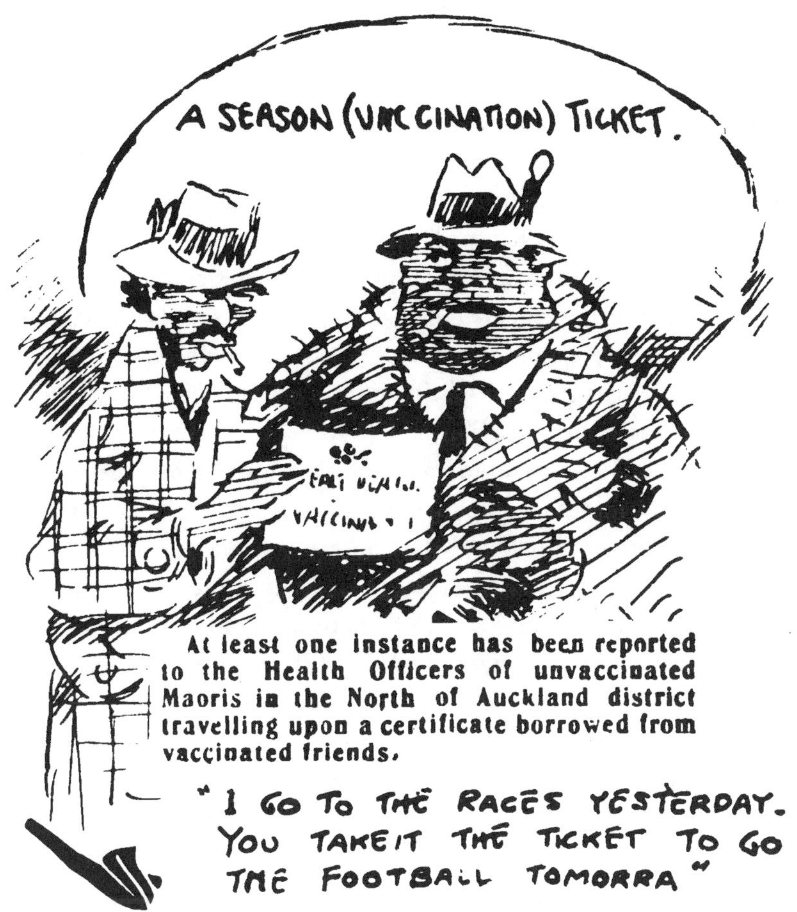

Despite Dr Makgill's testament to Maori co-operation during the 1913 smallpox epidemic, many Europeans thought differently. Such prejudices were fuelled by this cartoon of a Maori offering to lend his vaccination certificate to a friend. *ATL, N-P 423- (New Zealand Free Lance, 26 July 1913)*

inspectors encouraged communities to reduce the risk of typhoid by improving water supplies and erecting latrines. Their efforts were often frustrated by lack of funds, apathy or antagonism.[242] As for the Maori medical officers, Pomare and Buck did their best with the limited time and resources at their disposal. During his years in sole charge Pomare found it hard to be as proactive as he would have liked. In October 1903 Dr Herbert Barclay of Waimate reported that local Maori were upset because Pomare had not visited them despite the presence of widespread typhoid.

The district health officer had paid a visit at Barclay's instigation, 'but a few lectures from their own medical man would have been invaluable'.[243] Buck's appointment in 1905 helped relieve some of the pressure on Pomare. He later recalled how tact and appeals to tribal pride overcame resistance to typhoid inoculation.[244] The construction of the Araiteuru Pa at the 1906–7 Christchurch Exhibition helped reach a wider audience: 'As far as the visiting Maoris are concerned, it was a great object-lesson to see how the picturesque and artistic in their ancient villages could be preserved, and the modern conveniences of the pakeha in water-supply and sanitation added for the perfecting of the whole.'[245] Buck also invoked the custom of building latrines (paepae) in fighting pa to persuade tribal leaders of the benefits of sanitary measures.[246]

The containment or eradication of typhoid remained a major component of the Health Department's agenda for Maori even after the departure of Pomare, Buck and the sanitary inspectors. This was partly driven by Pakeha self-interest. In 1911 Makgill wrote to a colleague at Kawhia about the post-mortem confirmation of typhoid. He noted that the disease was rife among Maori, and generally occurred without medical attention or notification: 'I have no doubt there must be carriers of infection among them, and probably one had visited the kainga.'[247] The following day Makgill informed the Native Department Under-Secretary: 'As matters stand the Native race is a menace to the wellbeing of the European.'[248] His fears had some justification in relation to typhoid. In 1918 Maori or 'half-castes' accounted for 155 of the 351 typhoid cases in Auckland Province.[249]

The Maori health nurses appointed from 1911 were intended to rebuff this threat. Several speakers at the 1911 Hospitals' Conference stressed their importance in preventing the spread of typhoid from Maori to European communities.[250] Much of their time was devoted to nursing typhoid victims and giving advice on a suitable diet for them.[251] They were also expected to identify unreported cases, the majority of which occurred among Maori.[252] Their involvement in typhoid nursing fostered a mutual respect which was expressed very clearly in an anonymous contribution to *Kai Tiaki*: 'To see what Maori typhoids live through, and the conditions they are frequently found in, makes one utterly disbelieve the hackneyed saying that "the Maori has no stamina, and, like other dark races, cannot fight out an illness, etc."'[253] After less than a decade of Maori health nursing the Department claimed that typhoid camps run by nurses had helped overcome Maori repugnance at hospitalisation.[254] This was a marked improvement on the situation just five years earlier, when a district health officer reported that some Taumarunui Maori had assaulted Nurse Moore when she suggested hospitalisation. Noting that no action had been taken because the principal assailants had contracted typhoid and one had died, he concluded: 'Even the younger and better educated Natives learn but slowly and uncertainly to adopt sanitary methods, so the nurses have constant disappointments and difficulties.'[255]

In 1917 the Census and Statistics Office made the first attempt to collate New Zealand's health statistics. Despite the absence of reliable Maori data, the Office was able to draw some conclusions: 'cancer is rare as a cause of death among the Maori people, though unfortunately tuberculosis and typhoid are not.'[256] Nevertheless, official discussion of the tuberculosis problem in the first twenty years of the century rarely looked beyond the European population. James Mason's 1905 paper to the Auckland Branch of the NZBMA on 'The Relation of the State Towards Consumption' made no mention of Maori.[257] The discussion of the administrative control of tuberculosis directed by his successor, Valintine, at the 1911 Hospitals' Conference and the 1912 conference dedicated to this topic also ignored the Maori situation.[258] The government was still in denial in 1920 when Health Minister James Parr claimed that New Zealand, 'in comparison with other countries, is in a most fortunate position as regards tuberculosis', and Robert Makgill wrote at length on 'The Duty of the State in Regard to Tuberculosis' without referring once to Maori.[259]

Despite this official silence the threat to Maori posed by tuberculosis had long been recognised. New Zealand's approach to tuberculosis after 1900 adopted the United Kingdom practice of institutional care and was ill-suited to Maori needs.[260] Edwin Chill, an English physician, proposed such a policy for Maori during a visit to the colony in 1906: 'Surely they are a race worth preserving. A little outlay should procure them qualified and more accessible medical advice, and a sanatorium for the treatment of tuberculosis in place of their miserable tents. The great stumbling-block, one can conceive, is the inborn native superstition, but even this is not an insuperable difficulty.'[261]

Chill's plan may have been naive and over-optimistic, but it did not differ greatly from the strategies of Pomare and Buck. In 1903 Pomare advocated a Maori tuberculosis hospital staffed by Maori nurses or, at the very least, a special ward for Maori patients at Te Waikato Sanatorium near Cambridge.[262] The idea was repeated in his 1904 blueprint for Maori health.[263] For the next decade officials kept a watching brief on tuberculosis among Maori. When Buck attempted to downplay the incidence of the disease in 1908 he was contradicted by Pomare, who believed it to be significantly under-reported.[264] The differential between European and Maori was discounted by the Department in 1909: 'At a rough estimate, the whole population, including Maoris, would show a proportion of a little over 2 per thousand of tubercular cases, somewhat under the incidence among Natives alone.'[265] By 1912 there was mounting anxiety about the impact of tuberculosis on South Island Maori. Health officials complained that Maori almost always pleaded poverty when asked to make sanitary improvements.[266] Drs George Blackmore and Arthur Pearson of Christchurch were commissioned in June 1912 to investigate the prevalence of tuberculosis at Tuahiwi Park and report on the best course of action. The Department ordered a trial of weekly tuberculin injections, to be administered by James Crawshaw, a local GP, at Tuahiwi and Little River. Crawshaw was optimistic about the outcome, even though he conceded that tuberculin was no longer highly regarded.

As with typhoid, there was an element of Pakeha self-preservation about the Department's actions that was spelled out in Crawshaw's report: 'It behoves us very seriously to try and stamp out this disease amongst the Maori race, because by so doing we are removing a disease that is a menace to the white race in New Zealand.'[267]

The Tuahiwi scheme was labour-intensive and therefore too expensive for large-scale use.[268] Pomare had waxed eloquent in 1902 about the benefits of placarding Maori communities with posters admonishing them not to expectorate, in order to reduce the risk of infecting others. Maori health nurses continued this inexpensive preventive regime by advising Maori 'to use antiseptics, and to expectorate into tins, which are afterwards burned'.[269] The results were not encouraging. By 1920 tuberculosis was regarded as a 'serious menace in a Maori community'. District nurses were expected to compile registers of sufferers but found this difficult since they were reluctant to leave their families and seek admission to a sanatorium (always assuming places were available). As the Director-General of Health rather gloomily concluded in the same year, tuberculosis was difficult for Europeans but 'heart-breakingly more so in the case of Maoris'.[270] This was a statement at odds with the upbeat assessment of his Minister that was cited above.

Attempts were made during this period to assess the prevalence of infectious diseases in the Maori community through surveillance by NMOs, nurses, and schoolteachers. The scale of the problem was never properly ascertained and Maori were sometimes ignored in official deliberations. This happened in relation to tuberculosis, and again during the investigation of the 1918 influenza epidemic. Maori constituted more than a quarter of the 8,000 or so New Zealand victims, and their death rate of 42.3 per thousand was one of the highest in the world, yet no Maori appeared among the 111 witnesses to the subsequent Royal Commission.[271] On the other hand, Maori health was frequently debated in Parliament and Health Department officials attempted to grapple with the issues. Preventive measures were introduced and treatment provided where this was feasible, but the shortage of funds severely restricted such efforts.

The Health Department's lack of resources during the first two decades of this century obliged it to rely heavily upon other agencies, especially the Education Department's Native School teachers. In 1906 Edwin Chill praised the Jack-of-all-trades Native School master, 'who combines in his person the duties of lawyer, doctor, pastor, schoolmaster and friend'.[272] Shortly afterwards William Herries asked the Minister of Education to consider Native teacher salaries, citing their isolated position and 'onerous duties, which often include dispensing of medicine'. The Minister was able to reply that a new scale had already been approved.[273]

The expectations placed upon these teachers were daunting. In 1904 William Field mounted his first parliamentary attack on Maori infant mortality by calling for the appointment of salaried women (preferably with experience in rearing children) to visit and instruct Maori mothers. Richard Seddon replied that Native School teachers and their wives already educated communities about the care of the sick, and that his government proposed to train additional girls for this work.[274] Seven years later Buck lauded the impact of teachers on infant mortality rates.[275]

Teachers had, since the 1870s, been entrusted with dispensing medicines to the pupils in their care, a task which had helped make the schools into medical centres for their districts. In 1908 the Health Department issued a circular listing stock mixtures and their applications. The armamentarium included cough mixture, anti-fever mixture for children aged up to ten years, tonic, a cure for indigestion, children's diarrhoea powders, worm syrup, ointment for sores on skin not due to itch, ointment for itch, and a tonic for girls who were pale. In line with an official acceptance that teachers had some responsibility for the entire community, the circular also detailed two medicines specifically for adults, an aperient blood mixture and one to combat diarrhoea.[276] On taking over as CHO in 1909 Valintine claimed to be 'a little dubious as to the supply of medicines by Native School Teachers'. Although he considered this to be the best option in the current circumstances he believed Maori health needs would be better served by the pending introduction of district nurses.[277] In 1911 Valintine spelled out the proposed role of these nurses during the discussion of 'The Health of the Native Race' at the Hospitals' Conference: 'She shall pay visits of inspection to the Native schools, in which case copies of her reports will also be transmitted to the Education Department.'[278]

Amelia Bagley, Superintendent of Maori Health Nurses, visiting Te Araroa in 1912. *Kai Tiaki, July 1912*

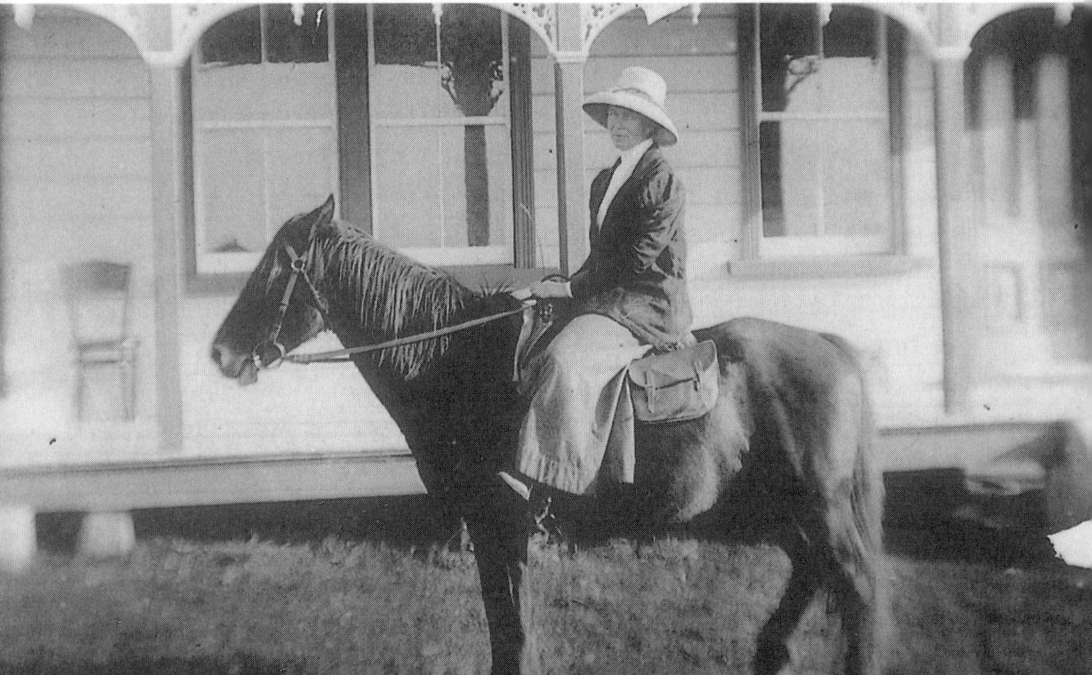

Despite this, many Maori continued to seek medical aid from teachers rather than health professionals, as Ngata reported to Parliament in 1912 in relation to districts overrun with typhoid.[279] The following year Health Minister Heaton Rhodes gave a cautious response to Ngata's appeal for medicines to be sent to the teacher at Te Waiti, Rotoiti: 'It cannot be expected that school-teachers of Maori schools should have sufficient technical knowledge to make the fullest use of the remedies which it has been the practice in the past to supply to them.' His Department now preferred the system to be overseen by the district nurses, though he acknowledged that this would not always be feasible.[280]

The problems associated with this policy were highlighted in 1919 when the Te Araroa teacher pleaded with the CHO to send a supply of medicines. No Maori health nurse had visited the school's 126 children for eight or nine months, and local Maori were reluctant to use Dr Wi Repa's services. Gisborne, the nearest large town, was three to four days distant in summer and anything up to three weeks in winter.[281]

While the Maori health nurses strengthened the overall provision of health services for Maori, their introduction was sometimes complicated or confounded by personality clashes. In 1915 Auckland's District Health Officer expressed concern at the number of Native School teachers who, while not actively opposing nurses and inspectors, 'appear to lose no opportunity of belittling their work, and wholly fail to make any effort to co-operate with them.' He attributed this to petty jealousy and asked that the matter be brought to the attention of the Secretary for Education.[282] Even so, many teachers supplied valuable and timely information to health officials. The infrastructure of some 250 Native School teachers by 1918, as opposed to only eighteen Maori health nurses, provided an important service to their local communities.[283]

4
'Betterment of the Maori Race' 1920–1940

'The fifth wheel': Maori health administration

The 1920s and 1930s brought increased pressure to provide or improve health services for Maori. Some of the strategies employed, such as the revival of Maori Councils expressly as Maori health councils, were a continuation of existing practices. Others broke new ground. The most significant of the latter was the creation in 1920 of a Division of Maori Hygiene headed by a Maori doctor. However, funding shortages and concerns about overlapping with the work of medical officers of health and district nurses were to lead to the disbanding of the Division in 1930, in an attempt to achieve a better-integrated health system.

The influenza epidemic of 1918 had important repercussions for the administration of Maori health. A Royal Commission was appointed in January 1919 to investigate the causes of the epidemic and recommend measures for dealing with future outbreaks. In an attempt to attribute blame for the disaster, several witnesses in Auckland complained about poor sanitary conditions among Maori.[1] The Royal Commission, worried by a threatened recrudescence of the epidemic, issued an interim report on 22 April. This contained a short paragraph recommending that the health authorities implement section 68 of the Public Health Act 1908 dealing with the sanitation of Maori settlements; it also suggested that

Europeans be appointed to assist Maori with this work.[2]

Health Minister George Russell had already been alerted to public sentiment on this issue. From mid February local authorities bombarded his Department with letters and memoranda demanding that action be taken to combat the menace posed to public health by 'insanitary pahs'. This concerted campaign had its origins in a widely circulated Tauranga Hospital Board memorandum of 13 February.[3] Some communications were sent directly to the Minister. Others went to the CHO, while Taumarunui's Town Clerk dispatched one to Maui Pomare as 'Minister for Native Councils.[4] One of the few correspondents to deal in specifics was the Wairoa County Clerk, who acknowledged on 18 March that the scattered nature of most settlements made it difficult to impose sanitary measures; he suggested that periodical inspections might be carried out by a 'Special Officer of the Department'.

The campaign achieved its purpose. On 28 April Russell informed Pomare that his 'expert officers' were investigating the matter, and that as a first step he planned to circularise Maori on sanitary standards. His letter concluded: 'I may add that the Department is taking steps to propose the appointment of a whole time Officer as Health Officer to Natives. One will, of course, be appointed who has the necessary knowledge and experience in dealing with the native race.' The phraseology revived memories of the appointment of Maui Pomare in 1901 'by reason of his nationality'. On the same day CHO Thomas Valintine asked the Public Service Commissioner whether there was any need to advertise the post, since no one could compete successfully with Peter Buck. The need for transparency ensured that the position was advertised even though the result was a foregone conclusion.[5] The promised circular was drawn up by mid May and distributed shortly afterwards with the addendum that 'Dr Te Rangihiroa has been appointed Medical Officer for Maoris, and he will devote his energies to bringing about an improvement in the sanitary condition of Maori villages.'[6]

This laudable intention received little encouragement from the deliberations of the Royal Commission investigating the epidemic. Its final report of 13 May 1919 virtually ignored Maori. One of the few references noted that the Canterbury health district, with 217,046 European residents and 1,047 Maori, was too large to be overseen by a single medical officer. It is possible that the choice of Canterbury rather than an area such as Auckland, which had a large Maori population, was a deliberate attempt to downplay Maori health requirements.[7] In any case, the Health Department followed the Royal Commission's lead in responding to its findings. On 20 June the *New Zealand Times* printed a detailed commentary by Russell and Valintine. Neither made any reference to Maori health.[8]

Despite this muted response, Valintine's summary of medical and nursing aid to Maori in the Health Department's annual report for 1918/19 promised that he would be 'guided and considerably assisted' in these endeavours by Buck. He also admitted that Maori health required 'greater attention from the Department than has been possible in the past.'[9] Buck himself was enthusiastic about the potential of his new role. In August 1920 he explained that the epidemic had revealed the 'urgent necessity of some organization amongst the Maoris themselves to assist Health officials and medical men'. Buck endorsed the planned introduction of model by-laws to strengthen the hand of the Maori Councils and place them under the Health Department. This would, claimed the new 'Medical Officer for the Maoris', result in 'much good'.[10]

Buck's position was clarified by the Health Act of 1920, which created a new administrative structure for the Health Department. 'Maori Hygiene' became one of seven distinct divisions, alongside Public Hygiene, Hospitals, Nursing, School Hygiene, Dental Hygiene, and Child Welfare.[11] Each was headed by a director answerable to the departmental head, a position retained by Valintine, whose title changed from Chief Health Officer to Director-General of Health. Despite his own title, Buck's position was somewhat ambiguous. He was based in Auckland rather than in the Department's Wellington headquarters and, according to Valintine's 1920 annual report, enjoyed the status of a district health officer.

One of Buck's first and most important duties was to oversee the revival of the Maori Councils, many of which now existed in name only. The Native Land Amendment and Native Land Claims Adjustment Act of 1919, an extension of existing legislation, empowered the Governor-General to create special districts within which the Maori Council 'shall be a Health Council, to advise the District Health Officer in all matters relating to the health of the Maori inhabitants'. Under the direction of the district health officer, these councils had powers to carry out 'sanitary works' and 'enforce

. . . sanitary rules and observances'. Section 66 of the Health Act 1920 gave the Director-General or the Director of Maori Hygiene the responsibility for approving such work. The revised legislation also confirmed the right to 'enforce such by-laws relating to health and sanitation as the Health Council may specify'.

One potential difficulty for Health Department officials was the old bugbear of divided responsibility. It was not until September 1920 that Cabinet approved the transfer of administrative control of the Maori Councils from the Native Department to Health.[12] Almost two years later the two bodies were still haggling over who should be responsible for appointments to the councils, with each trying to hand responsibility to the other.[13] In the end the buck was passed to the Health Department. By April 1921 the Director of Maori Hygiene had reorganised many of the existing councils and created some twenty new districts in the North Island.

The first meeting of the Takitimu Maori Council at Poho o Rawiri, Gisborne, on 10 June 1902. *ATL, F44563 1/2*

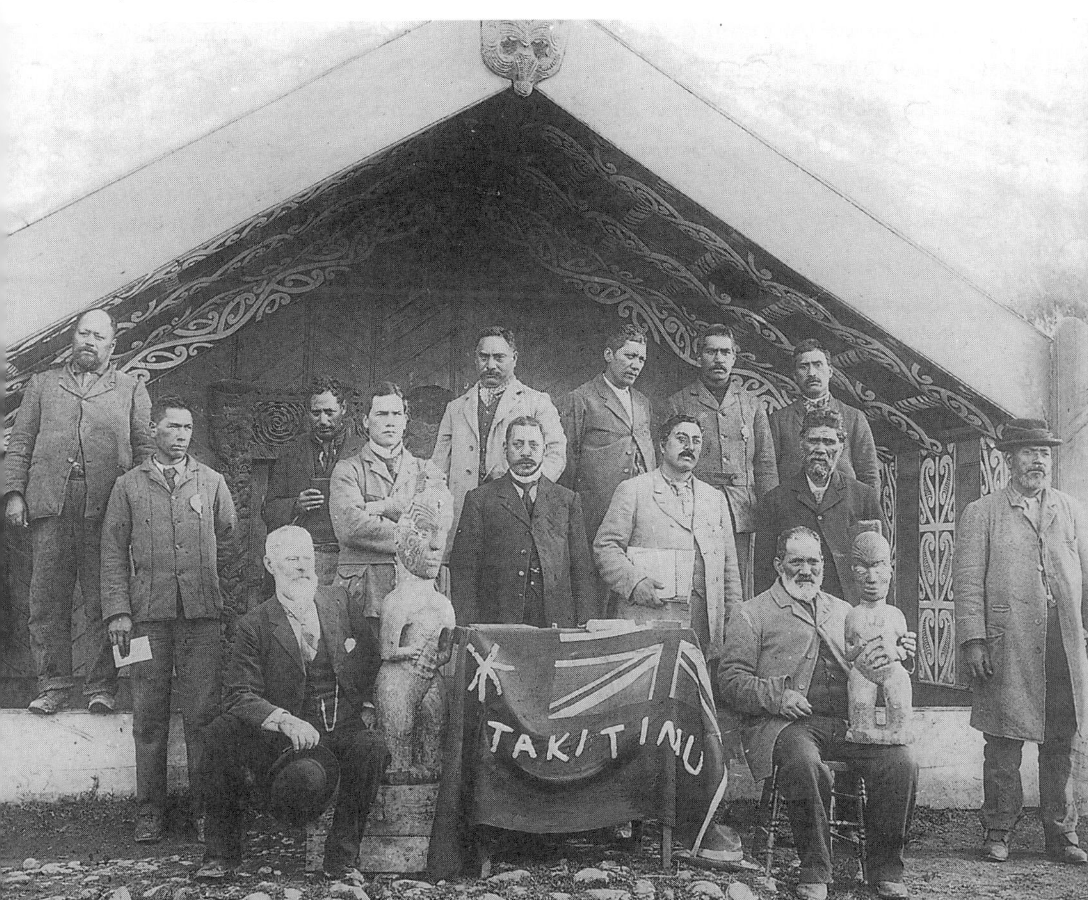

Seven councils had already adopted new by-laws, a process hindered by a lack of clerical staff to cope with the sheer volume of paperwork. Buck made no apology for giving priority to the North Island: 'There are three Councils only in the South Island, and as these Natives are living under very fair conditions I shall not deal with them other than in a formal manner until I have completed the whole of the North Island.'[14] Two years later he reported that all the councils were now in working order, with the exception of those in the South Island, which he had not been able to organise by correspondence.[15]

The three South Island councils (plus one for the Chatham Islands) were not gazetted until 1929. This reputedly completed the national network, with the exception of Waikato, which consistently refused to acknowledge the jurisdiction of the councils.[16] In 1930, Maori Health Inspector Harding Leaf sought the help of Auckland's Medical Officer of Health (MOH), Herbert Chesson, to form a Maori Health Council for Hauraki.[17] By 1931 there were 24 Maori Councils, each with seven members, and 260 village committees, each comprising five representatives. According to Dr Edward Pohau Ellison, Buck's successor as Director of Maori Hygiene, this amounted to a body of more than 1,400 'Maoris ever ready to assist in any emergency or cause the department may think necessary'.[18]

Ellison's statement, like Peter Buck's upbeat assessment in August 1920, glossed over a number of factors which limited the councils' effectiveness. Among Te Arawa, for instance, there were allegations in November 1920 that some hapu were not represented on the reconstituted council.[19] The following year the Director of Maori Hygiene pleaded with the medical officers of health (MOsH) to ensure the co-operation of influential Maori in the revived councils.[20] By 1928 Ellison was confident that the rise of a younger generation had brought about a marked improvement.[21] Not everyone believed this to be sufficient. Ten years later Emere Kaa, a 'well-born' Maori nurse who had helped develop health education for Maori in the mid 1930s, suggested to Whangarei's MOH that district nurses become ex officio council members. She also argued that women should be eligible for membership, since 'I do not consider that Maori men are competent to discuss health matters'.[22]

Crucially, the Maori Councils faced a perennial shortage of funds. The 1919 legislation authorised the Health Minister to meet the administrative costs of councils, and pay for approved sanitary work, while the Native Minister was permitted to offer subsidies from the Maori Civil List on a pound for pound basis. The Director of Maori Hygiene claimed in 1922 that the previously 'haphazard finances' had been replaced by a 'standard and objective' process for monitoring expenditure. Despite this improved accountability, he was soon to discover that extracting cash from the Native Department was easier said than done.[23]

Buck's annual report in 1924 described the Maori Councils as 'a potential factor that can be turned into an active force when special need arises', but he admitted that not all were equally active.[24] Financial considerations underlay much of the inactivity. Maori Council files at National Archives contain repeated complaints about the impossibility of achieving results without adequate funding. In 1929, for instance, the new chairman of the Kahungunu Maori Council explained that members' slackness and non-attendance was related to the failure to reimburse travelling expenses.[25]

Two years later Ron Ritchie, a European representative on the Wanganui Maori Council, reported to the Director-General that it had not functioned properly for years because of funding shortages and that many regarded the legislation as a dead letter.[26] Maori frustration with the scheme was summed up by Mangonui Maori Council chairman W. Kingi during a meeting with Labour Health Minister Peter Fraser in January 1938. The lack of expenses for council members, said Kingi, had been a drawback for the previous 30 years.[27]

One of the cornerstones of the Maori Councils Act 1900 was the power it conferred on each council to collect taxes or fines levied in relation to by-laws for the proper registration and control of dogs.[28] Intended to provide working capital, this power was something of a mixed blessing. In 1908 the Ngati Whatua chairman lamented that he was 'sick and tired of the dog-tax and of trying to collect it'.[29] These revenues were restored to local authorities in the early 1920s despite protests from Maori health officials. Buck, as Director of Maori Hygiene, failed in 1923 to persuade the Native Department to restore this tax in order to underwrite health improvements.[30] Seven years later his successor again deplored the loss of this revenue.[31] Agitation over the tax was widespread. In December 1932, for example, Ron Ritchie complained that the Wanganui Maori Council's lack of revenue had been exacerbated by the removal of the dog tax.[32] Six years later a conference of North Auckland councils met to express concern about their rumoured abolition. Delegates voiced their disappointment that inadequate funding prevented them from meeting to formulate uniform policies and suggested resurrecting their former right to collect the dog tax. Their plea met the same fate as all previous attempts.[33] The dog tax issue symbolised the financial ailments of the council system and the inability of the Health Department to provide adequate funding for this important attempt at self-help and limited self-government.

Although a lack of money lay at the heart of the Maori Councils' troubles, their influence on Maori health care was also affected by another recurring factor. The anti-tohunga sentiment of the early twentieth century became focused in the 1920s on the activities of Tahupotiki Wiremu Ratana and his followers, who were based at Ratana Pa near Wanganui. In May 1921 the Director of Maori Hygiene urged the Native Department to gazette the Wairoa Maori Council as soon as possible in order to control an imminent large gathering of Maori at Ratana Pa. This would, wrote Buck,

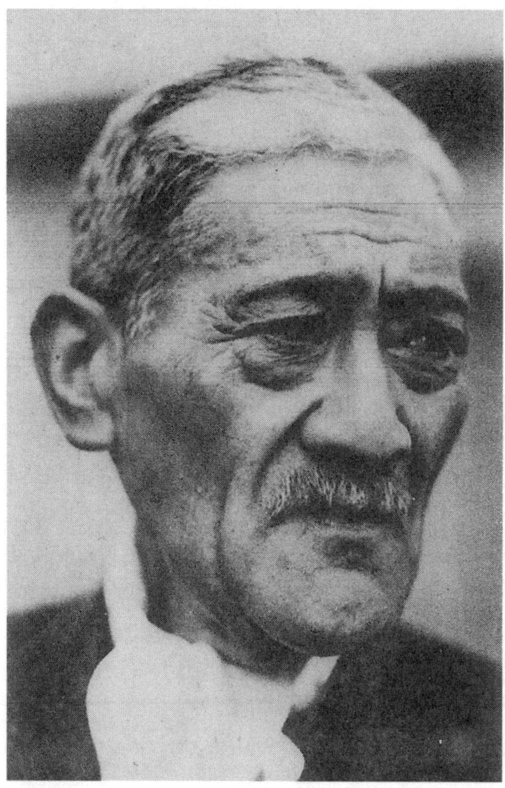

Tuhopotiki Wiremu Ratana (1873–1939), political leader, founder of the Ratana Church, and faith healer. *ATL, G-22120-1/2*

provide an opportunity to raise funds since breaches of council by-laws could be expected.[34]

Health Department concern with the Ratana movement during the next few years had three main components: sanitary conditions at Ratana Pa, the impact of Ratana's beliefs on the control of infectious disease and on the refusal to co-operate with district nurses, and their influence on the work of the Maori Councils. Departmental attitudes to all of these were shaped to some extent by political considerations and contained certain ambiguities.

The Health Department's principal file on Ratana Pa, which covers the years 1925–40, contains numerous and damning reports on its living conditions and health status by health inspectors and medical officers.[35] To a great extent these conditions stemmed from overcrowding and a lack of sanitary measures. Buck, as Director of Maori Hygiene, was ambivalent about pressing for large-scale improvements, arguing in 1926 that it was not in the best interests of Maori to turn the pa into a model village because the inhabitants would eventually drift back to their own districts as Ratana's influence waned.[36] After Buck's departure in 1927 Ellison adopted a very different stance. He advised the Mayor and councillors of Marton in July 1928 that Ratana leaders and residents had been persuaded to improve sanitation: 'In short it is hoped to make a model village there.'[37]

Departmental opinion was more clear-cut on the subject of infectious disease. In November 1921 Buck reported to Director-General Valintine that some of Ratana's followers objected to typhoid inoculation, a major part of the Department's work among Maori. Ratana himself apparently played no part in this campaign, wiring Buck with the message: 'No opposition. People can please themselves.'[38] Eight months later, in response to the death of a Maori pupil whose family had refused treatment because of their faith, Buck wrote to the Matauri Bay Native School's head teacher: 'I have always been opposed to Ratana as I dreaded the evils that would spring from his teaching.'[39] A few weeks later, following a report from MOH Herbert Chesson that Ratana supporters were concealing typhoid cases, Buck urged the Department to delay action until after the forthcoming general election. He explained that invoking the Tohunga Suppression Act might create a martyr: 'A dying cause is easily fanned into fresh life by opposition.'[40]

The Ratana influence on Maori Councils was a matter of concern to Buck and his colleagues, and one upon which they could act. In October 1925 Native Health Inspector Takiwaiora Hooper alerted Buck to the fact that Ratana's followers claimed to have 'constructed a registered Maori Council and have self-governing laws for the Native race of the Dominion'.[41] Buck went public in his annual report: 'As the Ratana movement is creeping into the work of our Councils and committees, I attend the meetings of these bodies so as to rebut the many wild statements being circulated amongst the people.'[42] The report was written just two days after Hooper informed him of a local desire to revive the Kurahaupo Maori Council to control the Ratana Camp.[43] Buck reacted swiftly and positively. On 11 June he suggested to Valintine that a new council of people who did not support Ratana should be established. Two weeks later he asked Hooper to supply seven candidates: 'We don't want any Ratanaites on the Council nor on any Komite Marae.'[44] Achieving this result required careful negotiation, but on 9 October a correspondent of the *Wanganui Chronicle* noted that the seven appointees were all men of high rank who had studied at Te Aute College. The majority were described as prosperous farmers. On 20 October a second correspondent, 'Pakeha Maori', praised the new members as a 'first class lot of young blood'.

By 1931 the Health Department was claiming publicly that the 'Ratana element which once harassed and obstructed the Maori Councils at every turn, now seeks representation on the Councils and Village Committees and assist in the work.'[45] Privately, officials continued to be critical of the allegedly divisive role played by Ratana members in some Maori Councils.[46]

In 1935 Ivan Sutherland of Wellington published an analysis of agriculture, education, health and other aspects of Maori life. While he regarded the Ratana movement as 'largely a spent force' he expressed admiration for the Maori Councils and 'the years of work done in the face of immense difficulties and discouragements in the Maori villages'.[47] Once again, departmental heads publicly concurred with this view. The Director-General, Dr Michael Watt, who had succeeded Valintine in 1930, stated in his 1934 annual report that the many Maori Councils which continued to function were of great help to his MOsH.[48] Two years later he revealed a rather different bias. His memorandum to new Health Minister Fraser on

Maori health expressed doubt as to whether the councils warranted retention in their present form; the matter required further investigation.[49]

In 1937 Dr Sylvester Lambert, the Pacific representative of the influential Rockefeller Foundation, prepared a confidential 'Survey of the Maori Situation' for the Labour government. His report included a statement that 'I did not see any direct evidence of Maori Councils and so I cannot discuss them.'[50] In 1940 Harold Turbott, formerly MOH for Gisborne and the East Cape, claimed that the councils had not functioned effectively since the control of infectious diseases had been entrusted to Pakeha health inspectors some twenty years earlier. He acknowledged that their failure was largely economic in origin—'The urgent need is for some form of income other than the distasteful and little-used method of fining their own people'—and suggested that with greater powers the councils 'could form excellent training-grounds in leadership for younger Maoris'.[51]

Whatever the shortcomings of the Maori Councils they outlasted both Peter Buck, the man charged with their revival in 1920, and the Division which he headed. In the 1920s they continued to suffer from the chronic underfunding which had bedevilled earlier initiatives in Maori health. Maori Hygiene in 1921/2 was allocated £4,750 from the Health Department budget of £214,205 (a figure which excluded hospital board costs). This sum included £1,200 to cover ongoing relief for the 1918 influenza victims and £2,000 for temporary camp hospitals used to house typhoid patients. Only £50 was set aside for the sanitation of Maori settlements. Other costs, including Maori Council administration, were met from the Civil List.[52]

For the year to March 1928 the total departmental budget had risen to almost £900,000, of which just £16,387 was dedicated to Maori Hygiene. This compared with almost twice that amount for Dental Hygiene and the £20,841 given to the School Medical Service.[53] Even this level of spending on Maori health was under threat. In February 1929 Valintine wrote to his Minister, Arthur Stallworthy, about a Native Department proposal which would reduce the Civil List contribution towards the cost of medical attendance on Maori. He noted that prior to 1917 his Department had received £3,000 as against an expenditure of £7,600, compared with the current contribution of £3,600 towards a total outlay of £16,000. Valintine was strongly opposed to any reduction, arguing that spending should actually be increased.[54] Health Minister Arthur Stallworthy later cited Valintine's figures in defence of his Department's record on Maori heath.[55]

During the 1930s the amount identified as Maori Hygiene expenditure fluctuated from year to year, partly as a result of the depression. By 1939 the net cost of £14,547 was still some way below the figure for 1928. The apparent reduction may have resulted in part from the changes to departmental administration which saw the demise of the Division of Maori Hygiene in 1930. This change was masterminded by Michael Watt, who had understudied Valintine for the previous five years. Watt had undertaken a study tour of America shortly after his appointment as Deputy Director-General. He returned with a vision of a better-integrated health programme, one that would remove 'all possible chance of over-lapping and waste of effort' and be centred on the MOsH.[56]

Launched in North Auckland in 1927, the scheme was extended to cover the entire country once Watt became Director-General in 1930. Watt's unpublished autobiography, written in the 1950s, extolled the advantages for Maori of this innovation: 'For the first time we began to obtain reliable information about the state of health of the Maori people and were able to plan a health programme suitable for their needs.'[57] In 1937, however, his summary of the Maori health situation had been more forthright. Then Watt condemned the Division of Maori Hygiene as 'only a name without any significance'. He alleged that Buck and Ellison were 'more or less free lances under the Director-General to do what they could for Maori health. . . . Generally speaking they only functioned when they were called in by the Medical Officer of Health to handle an epidemic which was beyond his capacity. The rest of the time they drifted round. They had no defined duties.'[58] This evaluation was at odds with his assessment of Maori Hygiene in 1925, when he was Acting Director-General: 'The work of the officers of this Division in the conquest of disease has undoubtedly helped to foment that spirit of good will and loyalty which so distinguish the Maori race.'[59]

Despite Watt's apparent support in 1925, Buck decided to leave the Department in 1927, three years before the Division was abolished. There was as much pull as push in Buck's decision. He was increasingly absorbed by his ethnographical and anthropological interests, which he hoped would aid the current and future prospects for Maori health. Buck's 1923 annual report floated the idea that Maori Councils might compile information on Maori culture and thus make use of the lessons of the past; he then concluded his next report with the following statement of intent: 'As the sciences of anthropology and hygiene must be intimately associated in working for the proper understanding and betterment of Native Races, I take it that it is the duty of the Division of Maori Hygiene to follow up the line of investigation already initiated by my division.'[60] This approach was approved by Valintine, who agreed in May 1924 that preventive medicine must of necessity encompass a wide field of investigation.[61]

By 1927 Buck was weary of burning the midnight oil to pursue his anthropological interests and had come to believe that someone else could 'do my health work equally well or better'.[62] Soon afterwards he resigned to take up a position at the Bishop Museum in Hawaii where he remained until his retirement. Valintine paid tribute to Buck's contribution and welcomed his replacement, Ellison, as one who 'bids fair to make an excellent successor to Dr Te Rangi Hiroa'.[63]

While the future prospects for the Division were undoubtedly damaged by Buck's departure, the writing may already have been on the wall. His correspondence with Apirana Ngata, shortly before the latter became Native Minister, is illuminating. Ngata described Ellison as lacking Buck's 'innate gift of making the fifth-wheel of the coach appear as an essential part of the show'. Some months later he provided Buck with a gloomy projection of the future under Ellison. The red-tape ethos of the current regime meant that MOsH and the Director-General were able to 'ride rough shod over the Division of Maori Hygiene, which they were always in a position to do, but for the personal factor they had to reckon with in yourself'. Buck's reply helped explain his resignation: 'It was only Valintine's deep rooted affection for me for the assistance I gave him and his department during the small pox epidemic in the North that helped me to keep the fifth wheel attached so long to a vehicle whose axles were already occupied. The realisation of the supernumerary nature of the wheel probably influenced me in making the decision that I did.'[64]

Ellison's paper on Maori and hygiene, written in 1930 before he too departed, acknowledged that the Division's 'problems bristle with difficulties'.[65] Within a year it seems they were regarded as insurmountable. As predicted by Buck and Ngata, the Division of Maori Hygiene did not survive the elevation of Michael Watt and the retrenchment in government spending in the early 1930s.

The Health Department's in-house historian, F.S. Maclean, who was recruited in 1927, claimed that Watt decided to abolish the division after Ellison resigned. Maclean described this as a wise decision which challenged MOsH to bring Maori health standards more into line with European.[66] Watt stated in 1937 that Ellison was transferred to the Cook Islands as part of the economies forced upon the government. He believed this might have been at the suggestion of Ngata, a fact confirmed by Ngata in a letter to Buck.[67] Watt represented the disbanding of Maori Hygiene as a positive benefit, for MOsH now displayed a personal interest in Maori health which had not been the case when they regarded this as the responsibility of Buck or Ellison.[68] This claim is at odds, however, with his statement of the previous year that the improvements expected from the transfer of responsibilities to medical officers and district nurses had been prevented by a lack of staff.[69]

Peter Buck's early efforts as Director of Maori Hygiene had drawn praise from his colleagues, including Auckland's District Health Officer, whose 1920 annual report had described the revival as one which promised much.[70]

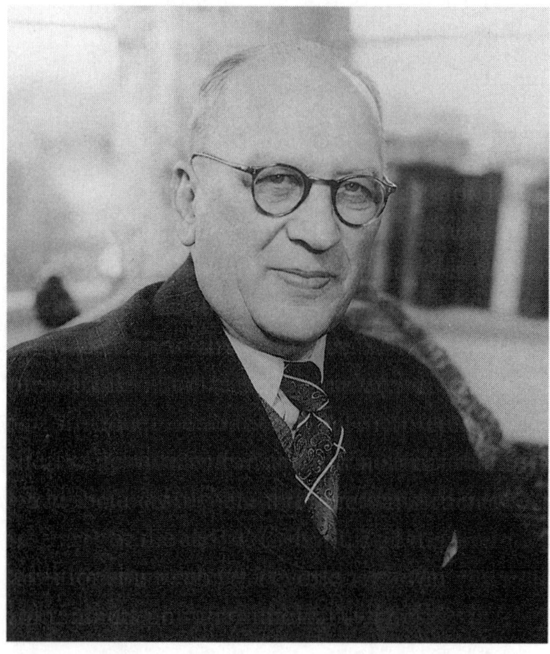

Edward Pohau ('Ned') Ellison (1884–1963) graduated MB ChB NZ in 1919. *Family collection*

Modern historians have been less generous in their appraisals. Keith Sorrenson, in his introduction to the Buck–Ngata correspondence, claimed that Buck showed little interest in Health Department work other than the reorganisation of the Maori Councils.[71] Mason Durie has criticised Buck for failing to instal Maori Councils as significant partners of the Health Department, thereby missing an opportunity to establish direct links with Maori health workers. He claimed that Buck's departure and the subsequent abolition of the Division ended 'the likelihood of a Maori health workforce closely linked to Maori communities skilled in Maori approaches to health, and able to offer effective Maori leadership.'[72]

This criticism seems somewhat harsh, given the dearth of Maori health professionals in New Zealand at this time.[73] It also ignores Buck's own perception of Maori health policy and administration. In 1949 he noted that 'Ned Ellison, also endowed with Maori blood, took my place in Maori Hygiene until the general advance in Maori understanding of health matters no longer needed a special ambassador of their own blood to help them to understand. . . . The European District Health Officers could now embark both races in the same ship and sail out on a calm sea.'[74] Consciously or otherwise, his remarks contained echoes of Pomare's much earlier image of Maori health being offloaded by the ship of state.

Buck's apparent faith in the health machinery of the 1930s was not shared by Sylvester Lambert, the author of the 1937 survey to which Watt's critical comments had been attached. Lambert was a close friend of Maui Pomare, whom he credited with advancing public health during his period as Health Minister from June 1923 until January 1926; he also had a high regard for Buck, Ngata and Ellison. Lambert's report to the Labour government recommended reinstating a Department of Maori Hygiene with properly selected and trained staff as a 'powerful means of creating an understanding between the races'. While Lambert considered New Zealand to be a world leader in controlling environmental hygiene for its European population he felt it lacked any preparation for dealing with the very specialised field of Maori health.[75] Labour did not respond to Lambert's recommendations.

'The same ratio': Maori and hospitals

In May 1919 the *Bay of Islands Luminary* reported local objections to a Health Department proposal that hospital boards should meet the costs of

Maori patients in the event of a recrudescence of the influenza epidemic. The Bay of Islands Hospital Board felt that this would be 'ruinous' and passed a resolution to the effect that 'the health of the Maoris is a national and not a local responsibility'.[76] This section focuses on four central aspects of the debate about Maori and hospitals during the 1920s and 1930s: the revival of earlier concerns about the burden on ratepayers and the feasibility of rating Maori land for this purpose; hospital fees and the question of 'indigence'; Maori attitudes towards the hospital system; and the impact these had upon Maori admission rates.

The most insistent calls for some alteration to the financing of Maori hospital care came from those hospital boards which considered themselves to be particularly hard done by. They were not necessarily the ones most affected by funding difficulties. In June 1920, 33 of the country's 43 hospital boards met to discuss common concerns. The four Bay of Islands boards,[77] Coromandel, Bay of Plenty and Tauranga, all of which had higher than average Maori populations, were not represented. The conference passed a resolution that taxes be imposed on all transfers of Maori land and that death duties be introduced on 'wealthy Native estates, for the purpose of reimbursing Hospital Boards for fees in connection with necessitous Natives'.[78]

The Health Department responded to this initiative with an editorial in the *New Zealand Journal of Health and Hospitals* which suggested the creation of fewer and larger hospital districts. The Department claimed that a streamlined structure would remove the burden on small hospital boards with large Maori populations and reduce the effects of large holdings of non-rateable Maori lands by distributing the impact across a wider area.[79] Successive generations of administrators were unable, however, to rationalise the hospital system in this way.[80]

A Hospitals Commission which reported in June 1921 recommended that non-rate-producing Maori land should be accorded the same status as Crown land. This would have excluded Maori land from the calculations which determined the contributions made by local authorities to hospital boards.[81] Again, this recommendation was never put into effect and individual boards continued to lobby for change. The Health Department suggested in 1922 that it might ease the burden on hospital boards by taking over their share of Maori medical and nursing services. As Deputy

Director-General Frengley pointed out, the Department's current annual expenditure of £13,431 on Maori health was approximately three times the estimated value of uncollected hospital rates on Maori land, and this 'should be sufficient to meet any agitation for a differential rate of subsidy owing to non-rate producing native lands'.[82] Twelve months later Valintine complained that there was still no definite policy to determine the respective contributions of his Department and the boards.[83]

This failure to establish clear guidelines had important implications for relations between the Department and the Hospital Boards Association (HBA) formed in October 1924. The latter's initial agenda contained a series of remits from the Mangonui, Whangarei and Tauranga boards on the cost of treating Maori. These included a plea for special subsidies to boards which treated large numbers of Maori 'and in whose district the Native-rates question is acute'.[84] This subject remained a core topic in the HBA's deliberations until the passage of the 1938 Social Security Act.

Health Department attempts to work with the HBA were sometimes hampered by other government agencies. In February 1926 the Director-General informed the Native Department that his Department currently spent £15,000 per annum on Maori health as against its £3,600. His plea for an increased contribution was summarily rebuffed: 'Logically there does not appear to be any good reason why the Native Department, as a Department of State, should make any contribution towards the health of the Maoris; your Department being charged with the administration of health matters for the Dominion, of which the Maoris are as much a part as the Pakeha.'[85]

In July 1927 E.A. Killick, long-time Secretary to the Health Department and its senior lay bureaucrat, produced a thirteen-page memorandum on the 'Treatment of Maoris in Hospitals'. This was a sequel to his exhaustive report of 1916 which had argued that the government had no legal obligation to provide a special medical service for Maori. In reviewing developments over the previous decade, Killick reminded Valintine that in 1922 Treasury had blocked any transfer of funds from the Native Civil List to reimburse the Health Department for the unexpectedly high cost of taking over 'outdoor' medical services for Maori (non-hospital medical and nursing care).[86]

There were also legal impediments preventing boards from seeking to recover costs from Maori. In April 1927 the Hokitika Hospital Board approached Health Minister James Young about the unpaid hospital bill of a Maori woman who had a considerable income from rents on Maori land. The board had obtained a court judgment only to discover that it could not legally take out a summons to recover this debt from rental income. Young encouraged the board to put up a specific case for him to take to the Native Minister, though any further action would be dependent on the goodwill of his colleague.[87] Later that year the Deputy Native Trustee confirmed that the Native Land Act 1909 forbade 'any deduction being made to this Office from rents paid to Natives to satisfy claims by Hospital Boards.'[88]

From this and other incidents it seems that the Health Department's political head was as powerless as his officials to effect change. James Young had been chairman of the Waikato Hospital Board at the time of the 1911 Hospitals' Conference and was sympathetic to the plight of the hospital authorities. In 1927 a number of local bodies in Waikato petitioned him about the way in which the large number of Maori in their locality placed an unfair burden on European ratepayers. The HBA then raised the matter with Prime Minister Gordon Coates, who held the Native Affairs portfolio. In response to these concerted demands that hospital care and charitable relief for Maori be placed on a dominion-wide basis, Young admitted that this 'very vexed' question required 'considerable investigation and consideration'. His reply to the Matamata Town Board also claimed that his Department's contributions to outdoor treatment and a subsidy for Maori typhoid patients meant that to some extent Maori health was already funded on a dominion-wide basis. Few were convinced by this argument.[89]

The defeat of Coates' Reform Party in 1928 brought new faces to the Health and Native Affairs portfolios but no significant change of policy. In August 1929 Native Minister Apirana Ngata informed Health Minister Arthur Stallworthy that he did not object to the government creating a special fund to reimburse hospital boards for treating Maori, if it could afford to do so. But Ngata strenuously opposed the suggestion that monies allocated as compensation for land confiscations or unfulfilled Crown contracts should be used to reimburse the boards. Two weeks later delegates from hospital boards which served 80 per cent of the Maori population met in Hamilton to discuss their position. The consensus was that regional population differences must be dealt with and the burden on ratepayers equalised.[90] Shortly afterwards the chairman of the Bay of Plenty Hospital Board, which had instigated the conference, and other HBA representatives, reported their concerns about the non-payment of hospital fees by Maori to Prime Minister Joseph Ward and Stallworthy. They also warned that boards might be forced to refuse admission to non-paying patients when accommodation was limited.[91]

Apirana Ngata responded to this veiled threat by reminding Ward that non-payment occurred in those districts which historically had suffered most from the loss of land, and that the state had done nothing to right this situation. He also drew attention to the fact that ever since 1900 the Health Department had urged the abandonment of tohungaism and Maori custom in favour of Western medicine. Ngata concluded with the comment that he had seriously considered advising Maori not to seek treatment in public hospitals unless they could afford to pay: 'The indigent of every race in the world it seems may claim the hospital service, but when those of the aboriginal race do so, they are made the subject of taunts and reproaches.'[92]

Other rural New Zealanders now entered the fray. Submissions from the Bay of Plenty branch of the New Zealand Farmers' Union about the increased burden on Pakeha ratepayers brought the sharp rejoinder from Stallworthy that 'those hospital districts which have relatively large Maori populations are not as a class the most heavily rated for hospital and charitable aid purposes'.[93] The Waikato Hospital Board continued to worry away at the issue, submitting remits to successive HBA conferences on the need for special subsidies to boards which treated large numbers of Maori patients.[94] The HBA, however, was disinclined to act. A report from its executive in October 1932 noted the difficulty of devising an equitable rating system and concluded that it could not recommend seeking further direct assistance from the government.[95]

Six months later the government appointed a committee to consider the entire issue of the rating of Maori land. Chaired by Alexander McLeod, the MHR for Wairarapa and a former Minister of Lands, the committee examined the question of 'Native Liability to Hospitals and Charitable Institutions'. Its report claimed that some European ratepayers were becoming overburdened as a result of Maori migration to districts possessing a suitable climate and a ready supply of food. It therefore recommended increased subsidies for districts with extensive Maori populations.[96] The Director-General agreed that some hospital boards were 'burdened' but rejected the proposed solution. Hospital boards with large Maori populations, he stated, did not compare unfavourably with others in terms of hospital or general rating, although he did concede that differing methods of calculating the figures made it hard to arrive at true comparisons. The Department did not think there was any justification for increased subsidies.[97]

The debate continued with reduced vigour until the introduction of hospital benefits under the 1938 Social Security Act. These benefits, which came into effect on 1 July 1939, ensured that both inpatient and outpatient services at public hospitals and the Plunket Society's Karitane hospitals became entirely free to patients. Hospitals were reimbursed at the rate of six shillings per day, a figure which was 'fixed as returning to Hospital Boards considerably more than they had succeeded in collecting from patients' fees in the past'. Never intended to cover the entire cost of hospital care, these payments were supplemented by levies on local ratepayers and by variable subsidies from general taxation, the latter intended to allow for areas of special need.[98] The implications for Maori were spelled out in the contribution of Harold Turbott, a future Director-General of Health, to Sutherland's *The Maori People Today* in 1940: 'Either nurse or doctor may send the Maori patient for free treatment at a public hospital, Hospital Boards in the various districts being charged with the provision of curative treatment as required.'[99]

Much of the anxiety and irritation over Maori and hospitals in the two decades covered by this chapter stemmed from hospital boards' frustration at their inability to collect fees from patients. The growing numbers of Maori patients, allied to the rating issue, meant that Maori were increasingly targeted by some boards. This trend may have been encouraged by a synopsis of hospital board affairs published in the Health Department's *Journal* in September 1920. This emphasised that the government had no obligation, either statutory or implied, to treat Maori patients on different terms to Europeans when it came to collecting hospital fees. When one hospital board discussed the question of defaulters in mid 1920 'a laugh was raised by the remark being passed that the liability to pay was not generally realized in some cases by Europeans as well as Natives.'[100]

Many hospital boards in the 1920s had trouble with the collection of fees from patients in general. The Health Department's annual report for 1924 advised them to be realistic about who could or could not pay, and to write debts off after a finite period.[101] Maori were clearly not alone in their failure to contribute. During 1926/7 Rawene Hospital admitted 292 Europeans who paid a little over one-third of their total debt of £2,403; the 150 Maori treated during the same period handed over just 6 per cent of the £1,248 they owed.[102] In some areas the bulk of the write-offs were generated by Europeans. Between 1924 and 1927, for example, the Hokitika Hospital Board had a shortfall of almost £1,800 in sums owed by sawmill workers; a deputation of board members also complained to the Minister that £68 had been lost on Maori patients during the year, and cited the example of a Mrs Tainui who collected quarterly rents in excess of £31 but still refused to pay her hospital bill.[103]

It is difficult to discern any clear pattern in patient debts, which depended on factors such as relative population size, use of hospital services and economic circumstances. The direct comparison by hospital boards of European and Maori payment rates rarely took these factors into account. The Waikato Board member who chaired the 1929 conference in Hamilton reported that it had recovered only 8.4 per cent of Maori patient fees, a figure matched by the Bay of Plenty. T.S. Houston of Mangonui then complained that his board retrieved only 3 per cent, compared with 50–60 per cent of European fees.[104]

The Cook Hospital Board, based in Gisborne, had expressed its concern to the 1921 Hospitals Commission about the financial hardships of boards which served a large Maori population. In 1935 it informed the Director-General that it had recovered little more than 7 per cent (£96 from £1,256) of the hospital fees owed by Maori for 1934/5, and that it had never succeeded in collecting more than 12 per cent of the debts incurred by Maori patients. This compared with the board's overall recovery rate of more than 27 per cent (£5,342 from £19,568) of the total fees incurred during the financial year.[105]

By 1936 other boards had joined the chorus of complaints about non-payment by Maori. The Waiapu Hospital Board, which had twice as many Maori as Pakeha patients, complained to the Native Minister in 1937 that Maori did not pay their share of the bill. The board admitted, however, that it was unclear if this resulted from unwillingness or from inability to pay.[106] Opinion varied on the answer to this question. E.A. Killick's 1927 memorandum alleged that most Maori expected to be considered as indigent when it came to hospital fees. He criticised 'lazy feckless Maori . . . [who are] prominent at race meetings, billiard saloons and owning possibly a motor-car' for bringing into disrepute their compatriots who met their obligations 'like Europeans'.[107] When Killick's views were echoed by a Mr Davey of Wairoa at the Hamilton conference he was quickly taken to task by William Wallace, chairman of both the Auckland Hospital Board and the HBA, who pointed out that well-to-do Pakeha were equally guilty of such practices.[108]

It is hard to assess to what extent the comments of Killick and Davey were representative of attitudes within the hospital and health sectors. Numerous observers acknowledged that many Maori were not in a position to pay for treatment. W.N. Dane, Native School master at Whangaroa, informed the Director of Maori Hygiene in October 1927 that 'the natives in these parts have very few guineas with which to pay'.[109] Some months later Ellison assured Valintine that he had always urged Maori to bear their share. He suggested that hospital boards might encourage Maori to pay by instalments rather than frighten them off by presenting the entire bill at once. Valintine agreed and arranged to draft a letter in Maori for circulation by individual boards.[110]

The financial difficulties were compounded by depression in the 1930s. F.S. Maclean, then MOH for Wellington, described conditions in Hawke's Bay in 1932: 'For reasons of poverty the Maoris very seldom consult private medical practitioners or dentists, and make use of the hospitals only when compelled to do so. In the aggregate there must be a vast amount of unnecessary suffering, crippling and mortality.'[111] Director-General Watt, in his 1937 survey, confirmed that the Department was aware of the problem. The increasing number of Maori who were treated at smaller public hospitals were supposed to contribute towards their care, 'but they cannot pay'.[112]

Various solutions to these problems were put forward. Some delegates to the 1929 conference advocated an extension of Maori farming activity to prevent pauperisation, a policy embraced by Apirana Ngata during his time as Native Minister.[113] In July 1932 the Mangonui Hospital Board suggested imposing a levy on Maori butterfat production to meet hospital fees. This was rejected by the Director-General as inequitable since it would affect the entire population, not just patients; Maori dairy farmers would be treated differently from other sectors of the community and from their Pakeha counterparts.[114] Later that year the HBA executive reported that hospital boards had incurred combined losses of £27,000 in treating Maori during the previous year. It expressed the hope that the farm settlement scheme to make Maori self-sufficient might solve the problem.[115] The Health Department sympathised with this view, believing that self-dependent farmers and improved housing were the keys to improved Maori health.[116]

Such discussions were a natural consequence of the increased use of hospitals by Maori in the 1920s and 1930s. This reflected changing Maori attitudes and gave some indication of the success of district nurses and others in promoting the benefits of Western medicine. It is difficult to quantify Maori admissions in this period, since many hospitals did not distinguish them from other patients, and others did so only when complaining about the burden imposed by increased usage. The remainder of this section examines altered Maori perceptions of the hospital and the effect this had upon Maori admissions.

Following Peter Buck's appointment as Director of Maori Hygiene there was an expectation among his colleagues that he would persuade Maori to embrace Western medicine. In 1921, for example, the Whangarei MOH asked Buck to visit a family which had suffered ten deaths in two years but refused to accept medical assistance, attend hospital 'or do anything in reason'. He wanted Buck to knock some sense into them. Buck promised to 'take a run up as soon as I can and see if anything further can be done', though he anticipated that little could be achieved with such stubborn individuals. It seems unlikely that any other divisional director would have taken, or would have been expected to take, such a personal interest.[117]

The main agents of persuasion were the district nurses. A number of medical students who undertook research projects on Maori health in the 1930s commented on the fact that many Maori refused to seek help until they were in extremis; their failure to recover served as a disincentive for the next prospective patient, and so the pattern continued. This vicious circle was eventually broken throughout the country. At Te Kuiti, for instance, Dr Cedric Isaac reported a 200 per cent rise in Maori admissions

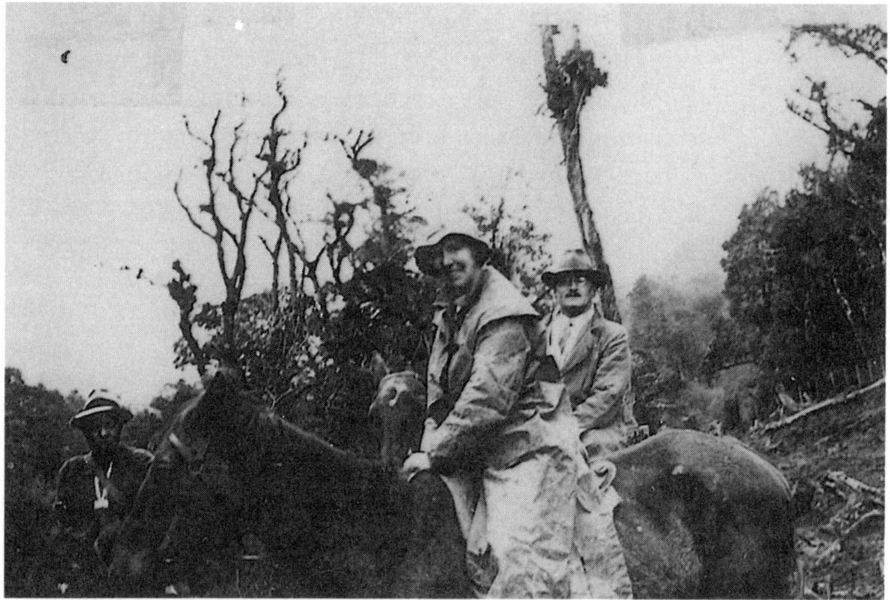

Nurse Pickett and Dr Wyn Irwin prepare to set off along the Maungapohatu Track in 1935.
Enid Pickett

from 1938 to 1940.[118] At the same time, the district nurse service was praised for preventing unnecessary hospitalisation.[119]

In the late 1920s Health Minister Young reacted to hospital board disquiet about the mounting burden of unpaid Maori hospital fees by describing this as a recent phenomenon which reflected growing Maori confidence in hospital treatment.[120] Others were less sanguine about this trend. The Bay of Plenty branch of the Farmers' Union considered that the swing away from tohunga had gone too far and that Maori now had 'rather too great a partiality for the comforts of the modern hospital'.[121] In reality, the position was less clear-cut. The claim made in 1933 by the government-appointed Committee on the Rating of Native Land that Maori now made 'full use' of hospital facilities was an exaggeration.[122] Old suspicions died hard. Michael Watt, shortly after becoming Director-General, portrayed the efforts to overcome Maori prejudice against hospitals as a 'long uphill fight'.[123] Taranaki MOH Wyn Irwin reported in 1936 that Hawera Hospital was still regarded as tapu by many Maori, 'and a place where only death can eventuate'.[124]

Quantifying the use made by Maori of hospital services is an exercise fraught with difficulties. According to the 1926 census the 63,670 Maori then resident in New Zealand constituted 4.5 per cent of the country's 1.4 million inhabitants. Two years later Frederick Bennett, described by Valintine as 'well known to the Department as one of the most zealous Maori clergymen', claimed that the Department was doing practically nothing for Maori. Valintine acted swiftly to rebut the claim, providing Bennett with statistics to show that in relation to population Maori received considerably more individual treatment and attention than Europeans from hospital and public health services.[125]

Valintine's calculations were based on departmental expenditure and selected staffing figures. It is questionable whether he could have supplied precise details of hospital admission rates, for many hospital boards seem to have supplied data only when they wished to register a protest. In 1929, for instance, a Waikato representative indicated that his organisation had treated 583 Maori patients over the previous two years. He did not place this in the context of the total of more than 6,000 treated, preferring to stress the fact that Waikato had 11,395 Maori, one in six of the country's total Maori population, and that the local hospital board therefore carried a disproportionate share of the burden.[126]

The proportion of Maori inpatients varied widely. The fact that Waiapu had twice as many Maori as European patients mirrored the population distribution within its catchment area. The Board approached the Minister in 1937 because the increase in patient numbers over the past five years had been made up entirely of Maori who could not or would not pay.[127] Hokianga Maori availed themselves of half the hospital services by the mid 1930s.[128] A similar situation existed with the neighbouring Bay of Islands Hospital Board, which informed the Health Department in 1937 that Maori constituted 46 per cent of the population 'and Natives are using the hospitals in approximately the same ratio'.[129]

Proportionality did not apply everywhere. The Cook Hospital Board's district contained a large number of Maori yet they accounted for only 7.4 per cent of its 1,939 patients in 1935.[130] Taranaki Maori, who had been amongst the first to benefit from Governor Grey's 1840s hospitals, were another group to make limited use of hospitals in the 1930s. Although New Plymouth Hospital trebled its Maori inpatients from 60 in 1932 to 180 in 1937, even this higher figure amounted to only 7 per cent of all admissions.[131] At Dannevirke Hospital the 350 Maori admitted from

1934–9 constituted about 6 per cent of inpatients.[132] Some hospitals in areas with larger than average Maori populations fell far short of this figure, which roughly corresponded to the percentage of Maori in the total population (5.2 per cent in 1936). Wanganui Hospital had been one of the first nineteenth century hospitals to concentrate its efforts on European rather than Maori patients, a trend which apparently continued into the 1930s. A survey conducted in 1935 identified only 135 Maori admissions since 1932, a period during which almost 7,000 patients had passed through the institution. The author concluded that Maori, who accounted for only 2 per cent of admissions, had to be made more aware of the many health facilities at their disposal.[133]

The reliability of these Maori patient statistics is open to question. The collection of data was encouraged in the late 1930s by Otago University's Professor of Public Health, Charles Hercus, who had worked for the Health Department in the early 1920s and retained links with his former colleagues. The students who had most success in this sphere were the offspring of public health officials. Margaret Beedie was the daughter of Dannevirke's Medical Superintendent. Her thesis acknowledged the difficulty of identifying Maori, many of whom had Pakeha names. She and her co-author therefore relied on their personal knowledge of the district to ensure accuracy.[134] Richard Dawson, the son of New Plymouth MOH Frederick Dawson, seems to have been less au fait with his cohort. He distinguished Maori from Pakeha in the New Plymouth and Hawera Hospital records on the basis of names but claimed that his findings for 1933–6 were validated by a comparison with data for 1937, when the hospital registers did include details of ethnicity.[135]

While there is uncertainty about the accuracy of the hospital statistics, and many omissions in the figures provided, it is possible to reach some conclusions. Before the 1936 conference on Maori welfare, Health Department officials opposed the creation of separate institutions because Maori were now less reluctant to enter public hospitals and boards and their staff displayed more sympathy towards Maori who sought admission. This claim was made public by Director-General Watt during the conference.[136]

The most significant influence in the later 1930s was the introduction of the Labour government's social security scheme. This coincided with greater use of hospitals by Maori. In August 1938 the Wairoa Hospital Board, a third of whose beds were occupied by Maori, sought urgent assistance with capital expenditure to enable it 'to cope effectively with the ever increasing amount of treatment of natives in addition to Europeans'. A follow-up letter from the Board expressed its fears that it would be unable to comply with the terms of the Social Security Act because of overcrowding. When the Health Department argued that this was essentially the responsibility of the Native Department, Internal Affairs and Treasury, the Acting Native Minister swiftly turned the tables by stating that the matter was 'entirely one for consideration by my colleague, the Hon Minister of Health'. The episode highlighted yet again the lack of any clear-cut definition of responsibility for Maori health.[137]

Writing in 1940, Harold Turbott dampened the earlier optimism of some of his colleagues. Although Maori were displaying a growing confidence in hospitals, a majority were either still totally averse to seeking admission or delayed until 'hope seems lost'. Turbott also criticised the racial antipathy which characterised certain hospitals and some staff: 'Such institutions hinder preventive health, for free use of base hospitals is the pivot around which health work revolves.'[138] Despite the changes which had already taken place, Maori still had some way to go to gain maximum advantage from the hospital system.

'Natural adjustment': subsidised doctors

In this period the Health Department became increasingly concerned at inequities in the system of subsidised doctors. There were almost equal numbers of appointees in the North and South Islands even though the two had very different Maori populations. Following the introduction of fee for service payments in the late 1930s their responsibilities were to be largely assumed by MOsH, district nurses and hospital boards. In the 1920s and 1930s the number of rural doctors remained virtually static at around 260. The proportion of rural doctors fell from 27 per cent of the total medical workforce in 1922 to 18 per cent in 1941. The Maori population, which was still concentrated in rural areas, had risen to 82,326 by 1936.[139]

The needs of people who lived in the backblocks, both European and Maori, had exercised politicians and officials since the turn of the century. In 1900 Walter Symes, the MHR for Egmont, raised the question of

Maori Population and Number of NMOs

Date	Maori Population	Number of NMOs
1858	56,049	–
1866	–	29
1874–5	47,330	18
1895–6	42,113	27
1906	50,309	35
1911	52,723	c.46
1921–2	56,987	42
1926	63,670	c.40
1936	82,326	c.40

subsidies for doctors to 'poor and struggling settlers', noting that 'no sane person would expect a medical man to go and live in the back blocks of the country'. The Minister of Lands promised to consider such a scheme, but warned that its costs would be high and that it might be difficult to implement.[140] Symes' cry was periodically taken up by other parliamentarians. During the Health Department Supply debate in 1907 William Herries (Bay of Plenty) appealed for increased spending on Maori health services since 'Europeans and Maoris alike were crying out for medical officers for the backblocks'.[141]

The Health Department cautiously supported this appeal. Its annual report for 1912 agreed that a subsidised medical service for the backblocks could be established with little or no alteration to the hospital machinery. More importantly, 'if administered with discretion it would not prove a costly venture'; patients should pay according to their means, as they did with the public hospitals.[142] Some communities formed medical associations which guaranteed a certain income to doctors who settled in the district. On at least one occasion the Health Minister offered financial assistance without consulting his officials. A departmental note appended to the Pongaroa Medical Association file in 1914 stated: 'Started by Department in error 1911. Buddo's Blunder.'[143] From its foundation in 1917 the departmental journal publicised medical association vacancies, with the first issue containing an advertisement for Pongaroa in Wairarapa. This offered a guarantee of £400 per annum and estimated that £500 could be earned from outside practice.[144]

The Public Health Amendment Act 1918 empowered the Health Minister to appoint at the request of any local authority 'resident medical practitioners' who would be permitted to charge prescribed fees or give free medical attention in 'necessitous cases'. The scheme was greeted with some scepticism by hospital boards. At Stratford, for instance, the chairman ridiculed this 'wonderful scheme' that had to be paid for by the people living in the hospital districts.[145] It was short-lived; the relevant sections were not carried over to the 1920 Health Act.[146]

Dr William Young's 1922 presidential address to the NZBMA included an assessment of the government's initiatives to meet the health needs of rural communities; these initiatives included subsidies for doctors to ensure medical services for Maori and in backblocks districts, district nurses and 'Native' or 'Maori' health nurses. While all had proved 'most useful and a boon' to the districts in which they were operating, Young lamented that there simply were not enough of them.[147]

The 46 NMOs of 1909 marked the high point of the service both absolutely and, given the upturn in the Maori population from the nadir of 1896, in relative terms. The introduction at the same time of district nursing services had signalled a change in policy and attitude, the repercussions of which would be felt throughout the next three decades. While these changes had begun before 1914 it was not until the country had settled down after the 1918 Armistice and shaken off the effects of the influenza epidemic that attention was again focused on the subsidised medical scheme.

Peter Buck had been critical in 1910 of what he believed to be the money wasted each year on subsidised NMOs.[148] A decade later, as Director of Maori Hygiene, his assessment was equally unfavourable. His first report in 1920 stated that it had been necessary to 'define their working-radius, as different conditions exist in various districts.'[149] By the following year Buck's attitude had hardened. It was now time to review the 'whole question' of NMOs, since Maori 'are not receiving the attention they should, and accordingly the Department not getting value for the money so expended'. This approach was supported by the Director-General, who noted that the services rendered by some NMOs were 'of a very perfunctory nature'. Valintine also took the opportunity to endorse his own policy of replacing some doctors with nurses, which he believed had brought an exceedingly satisfactory outcome.[150]

Buck again questioned the very essence of the subsidised scheme in his annual report in 1922. He now believed that Maori ought to pay for medical attention and that general practitioners must accept the risk of bad debts, as they already did with Pakeha patients. He added: 'In districts where subsidies were not given the natural adjustment took place long ago.'[151] Buck then claimed that the number of NMOs had already been reduced. This statement was at odds with the information given by the Deputy Director-General to the Health Minister later that year, which indicated that the Department had made payments to 42 part-time medical officers and 24 full-time nurses.[152]

By the time of his departure in 1927 Buck had achieved a reduction of a third in the number of NMOs.[153] E.P. Ellison, the new Director of Maori Hygiene, announced in 1929 that he meant to replace more NMOs with district nurses after conducting a full survey of the scheme. He had already submitted a report on Nelson–Marlborough and was now working on the North Island, where the medical officers were on the whole 'giving splendid service'.[154] By the following year Ellison was singing a rather different tune. During discussions between the Department and the Native Trustee about the situation in Nelson and Marlborough he commented: 'Personally, I think the time is ripe when all of these doctors' subsidies should be withdrawn & one or two district nurses appointed for more effective preventive work.'[155] Ellison submitted his final report as Director of Maori Hygiene in 1931, by which time the number of NMOs was back up to 40. While some did 'exceedingly good work and far in excess of the subsidy they receive ... others do not appear enthusiastic'. The report made no specific recommendations, leaving the way clear for Watt, Valintine's successor, to consider alternatives.[156]

The disbanding of the Division of Maori Hygiene in 1930 placed the responsibility for Maori health squarely on the shoulders of the MOsH. In August 1932 Watt asked these officers to report on the operation of the NMO scheme. The replies confirmed the continued existence of the discrepancies which had affected it for decades. F.S. Maclean of Wellington, for example, reported that the 309 Maori living in Patea Borough and its immediate environs received subsidised medical care from Wilfred Simmons, the Medical Superintendent of the local hospital. The remaining

8,000 Maori within the Wanganui-Horowhenua and Wairarapa-Hawke's Bay Health Districts were denied such treatment.[157] The most significant factor, however, was the gulf separating the North and South Islands. As Maclean pointed out, the former had eighteen NMOs for a population of almost 61,000, while the latter's 22 NMOs had only 2,800 prospective patients between them. The subsidies paid in the two islands totalled £915 and £973 respectively.[158] Whangarei MOH Duncan Cook used these figures to argue that there was no logic to the system.[159]

Several of the MOsH supplied detailed commentaries on the practical effects of these disparities. Maclean had admitted earlier in the year that his attempts to tackle poor Maori health in the lower North Island were hampered by a shortage of district nurses and the fact that there was only one subsidised doctor in the Wanganui–Horowhenua and Wairarapa–Hawke's Bay districts.[160] In contrast, Nelson–Marlborough had six doctors for fewer than 700 Maori.[161] (This was less generous than the position four years earlier, when Maclean's predecessor, William Mercer, calculated that the six doctors received £355 for attending 82 families comprising some 400 individuals.)[162]

Identifying the problem was straightforward, but resolving it had always been another matter. When asked to comment in 1920 on a request for an additional NMO for Kaka Point, a coastal settlement near the mouth of the Clutha River, Buck expressed strong opposition in principle to any further appointments, since neither the Department nor Maori received value for money. But with respect to the South Island, he added, this was a policy question on which he was not in a position to give an opinion.[163] Many South Island Maori claimed rights to medical treatment and other social services under the 'tenths' provisions of the nineteenth century land sales. In 1921 the Health Department asserted that the Ngai Tahu tenths contained no express provision for hospital or medical treatment.[164] Nevertheless, at the time of the 1932 survey Wellington MOH William Findlay warned against provoking the resignation of Dr Edward Bydder of Takaka by reducing his salary, since this would generate 'the usual protest from the Maoris to high authority re their right to favour from the Tenths'.[165]

Most of the MOsH who responded in 1932 favoured an extension of the district nursing programme at the expense of the NMOs, with doctors receiving fees for approved consultations instead of an annual payment. In answer to the Director-General's question as to whether the NMO scheme ought to be extended or reduced, Duncan Cook replied that the Department's aim should be 'the ultimate extinction' of these positions.[166] Watt concurred. After deliberating for some months he informed the MOsH for Auckland, Whangarei and Gisborne that he was considering cancelling the NMOs in areas which had ready access to public hospital or nursing services. This was greeted by Harold Turbott of Gisborne as a welcome extension of choice, removing the constraint which in the past obliged the MOH to use the nominated doctor even though he might be technically unsuitable or lack mana in the local community. The replies to the Director-General cautioned him to pay due heed to individual circumstance. John Boyd of Auckland advised that the cancellation of the existing appointments at Morrinsville, Te Kuiti and Taumarunui would entail no hardship since hospital and nursing facilities there were sufficient—'if availed of by them'—but Kawhia should be allowed to keep its subsidy since it had only a small cottage hospital and a matron with no maternity experience.[167]

In December 1933 the Director-General sent an outline of his proposed scheme to the NZBMA for consideration. All existing subsidies were to be cancelled and Maori encouraged to use public hospitals. District nurses would be authorised to engage a doctor when necessary, with patients given freedom of choice of medical attendant where possible. Watt stressed that the proposed changes were not an economy measure but were intended to spread the benefits of medical services to all Maori.[168] This was the sighting shot in what proved to be an extended debate.

Eleven representatives from Health, two from Education and one from the Native Department attended a Maori hygiene conference in May 1934. They endorsed Watt's agenda. He then informed the Health Minister that he would soon be in a position to submit definite proposals 'for the betterment of the Maori race from the point of view of this Department'.[169] Such hopes were premature. The NZBMA council and divisions favoured acceptance of the Department's plan, though some wanted modifications to allow for local conditions.[170] The process then seems to have ground to a halt.

Five months after New Zealand's first Labour government took office in December 1935 the Director-General sent a copy of the plan, virtually unchanged from that of 1934, to Health Minister Peter Fraser. Watt's letter hinted that negotiations with the medical profession may have contributed to the delay. He noted that a scale of fees had been agreed with the NZBMA and that he had rejected an offer from a group of doctors to work at a lower rate for fear that failure to adopt a universal scale would lead to friction. Fraser signalled his approval and Watt asked his MOsH to update their previous recommendations.[171]

The replies revealed further obstacles to a smooth transition. Dunedin's Thomas McKibbin stated that there were few Maori 'living under native conditions' in his health district. Areas such as Bluff, whose doctor currently received £50 a year, would not merit the full-time services of a Maori nurse. McKibbin advised the retention of the NMO in such circumstances, adding that the payments were not over-liberal considering the workload and the doctor's secondary role as a dispenser of medicines. This echoed F.S.

Despite Thomas McKibbin's assurances about the situation in Otago, housing conditions for many Maori in the mid 1930s were not much changed from those of the nineteenth century. *ATL, F37893 1/2*

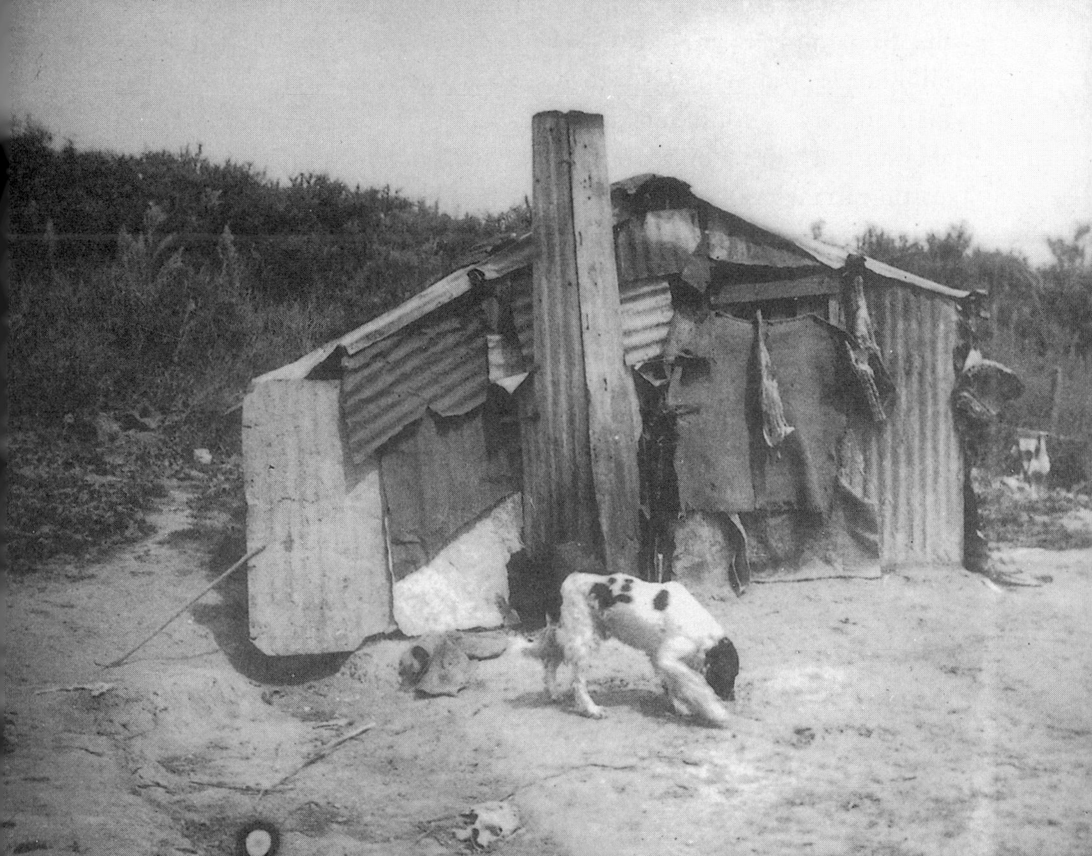

Maclean's earlier findings that the scattered nature of the Maori population in Wairarapa made it impracticable to appoint a district nurse to cover the entire area. McKibbin also identified another potential impediment. Some doctors were actively opposed to the district nurse scheme; this would presumably create tension if a doctor had to be called in.[172]

One South Island official foresaw other difficulties. Christchurch's MOH reminded the Director-General that the Department would not be keeping faith with local Maori if it abandoned subsidies in the areas covered by the Selwyn and Ahaura tenths. Watt's response noted that subsidised doctors in the Canterbury and West Coast Health District were disproportionately expensive.[173] This had always been the case, but officials now seemed determined to rectify the situation. Wyn Irwin, MOH for Wairarapa–Hawke's Bay, challenged Maclean's view that the Department had no power to cancel the payments to the eight Nelson–Marlborough NMOs from the Maori Trust Fund, explaining that the Deputy Native Trustee had confirmed that these funds could go instead to the district nurses.[174] Watt's reaction is not recorded.

Departmental annual reports in the later 1930s contain no reference to the dismantling of the NMO scheme. The Department had received ministerial approval in May 1936 for a scale of fees which paid five shillings for a surgery consultation or domiciliary visit, plus a one-way travel allowance of four shillings per mile for visits, but it took time to cancel the existing arrangements and implement this new system.[175] Even then, the Department had some reservations about a wholesale dismantling of the prevailing structure.

James Wadmore had been appointed NMO for Whakatane in 1908. Turbott's report to the Director-General in 1932 described Wadmore, who saw himself as the government official charged with 'the supervision of the Maori health (curative)', as the only one of the five East Cape NMOs to take his position seriously. Although he favoured the transfer of NMO funding to the district nurses, Turbott had some sympathy with Wadmore's situation.[176] Four years later Wadmore was informed of the decision to cancel his appointment with effect from 31 March 1937. He wrote immediately to express dismay at the loss of his very small salary. Wadmore was particularly upset by the lack of appreciation of his long and faithful service. This had, he claimed, included pioneering the use of anti-typhoid inoculation for North Island Maori, a practice which had saved the Department hundreds of pounds. Wadmore also attributed deficiencies in medical attendance on Maori to a lack of co-operation from district nurses.[177] Unwilling to let the matter rest, he then contacted his local MHR, stressing that he saw about 45 Maori each month and that the commitments of the other local doctors meant they were not free to visit Maori.[178] Health Minister Fraser's reply to the MHR explained that the new policy rested on use of the district nurse in the first instance. Patients would be encouraged to use public hospitals where appropriate and would be free to choose their doctor provided this entailed no additional expense. NMOs were to be retained only where there was no district nurse; regretfully, this meant that Wadmore's appointment could not be renewed.[179] This new policy was welcomed later that year by Apirana Ngata, who commented during the Health Supply debate that the £1,380 currently spent on NMOs (from a departmental budget of £1.141m) would be better spent on improving Maori housing, which lay at the heart of the health problem.[180]

The need to assess individual circumstances slowed the process of change. It was not until July 1938 that subsidies paid to doctors in North Auckland were replaced by a fee for attendance on Maori. The Whangaroa Hospital Board accepted this change as inevitable, but was anxious that some members of the large and scattered Maori population would miss out because of problems in obtaining authorisation to call in a doctor.[181] Departmental officers were also concerned about the mechanics of the new system. Whangarei's MOH, Carlyle Gilberd, feared that some doctors would refuse to take part in the planned roster, and that Maori reluctance to express a preference for a specific doctor would complicate matters further.[182]

By 1940 the Department was considering alternatives to the fee for service system. Golan Maaka, a Maori doctor, had recently returned to New Zealand from an International Red Cross posting in China, where he had gained experience in treating civilians infected with venereal disease.[183] He was recruited by the Health Department to deal with the high incidence of syphilis among Bay of Plenty Maori. The extension of his duties to include general practice raised questions in the Director-General's mind as to whether the concept of full-time 'Maori' GPs should be extended to other regions. He was encouraged in this direction by one MOH, Gordon

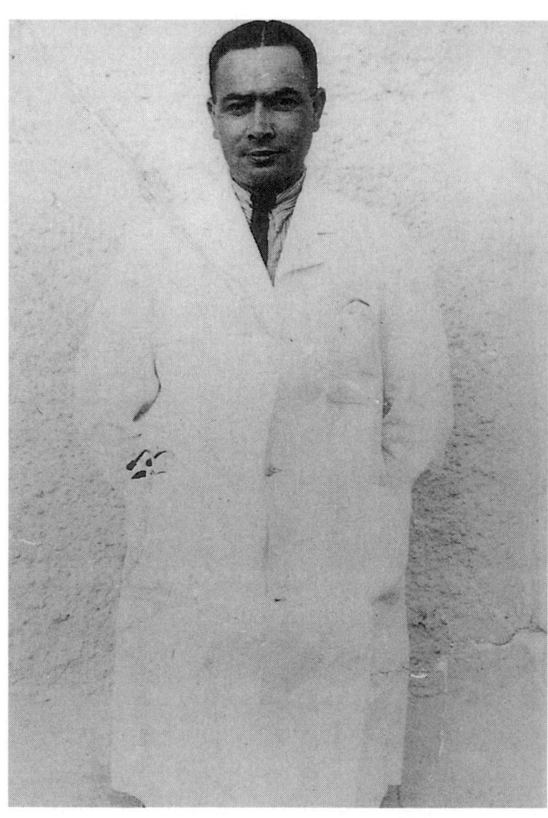

Dr Golan Maaka (1904–78) MB ChB 1932, photographed while serving with the Red Cross in China during the Sino–Japanese War in 1938. *Photograph by permission of Brad Haami*

Dempster, who believed this would be a more effective way to spend the £1,400 disbursed each year on treating indigent Maori. Watt therefore sought guidance from the MOsH in Hamilton, Gisborne, Palmerston North and Auckland, while warning that he did not know if the government would sanction such appointments, or if the Department could find doctors to accept them.

The replies confirmed the need for services in certain locations. Hubert Smith (Auckland) identified Tauranga, whose 3,000 Maori constituted 25 per cent of the population, as the only location within the Auckland district meriting a full-time appointment. Kenneth Davis (Gisborne) cited the dearth of doctors in the East Cape, the high incidence of tuberculosis, and the large Maori population who could not adequately reimburse a private practitioner as ample justification for a full-time post. Duncan Cook (Palmerston North) argued that the lack of any preventive element in the fee for service scheme impeded lessons being learned from the shocking health conditions. He suggested that full-time doctors should work in tandem with district nurses since Maori would not accept the word of a female nurse alone, and the 'manifold duties' now performed by the MOsH meant they were no longer in a position to offer therapeutic or preventive care. Cook identified Wanganui as one place where a full-time officer was an 'urgent necessity'. No action was taken because of the pressures of war.[184]

Cook's thoughtful and detailed submission described the continuing retainer paid to Wilfred Simmons of Patea as a 'legacy of the past'. Other remnants of former structures survived into the 1940s. The Native Trust Office still maintained posts at Nelson, Takaka, Havelock, Motueka, Picton, Petone and Johnsonville.[185] Most Maori, however, did not have access to such services after the introduction of health benefits in 1939.

In attempting to provide an overview of the policy decisions which shaped the NMO scheme it is easy to lose sight of the individuals involved. Yet the attitudes of providers and their relationships with patients did much to determine the ultimate fate of the venture. Departmental officials sometimes had to tread carefully and act persuasively in order to retain or recruit doctors. A number of doctors resigned in the 1920s because they felt abused by the system. Some became increasingly dissatisfied with the requirement to treat patients whom they did not regard as indigent. Albert McClymont of Havelock, who had graduated from Otago in 1920, typified this group. The majority of local Maori lived far from his surgery; in June 1922 he refused to undertake home visits on the grounds that they could always find money for a car to come into town to get drunk. He therefore felt no obligation to offer them preferential treatment. The Department attempted to appease him by specifying that his retainer of £30 per annum covered visits within a five-mile radius, but only for acute illnesses. It also stipulated that non-indigent patients should be charged at a rate agreed between the 'Medical Practitioner and the Native'. This proposed compromise soon foundered. McClymont resigned in 1923, complaining that Maori came to Havelock, had a few drinks, then visited him with imaginary disorders as 'part of the normal round of entertainment'. Any suggestion of a fee, he reported, was met with a 'torrent of filthy abuse'.[186] His experience was not unique.[187]

On occasion the Department was drawn into territorial disputes between rival doctors. In 1924 John Gregg complained to Health Minister Maui Pomare that 'a bounder Dr C Russell' had set up in opposition to him and was using unprofessional conduct to obtain Gregg's position as NMO. Cedric Russell, an ex-Army doctor, had recently settled in Picton and was currently the 'popular Medical man of the Town', according to a departmental informant. Both the Minister and the Director of Maori Hygiene advised Valintine to transfer the subsidy to Russell since 'once Maories lose confidence in a medical man they cease to go to him and the subsidy is wasted'.[188] When Gregg aired his grievance in the pages of the *NZMJ* the Director-General explained that it had been a 'case of sentiment on the part of the Maoris', whose wishes had to be respected since they funded part of the subsidy (through the Native Trustee).[189]

A later dispute at Takaka raised even more complex issues. Local Maori petitioned the Minister of Native Affairs in 1936 to have Edward Bydder replaced as NMO by Louis Potaka, who had acted on Bydder's recommendation while the latter visited Britain. The Director-General was reluctant to comply. Potaka was an unknown quantity and should he depart within a short time it might be difficult to persuade Bydder to resume. The local health inspector was unwilling to be intercede since he was personally friendly with both men. Wyn Irwin, MOH for Wairarapa–Hawke's Bay, was convinced that the transfer would be an injustice to Bydder and queried the growing tendency of Maori to seek change: 'To my mind the Maoris are, whether as a result of nationalistic propaganda or no, becoming far too aggressive and bumptious in their attitude in these matters.' The issue was further complicated by the revelation that Potaka planned to take an action in the Supreme Court against Bydder. At the same time the NZMBA was intent on prosecuting Potaka for breaching medical ethics. The matter was resolved by the death of Potaka before the matter came to court.[190]

The Bydder–Potaka dispute had an additional dimension: Potaka was the son of a Maori farmer. In 1929 Dr Assid Corban, the Auckland-born son of Lebanese winemakers, had urged the Minister of Health to appoint more Maori doctors since Ellison could not cover everything and some Maori were reluctant to attend Pakeha doctors. He referred to the attempted establishment of a travelling clinic by Tutere Wi Repa, Peter Buck's near-contemporary, as an example of what might be done.[191] However admirable in principle, Corban's aim was unrealistic because of the almost total lack of Maori doctors.

In 1994 Mason Durie published a list of Maori doctors and nurses, almost all of whom had qualified after 1940. The only doctor to spend any time in general practice prior to 1930 was Wi Repa, whom he praised for having 'devoted his entire professional life to unselfish commitment as a general practitioner at Te Araroa', where he demonstrated 'the effectiveness that Maori professionals could have among their own people'.[192] This assessment was one with which few Health Department doctors would have agreed. The Department's extended correspondence with and about Wi Repa for the years 1908–46 reveals him as a somewhat erratic individual who alternated between medicine and farming in the 1920s and voluntarily removed himself from the Medical Register for part of this time. A number of Health Department assessments concluded that he was unpopular with both Maori and European patients. As a role model for prospective Maori doctors he was less suitable than Pomare, Buck or Ellison.[193] Despite these shortcomings, the Labour Party's Maori conference resolved in 1936 that 'in respect to the medical professions the scholarships that assisted doctor Wi Repa and doctor Buck [should] be restored'.[194]

The lack of Maori physicians placed the onus squarely on the shoulders of European doctors. One in six of all rural medical practitioners held appointments as NMOs, a proportion which had remained relatively constant since the 1890s. As has been indicated, some were more fully committed than others. The replacement of the NMOs by a fee for service arrangement was an attempt to spread the burden more evenly and integrate Maori more fully into mainstream medical practice. While the focus in this section has been on the formal system of NMOs, we must not forget the role of other local doctors in treating Maori. As Beedie and Hunter concluded in their 1942 survey of Maori health in Southern Hawke's Bay: 'These doctors attend Maori patients in the course of their practice. Some Maoris consult them of their own initiative and others when advised to do so by the District Nurse, but there is no routine supervision of Maori health by a local medical practitioner. Much of their attendance receives no pecuniary reward, but the doctors are resigned to the situation and accept their responsibilities without complaint.'[195]

'Two principal scourges': fighting infection

When Peter Buck was reappointed to the Health Department in 1919 it was with the express purpose of improving sanitary conditions in Maori communities.[196] This response to questions raised by the 1918 influenza epidemic echoed the concept of a Maori 'sanitary commissioner' that had been approved by Cabinet at the height of the 1900 plague scare. Buck's proposal to restore the sanitary inspectors, which he had mooted without success after the 1913 smallpox epidemic, offered further parallels with Maui Pomare's earlier tenure.

The 'two principal scourges' of typhoid and tuberculosis were acknowledged as major public health problems, to be tackled by a combination of treatment and preventive measures. The sanitary improvement of Maori communities, however, was to be hindered by a lack of both money and trained Maori health personnel. Attempts to obtain external funding, principally through the Rockefeller Foundation, were unsuccessful.

With the benefit of hindsight, Buck was able to specify in 1920 that the new breed of Maori health inspectors should be young, energetic and educated, rather than the chiefly figures who had formed the original group in the early 1900s.[197] The first to be engaged was Harding Leaf, who had impressed Buck during war service with the Maori Battalion.[198] Valintine clearly had high hopes for the new system; he predicted in 1920 that within a few years Maori standards of sanitation would approximate those of Europeans.[199] This was never a realistic goal given the inadequate funding and the economic circumstances of most Maori.

Buck still believed in 1921 that the Maori health councils, in combination with district nurses and sanitary inspectors, would effect a great improvement in 'all matters incidental to Native health'.[200] He was to be disappointed. Departmental files contain numerous references to councils applying for inspectors only to be rejected on grounds of financial stringency. Maui Pomare, shortly before assuming the health portfolio in 1923, urged his predecessor to appoint such inspectors, citing the current Ratana activity as justification for treating this as a priority. He was no more successful than Buck had been.[201] In 1924 there was still only one Maori inspector, who also had to undertake a considerable amount of work among Europeans.[202]

European health inspectors did their best to serve Maori communities but had limited success. By 1926 the number of Maori inspectors had doubled to two, with Buck stressing that they were experts in Maori lore and therefore in a position to be effective.[203] Their activities, however, were restricted to pa and kainga dwellers.[204] There were three North Island inspectors in 1928, one for every 20,000 Maori. Their numbers reached a peak of four nationwide in the late 1920s, before falling to just two.[205] These inspectors acted as intermediaries between Maori and the health bureaucracy. Takiwaiora Hooper, for example, informed Dr Ellison in 1929 that Ratana's followers would confide in him but would not disclose their troubles to Pakeha.[206] The system involved political as well as health considerations; Hooper in 1926 defended his right as a local Maori to challenge Ratana's failings without consulting Health Department officials.[207]

Michael Watt, the Director-General from 1930, had little regard for the abilities of the Maori inspectors, whom he discarded in 1931 as part of the reorganisation of Maori health care. His summary of the Maori health situation in Sylvester Lambert's 1937 report noted the existence of 'about four so-called Maori Inspectors, that is, men of Maori blood'. Watt was sceptical of their achievements, claiming that they were untrained and had 'scoured up and down the country, running up expenses and achieving very little'.[208] This evaluation was endorsed in 1938 by one of the first social scientists to study New Zealand's public health system. D.F.B. Eyres, in assessing Pomare's fourteen-point 1904 blueprint for Maori health, concluded that only the employment of Maori health inspectors had proved of doubtful value.[209]

Despite's Watt's change of direction, Wanganui Maori achieved something of a coup in 1932 when they successfully applied to have Te Rakaherea Woodbine Pomare, Maui's son, appointed as Native Inspector of Health to the upriver regions. Their request revealed one weakness in Buck's dream of an educated inspectorate. The applicants acknowledged that Pomare, who had enjoyed all the advantages of a European education, would have to learn Maori language and custom in order to succeed. The prospect of failure made them hedge their bets: 'The work we are advocating for him can be temporary and if he does not prove himself worthy then he can be dropped.'[210] The venture was successful. Pomare served as a Maori health inspector from 1932 until the outbreak of war in 1939. He later rose to be a tutor inspector and took charge of the national training scheme for health inspectors in the early 1960s.[211]

Staffing policies were only one element in the drive to improve Maori sanitation after 1920. At the time of the 1918 influenza epidemic the Huntly Town Council had complained to the Minister of Health that many Maori pa were entirely without sanitary conveniences or drainage.[212] During his seven years in office Buck repeatedly commented on the improvements which were taking place, describing a water supply in 1926 as one of the 'most potent factors towards establishing good health'. These achievements were attributed to a combination of self-help and government subsidy, the latter controlled by the Native Department. All in all, the scale of operations was modest, with Buck's 1924 annual report including a plea for just £500 to assist impoverished Maori Councils to install latrines at meeting houses.[213] One of the most ambitious projects was the attempt to create model Maori villages at Ohinemutu and Whakarewarewa, Rotorua, following a 1926 Commission of Inquiry.[214] Other successes rested on local initiatives. In 1921 the *Opotiki Herald* reported that district nurse Robina Cameron, who later founded the Women's Health League, had organised a competition to determine which of five local pa had made the greatest sanitary progress. The *Herald* contrasted the success of this 'comparatively humble official' with the alleged inaction of 'native health experts' in Wellington.[215]

The majority of these schemes in the 1920s involved communal effort.[216] One barrier to progress was the requirement that Maori themselves find half the money; many communities simply could not do so. The old bugbear of departmental responsibility also entered the equation. Acting Director-General Watt asked in 1929 who would fund communal conveniences in heavily used pa: 'Will the Native Department provide funds for work of this sort or must it all come out of the Health vote?' Ellison identified a number of possible sources of funding, including the Maori Purposes Fund, the balance of the Native Civil List £7,000, the Native Trust Fund (of which £425 per annum was already administered by the Health Department), the Arawa Trust Fund, and the Tuwharetoa Trust Fund.[217]

As Native Minister from 1928 to 1934, Apirana Ngata was very conscious of the sanitary defects of Maori communities. In 1931 he questioned Sylvester Lambert of the Rockefeller Foundation about his organisation's lack of interest in Maori. Lambert invited him to submit a specific proposal, 'no matter how big'. Ngata's response, costed at more than £160,000, included sanitation, water supply, the eradication of tuberculosis, and a university chair in Maori earmarked for someone like Peter Buck.[218] Nothing came of this proposal. In January 1933 Ngata informed Buck of another meeting with Lambert, who had recently initiated a soil sanitation project in Rarotonga. Five months later he reported that the Rarotongan supervisor had visited New Zealand to advise on the construction of concrete privies and related matters. Ngata intended this scheme to proceed in tandem with the current improvements in water supplies, which were part of the Native Department's land development programme.[219]

In 1934 Ngata had further talks with Lambert's superior, Dr Victor Heiser. His main concern was whether the New Zealand government would offer matching funding for any project approved by Heiser, as required under Rockefeller regulations. Once again, the discussions brought no tangible result, and later that year Ngata resigned from office amidst allegations of irregularities in the land development scheme accounts.[220]

When Lambert reported to the Labour government in 1937 he was sharply critical of the poor soil sanitation in Maori settlements and the stark contrast between European and Maori water supply and latrines. He defined the latter as the foundation of public health, however embarrassing or distasteful the subject was to health inspectors. Watt, presumably forewarned of this attack, defended his Department's inaction on soil and water sanitation, pleading a total absence of funds for this purpose.[221] Later that year he contacted the Native Department about Ngata's suggestion that a government fund be established to provide financial advances for the installation of water supplies in Maori settlements. Watt was anxious to ensure that the proposal would not place any additional burden on his budget: 'Presumably the fund suggested would be administered by the Native Department.' It was yet another example of the buck-passing which had bedevilled Maori health policy for so long.[222]

Harold Turbott, the MOH for Gisborne, had noted in 1929 that Maori were moving away from pa and occupying better housing, with tanked water supplies and individual privies.[223] A decade later he was less optimistic. His 1940 survey of health and social welfare was highly critical of the sanitation of the majority of Maori homes and settlements. Water supplies were unsafe, with over 80 per cent classified as unsatisfactory in a 1938 South Auckland Health District survey. Arrangements for the disposal of human waste were equally defective, contributing to high mortality and morbidity.[224] The implications were summed up by K.R. Taylor, whose thesis on health administration in New Zealand was one of a number of studies to emerge in the wake of the social security debate in the 1930s. Taylor's conclusion was sombre: 'It seems that, until better housing and sanitation can be arranged, and those infected can be restrained from participating in the close communal life led by the Maori, very little change can be expected in the death rate.'[225]

The main 'filth' disease to afflict Maori during this period was typhoid or enteric fever. The concealment of Maori sufferers led to questions in Parliament. In 1921 Health Minister James Parr responded to one inquiry by announcing that Valintine and Buck intended to 'comb out these villages from Waikanae north' to ascertain the extent of an outbreak which had begun in a pa near Levin.[226] Such concealment hampered strategies for both treatment and prevention. Dr Frances Preston, who worked in Hokianga in the early 1920s, later recalled that Maori hid typhoid cases

A temporary typhoid hospital at Maungapohatu, Rua Kenana's kainga in the Urewera, 1924. The Presbyterian missionary John Laughton stands at left. *ATL, F30884 1/2*

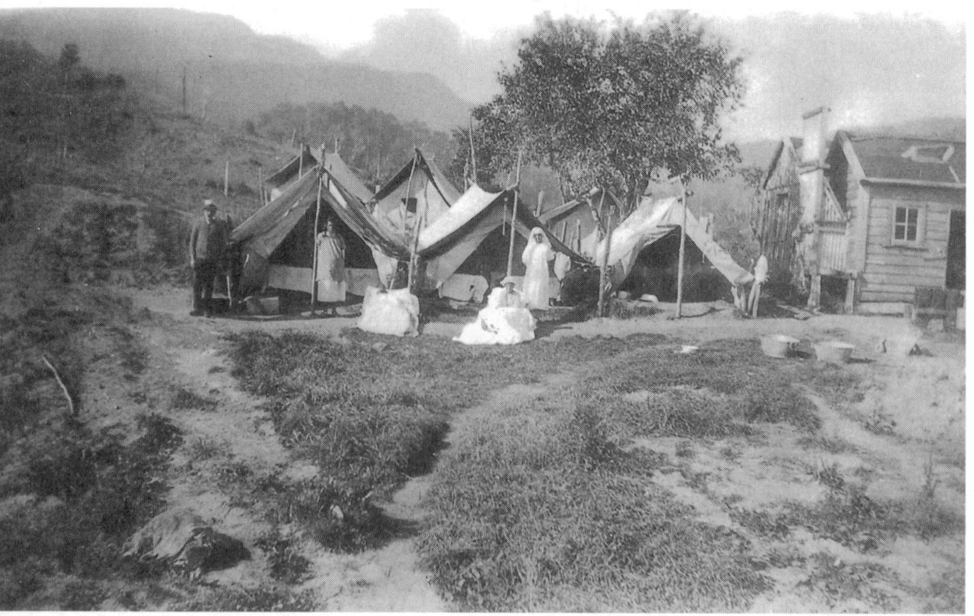

since they regarded hospitals as places in which to die and that it was the nurses' 'unenviable job to seek out these truants'.[227] Temporary typhoid camps or hospitals were set up as halfway houses to isolate cases within their own localities. In some instances the outbreak was too far from the nearest hospital to contemplate admitting those afflicted.[228] The nurses who ran these camps helped overcome Maori repugnance at hospitalisation and the resulting separation from relatives.[229]

Convincing Maori to attend hospital was only one side of the equation. The Health Department also had to ensure that hospitals were able and willing to accept Maori typhoid patients. G.M. Smith's concerns about admissions to Rawene Hospital in 1915 were echoed seven years later when Deputy Director-General Frengley warned of the need to take special measures to deal with its current swamping by enteric cases.[230] The government then agreed to reimburse hospital boards at the rate of £1 per Maori typhoid patient per week.[231] Actually claiming this sum was not always straightforward. In 1934 Watt explained to Health Minister James Young that the policy had been introduced to help districts with a large Maori population and repeated typhoid, not those 'living practically in European style'. In recent years it had been invoked only by the Wairoa and Tauranga Hospital Boards. He therefore advised Young to deny a request for assistance from the Nelson Hospital Board, where most Maori were beneficiaries under the tenths fund. Young concurred, instructing the Nelson board on its 'recognised function and duty' to provide care for infectious diseases and reminding it that costs could be recovered under Section 51 of the Destitute Persons Act 1910.[232]

Treatment was an essential part of the fight against typhoid but prevention was the Department's primary aim. Officials recognised the difficulties of implementing sanitary improvement and therefore adopted anti-typhoid inoculation as the first line of defence, a measure which Buck described in 1922 as 'our sheet anchor'.[233] He was hopeful that this would render typhoid a disease of the past, or at least minimise its impact.[234] Resistance to inoculation from Ratana followers and others continued to hamper departmental efforts for the remainder of the decade. This opposition was encouraged by some European anti-vaccinationists, who were castigated by Buck in 1922 as 'ignorant pakehas' and in 1927 as 'interfering Europeans'.[235] By 1930 this opposition was on the wane and officials were more confident that their views would prevail.[236]

The tactics used by departmental officers to implement the inoculation programme pushed up to and beyond the bounds of ethical practice. In 1922 Buck issued a confidential circular on Maori resistance to anti-typhoid inoculation in which he argued that the benefits justified bluff or persuasion. He urged caution since immunisation was not compulsory, but concluded: 'Personally, I always take it for granted that the parents of school children have consented to inoculation. This attitude is all right when you have the co-operation of the Native School Teacher. Maori parents are hardly likely to bring a charge of assault against the nurses and the School Teachers. Where however the School Teacher has doubts because some of the parents object, then it is safer to postpone operations and report.'[237] This cavalier approach was also evident in Dr Watt's 1936 circular to MOsH. Watt stressed that 'under no circumstances are European children to be inoculated unless the prior consent of the parents has been obtained'. When it came to Maori, the rights of individual parents were outweighed by direct agreement between the Department and community leaders: 'the present system of carrying out the work with the general knowledge and consent of the leading members of the particular communities is to be continued.'[238]

The routine inoculation of all Maori schoolchildren every two years which began in the late 1920s brought a rapid decline in the incidence of typhoid. The Maori death rate from typhoid was estimated to be around a hundred times that for Europeans in the mid 1920s. By 1937 it had dropped to about 40 per cent of its earlier level. Officials clearly felt that the ends justified the means.[239]

The second major infectious disease to afflict Maori in this period was tuberculosis, the threat from which was well known by 1920. Despite this awareness, both European and Maori health professionals were reluctant to acknowledge the full extent of the problem or engage in debate about how best to tackle it. Buck downplayed the threat by claiming in 1926 that 'improved conditions of living are lessening this illness materially', but produced no data to support his contention.[240] Maori health was almost entirely ignored at the 1927 Australasian Medical Congress held in Dunedin, even in the discussions relating to tuberculosis.[241] Professor Charles Hercus went so far as to claim that New Zealand's tuberculosis death rate would be the world's lowest 'but for the white population of South Africa'.[242] He seemed to find nothing incongruous in omitting New Zealand's non-white citizens from his calculation in order to reach this conclusion. The Health Department followed suit with claims that New Zealand did indeed have the world's lowest tuberculosis death rate.[243]

The 1928 Committee of Inquiry on the Prevention and Treatment of Pulmonary Tuberculosis in New Zealand also excluded Maori from its statistics for the period from 1872, because of the unreliability of the data. It did, however, note that the data for 1920–4 recorded Maori death rates of 28 per 10,000 as against 5 per 10,000 for the 'general population'.[244] Dr William Aitken, writing on the reduction in tuberculosis since 1880, also excluded Maori statistics where possible and made no other reference to this sector of the population.[245] Both accurate data collection and effective treatment were hindered by the failure to seek medical assistance, concealment through fear of being sent to a hospital or sanatorium, and deficient reporting by some doctors.[246] The number of Maori with European names also made it hard to distinguish Maori from Pakeha cases, according to the Director-General of Health.[247] By 1935 tuberculosis was acknowledged to be about ten times as prevalent among Maori as it was among Pakeha.[248] Two years later the figures had been dramatically revised upwards. Health Minister Peter Fraser admitted to a Hospital Boards' Association delegation that he had been shocked to learn that Maori were 30 times more susceptible than Europeans. He repeated this sentiment at a second meeting some months later.[249]

Local observers identified poor housing and diet as two major obstacles to improvement.[250] At least one overseas expert queried this interpretation. Sylvester Lambert of the Rockefeller Foundation was 'not agitated by the housing conditions', pointing out that New Zealand's tuberculosis rates were still lower than those in the Pacific Islands, where the inhabitants had much larger houses and unlimited food supplies.[251]

In 1937, following earlier surveys in the East Cape district by MOH Harold Turbott, the government provided portable tuberculosis shelters or hutments for Maori patients, but only after a plan to construct cottages had been opposed by Apirana Ngata on the grounds that this would be five times as expensive.[252] The scheme was extended to Waikato in 1939. Turbott extolled the virtues of this practice, which the Department intended to expand over the ensuing decade: 'The scheme seemed to work

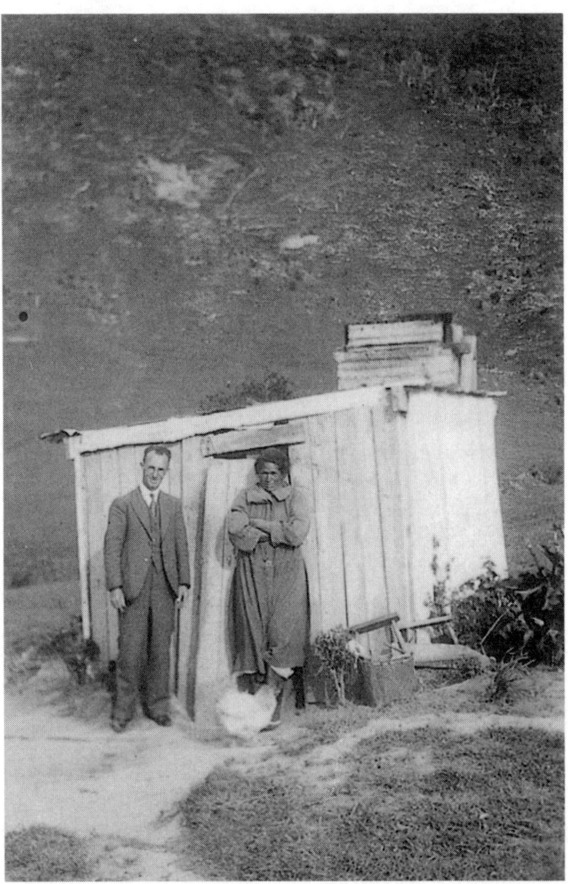

Health inspector Fogarty and 'Mihi', photographed by Miss Pickett during a tuberculosis campaign on the East Coast in the 1930s. *Enid Pickett*

successfully, it operated happily as regards the Maoris, and it was very cheap.'[253] Such approval was not universal. Ngata cast doubts upon the policy, stating that local opinion favoured centralised institutional care rather than itinerant nursing in local hutments; to this end the Waiapu Hospital Board was seeking special funds from the Health Department to construct a tuberculosis annexe. The Minister asked officials to investigate this request in the context of the difficulty encountered in collecting rates on Maori land. By 1940 the Department was considering making grants to hospital boards for this purpose.[254]

These initiatives appear to have had their origin in the report of the 1928 committee, which recommended that 'more active measures' be taken to control tuberculosis in Maori districts. The report made particular reference to the new East Cape health district, which contained almost one-third of the entire Maori population.[255] This recommendation was to pave the way for pioneering work by Dr Turbott which is described below. The development of these measures was interrupted, first by the depression of the 1930s and then by the outbreak of World War II. In 1943 Dr Norman Edson published an article in the *NZMJ* on Maori tuberculosis mortality which urged action by the government and the community to alleviate the problem.[256] The next issue contained a response from the Health Department's recently appointed Director of Tuberculosis, Dr Claude Taylor: 'Now we must concentrate on the incidence of tuberculosis in the Maori if his race is to be helped'.[257] Little could be achieved while war continued to rage, but Maori were targeted as a priority group when BCG vaccine was adopted in New Zealand in the late 1940s.

The Department's previous reluctance to introduce BCG may have reflected a growing sense of caution in dealing with Maori health issues. More than 30 years earlier the doctor responsible for the 1912 tuberculin trial had claimed that this untried treatment was justified: 'Although it is stated that tuberculin is not so effectual in pulmonary phthisis as in other forms of tuberculosis, I am strongly of opinion that the injections of tuberculin have been beneficial to the Maori race at Tuahiwi, and I feel that, if we are really sincere about preserving the Maori race, this injection of tuberculin will be found to be one of the factors at our disposal.'[258] The same rationale was not applied to BCG. Dr George Blackmore, who had initiated the tuberculin scheme in 1912, made reference at the 1927 Australasian Medical Congress to the importation of BCG vaccine to New Zealand for experimental purposes.[259] Developed in France in the early 1920s as a preventative for tuberculosis, BCG was systematically administered to high-risk groups in Scandinavia from 1927 onwards. It was not adopted in Britain until 1949 and never gained credibility in America.[260] New Zealand's health officials took the same cautious approach as their British counterparts. Director-General Watt outlined their philosophy in a letter to the Otaki Sanatorium's Medical Superintendent in 1936: 'The use of B.C.G. on Maori infants has been considered at various times in the past, but we all feel somewhat fearful about using it in this country.' Watt explained that the MOsH who had most to do with Maori believed that the risks were so great as to 'put it out of court for the time being'.[261] Attempts in 1938–9 by Apirana Ngata, whose own daughter had tuberculosis, to convince the Department and Health Minister Fraser of the merits of BCG proved equally fruitless, and another decade passed before its introduction.[262]

'A model for all'?: child health

In 1936 Victor Heiser, head of the Rockefeller Foundation's operations in the South Pacific, lauded New Zealand's unrivalled low infant death rate, claiming: 'Its system of child hygiene has been regarded as a model for all to follow.'[263] Heiser's comment was based upon repeated statements during the previous decade and a half by New Zealand health officials and others.[264] The tone was set year after year in the Health Department's annual report. In 1927 this boasted that newborn New Zealanders had an expectation of life greater than any other country's. Two years later infant mortality allegedly constituted a 'low record for New Zealand and also for the world'.[265] All of these claims omitted to mention that Maori were excluded from the statistics. For them, the position was very different.

Pakeha infant mortality (deaths in the first year of life) had fluctuated between 62 and 89 per 1,000 live births in the first decade of the twentieth century. After 1914 the rate did not exceed 52 per 1,000 and from 1921 onwards it never topped 50. In 1925 the rate dropped below 40 per 1,000, and it subsequently remained at or below this level. The contrast with Maori is striking.[266] No data are available for the first quarter of the twentieth century, but the estimates of government officials made grim reading. Pomare claimed in 1903 that more than half of all Maori died before reaching four years of age; 'one is not surprised to find this state of affairs when inquiry is made into the infant life of the Maoris'.[267] Five years later he was still lamenting the 'terrible' but unspecified level of infant mortality.[268] It was not until 1925 that the Health Department was in a position to enumerate Maori infant mortality. In 1931 Ellison published two graphs comparing Maori and Pakeha rates from 1925 to 1929 but did not supply precise figures.[269] Such data were available but appeared in different sections of the Health Department's annual report. The comparisons are sobering.

In 1925 the recorded Maori infant mortality rate was 107 per 1,000, almost three times that for Pakeha. In 1927 it shot up to 157.8 before plummeting to 78.5 in 1929. By the early 1930s it had climbed back to the mid 90s. A slight drop in 1933 allowed the Director-General to express the hope that the recent publication in English and Maori of a pamphlet on maternal and infant welfare would herald a further reduction 'and so in time bring this high figure more in line with the rate for Europeans'.[270] His hope was not realised. The Maori rate remained above 100 per 1,000 for most of the 1930s, with marked variations from year to year that were in sharp contrast to its stable or declining European equivalent. There was no sustained reduction until after World War II, and even then the Maori figures remained at least three times as high as those for Pakeha.[271] This section examines some of the reasons for this difference in infant mortality and the steps taken to counteract it.

Parental incompetence or neglect had been blamed for high Maori infant mortality almost from the beginning of European contact. Dr Arthur Thomson commented in 1859, in relation to the declining population: 'It is among infants that inattention to the sick, the first of these causes of decay, is most injurious.'[272] A later statement by Edward Williams, the Resident Magistrate at Waimate North, typified a common attitude amongst government officials in the second half of the nineteenth century: 'It is difficult to account for the rarity of large families amongst the Natives. The mortality amongst the children is more easily accounted for, and may be traced to the utter disregard manifested by the parents towards the health of their offspring.'[273]

James Pope's *Health for the Maori*, with its emphasis on sanitary improvement, the inculcation of a Protestant work ethic and the dangers of tohunga, made little attempt to engage with the problem of infant mortality. It was not until Maui Pomare joined the new Health Department in 1901 that any real effort was made to promote infant welfare. Pomare repeatedly stressed the need to educate mothers by sending out 'hygienic lady missionaries' who would target infant feeding as the key to change. Pomare recognised that most Maori infants were breastfed and correctly pinpointed inappropriate diet after weaning as a major contributor to high mortality rates.[274] His infant care manual, which first appeared in 1909, tackled this problem. Seven years later it was reissued in a greatly expanded form, with additional comments by district nurses.[275] Pomare's colleague, Peter Buck, also took a keen interest in this topic. He was particularly concerned at the abandoning of breastfeeding, in imitation of European trends: 'The introduction of the feeding-bottle into the Maori home has caused as many deaths as the guns of Hongi'. In order to combat this trend Buck wanted infant feeding and training to become an integral part of the training of nurses at the state-owned St Helens maternity hospitals.[276] Buck revisited the crucial topic of infant feeding in the section of his MD thesis which dealt with the present condition of the Maori race.

The endeavours of these two Maori doctors were supported by some parliamentarians, most notably Otaki's William Field. Responsibility for conveying Pomare's message was placed firmly on the shoulders of the district nurses.[277] The need for better education was also endorsed by the 1911 Hospitals' Conference, which resolved: 'That, in order to conserve the Maori race, the question of maternity and infant mortality be dealt with directly by the responsible officers of the Hospital and Charitable Aid Boards.' This suggestion was reinforced by Valintine's statement to the delegates.[278]

Those charged with implementing child health policies during the inter-war years faced an uphill struggle. There were never enough district nurses to provide adequate coverage. This shortage allowed many who could have benefited from their services to fall through the cracks. In 1927 Whangaroa's Native School teacher reported that Maori babies in his area frequently died through lack of care or knowledge. The 900-strong local Maori population therefore wished to obtain a district nurse who would, he promised, be supported wholeheartedly by both parents and the three Native School teachers in the vicinity.[279]

On 30 July 1931 the *New Zealand Herald* reported on the trial of an Ahipara mother who had been charged with failing to provide food and medical attention for her deceased seven month old child. The judge, who imposed a lenient sentence after a recommendation to mercy, stated that Maori were not receiving the medical attention to which they were entitled. His hope that the prosecution might 'bring home to the minds of native mothers the duty of procuring Government medical assistance for their children' in the person of the district nurse failed to recognise the limitations of the system.

In 1932 the Department's twenty district nurses undertook 23,790 home visits, paid 2,479 visits to kainga and attended Native Schools on 849

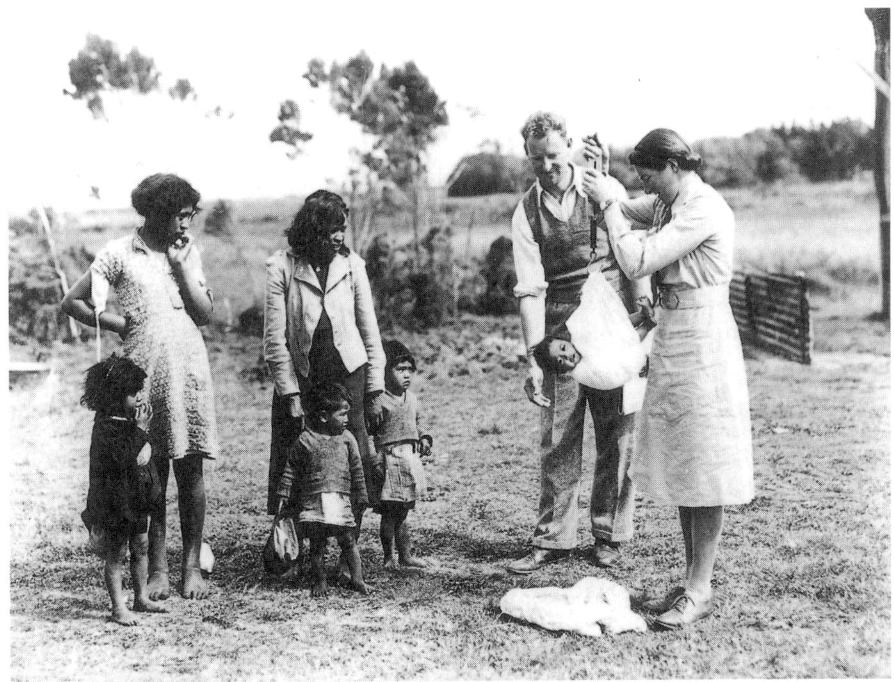

A district nurse at work in Northland during the 1930s. *ATL, F133316*

occasions. The 1931/2 annual report confirmed that maternity and infant welfare among Maori constituted 'a large part of their work'.[280] The Department also anticipated that the Maori Councils would provide advice on such matters as infant and maternal mortality.[281] In December 1932 Wellington's MOH, F.S. Maclean, suggested that district nurses should have a workload of 1,000–1,500 patients rather than the 2,500 or more in his own district in order to combat the ongoing problem of malnutrition, which most commonly coincided with weaning.[282]

In 1937 Sylvester Lambert described the Native Schools as 'most valuable adjuncts to the Medical Department'.[283] This was borne out by the results of a questionnaire completed by the heads of 135 Native Schools in 1934. The Director of Education forwarded these to the Health Department with the comment: 'Forty-five (45) headteachers state that the cases of sickness treated by them are too numerous to mention. The average number of cases treated by the remaining headteachers is fifty-eight (58).' A further 874 pupils had been visited by the head teachers in their own homes.[284] For many teachers the expectations of their pupils were daunting. 'Hamilton

Grieve', a Cantabrian who took up a North Auckland teaching post in the early 1930s, later recorded her panic on first sighting the school medicine chest and its staple ingredients of Epsom salts and castor oil.[285]

Lambert also claimed in 1937 that the development of preventive medicine had turned the Native Schools into centres for maternal, infant and child welfare.[286] This edifice, however, rested on shaky foundations. 'Hamilton Grieve', for instance, described how she was expected to act as a baby welfare expert despite knowing next to nothing about babies—though she did claim to be better informed than Maori mothers.[287] Greater experience was no guarantee of influence. Marjorie Childe, head teacher at Ohautira Native School near Raglan, informed the Director of School Hygiene in 1932 that the treatment of babies in her locality was 'absolutely inhuman', with three deaths from neglect in the previous month. Although Childe had two children of her own and had spent a month at a Plunket Society Karitane hospital for babies to gain experience, the local children were no longer entrusted to her. She attributed this to the influence of tohunga. The local Maori Welfare Officer advised the Under-Secretary of the Native Department that prosecution under the Tohunga Suppression Act would lead only to a blank wall because of the intertwined nature of Maori life and tohungaism, an opinion that was supported by the MOH.[288]

The second agency enlisted by the Health Department to help overcome its own shortcomings was the Plunket Society, founded by Dr Frederic Truby King in 1907 to promote the health of New Zealand's women and children. As early as 1906 Buck had recommended that the Department instigate a scheme for Maori along the lines of Truby King's fledgling venture.[289] The potential need for a separate but parallel development was demonstrated in 1908, when an editorial in the *NZMJ* supported Plunket Society work on the basis that it was essential to the 'permanence of what we believe to be the finest race that the world has ever produced—we mean the Anglo-Saxon race'.[290] The continued existence of such attitudes in the 1920s and 1930s found expression in the reluctance of some local Plunket committees to include Maori within the society's operations.[291]

Despite such deterrents the Department announced in 1930 that many Maori mothers were now accepting advice from Plunket nurses and that adaptations of Truby King's writings were to be translated into Maori.[292]

These claims were repeated in Ellison's 1931 summary of Maori health.[293] Two years later the Department's annual report promised 'special educational endeavours', including the production of pamphlets on feeding and clothing, to close the gap between Maori and European infant mortality.[294] The wish became reality shortly after the Conference on Native Education held in May 1934, when the Department produced an infant welfare curriculum for circulation among Native School teachers. Based on Mary King's *Mothercraft*, with a translation into Maori, the teacher's textbook had been introduced to most Maori schools by 1939.[295]

Doubts were expressed at the time about the effectiveness of Plunket. F.S. Maclean stated in 1932 that Maori mothers either did not consult Plunket nurses at all, or else did so too late to receive timely advice. He believed the community would be best served by ensuring that district nurses received both Plunket and midwifery training.[296] In 1937, to help close some of the gaps in Health Department coverage, it was agreed to permit Plunket nurses to employ a doctor at departmental expense in an emergency, or where the child of an indigent Maori family was ill.[297]

Some participants in Maori infant welfare work remained sceptical about the effectiveness of Plunket personnel. 'Hamilton Grieve' blamed the Maori rejection of breastfeeding, a mainstay of Plunket philosophy, on the

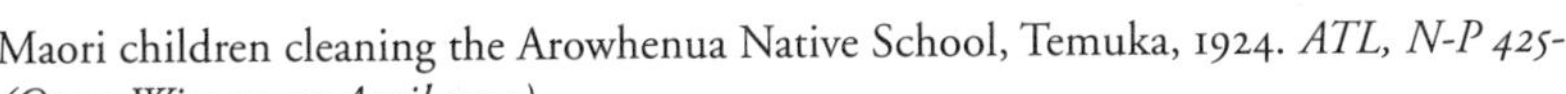
Maori children cleaning the Arowhenua Native School, Temuka, 1924. *ATL, N-P 425-(Otago Witness, 22 April 1924)*

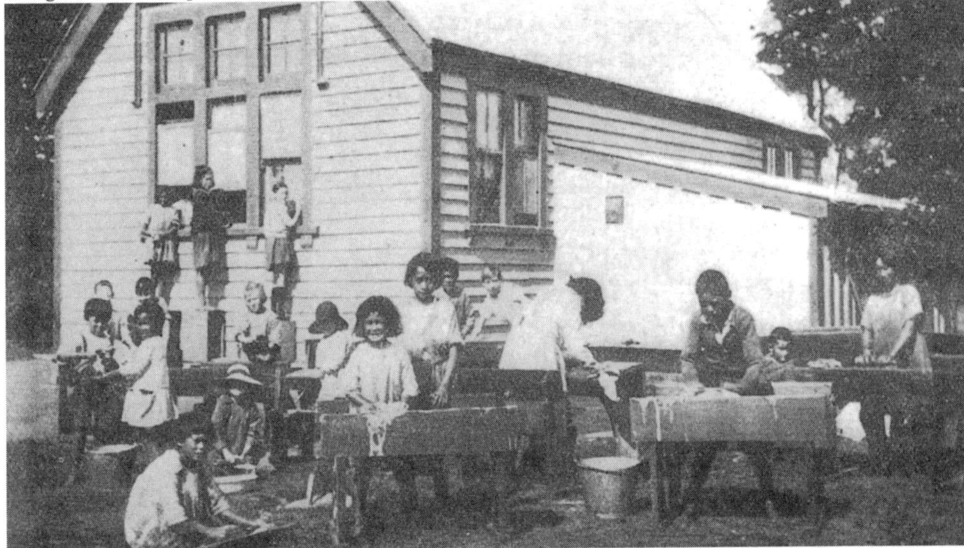

tendency for the entire community to involve itself in child rearing; she also claimed that any Plunket nurse sent to her particular settlement 'would be reduced to the gibbers in a week'. Grieve nevertheless attended local women's institute meetings both to exhibit her own baby and to espouse Plunket principles.[298]

These Maori women's institutes formed the third agency recruited by the Health Department to help meet its commitment to Maori infant and child health. The concept of networks of rural women had been initiated in Canada and taken up in England and Scotland. It was embraced during World War I by Besse Spencer, a New Zealand schoolteacher whose father was a Napier doctor. She established the first New Zealand institute in 1921 and by 1936 there were almost 900 branches around the country. The organisation's official history records that the focus on home-making, co-operation and citizenship as key elements of family life evoked a ready response from Maori women who 'thought highly of these values'. During the first decade they were encouraged by teachers and district nurses to join existing branches. The first Maori Women's Institute (Te Awapuni) was founded in May 1929 at Kohupatiki, near Hastings.[299] The movement was fostered in the early 1930s by Mrs Johnstone, a Native School teacher; the institutes were welcomed by Ivan Sutherland as a 'most promising movement'.[300] By 1937 district nurses were supervising about 40 branches in North Auckland alone, and Sylvester Lambert was inspired to predict that they would inculcate the 'new domestic culture so necessary for better health'.[301] Within a short time, however, relations had become strained as the organisation's Dominion organiser, Miss Kelso, clashed with certain MOsH over the future direction of the institutes.[302]

Harold Turbott, one of those involved in this dispute, claimed in 1940 that the women's institutes had failed to capture the Maori imagination. He predicted a brighter future for the 'Maori Health League', formed on tribal lines by Te Arawa women of the Rotorua district.[303] The Women's Health League had been founded in 1937 by Robina Cameron, a Health Department district nurse who had been based in Rotorua since 1931. Its patroness was Mrs Tai Mitchell, wife of the chairman of Te Arawa District Trust Board, who himself had been actively involved in health issues for many years.[304] Departmental officers appear to have regarded the League more favourably than they did the institutes.[305] Despite this, the institutes survived into the early 1950s; there were still about 42 branches in 1950, but many members then transferred their allegiance to the new Maori Women's Welfare League.[306]

After 1920 the monitoring of children's health beyond the pre-school years was the responsibility of the Health Department's School Medical Service. The mainstay of this work was the routine medical inspection of all schoolchildren, initiated in 1912.[307] In fact the inspection of Native Schools, which catered for about half of all Maori pupils between 1890 and 1940, had begun some time earlier as a joint venture between NMOs and teachers. In 1908 Buck called for this to be put on a more formal footing, with annual examinations and accurate record keeping.[308] Twelve months later his superior, Maui Pomare, admitted the impossibility of achieving systematic inspection: 'Our staff at present is too small to carry this useful work on in a regular manner.'[309]

Any hopes that the expansion of the School Medical Service after 1920 would benefit Maori were soon dashed. Valintine was also forced to concede in his annual report that the Health Department's 'irreducible minimum' was not achievable in the case of Maori schools.[310] (This standard was based on that set by George Newman, successively Chief Medical Officer of England's Board of Education from 1907 to 1919 and of the Ministry of Health from 1919 to 1935.) Valintine explained the position to his counterpart in the Education Department: 'While recognising the desirability of ultimately extending the full benefits of both the school Medical and Dental Services to Native Schools I regret that with the present staff available it is not practicable to do so.' Currently, he added, the school medical officers were unable to cover all the small country schools, whether they were Native or European.[311] Ada Paterson, the Health Department's Director of School Hygiene from 1924 to 1937, believed that school inspection should treat Maori and Europeans equally, but in 1925 she too had to acknowledge the impossibility of attaining this with the limited number of school medical officers. Once again, the district nurses were held up as a temporary solution, though Buck warned that the sheer size of some nurses' districts would create problems. Further discussions at ministerial level exhibited the same resignation.[312]

There was little discernible improvement during the remainder of the decade. The Health Department continued to admit its inability to provide a full inspection service for the 6,979 pupils who attended the 137 Native Schools in 1929, though staff were delegated to visit and offer advice on 'special problems'; this was generally restricted to the containment of infectious diseases.[313] The expansion in the 1930s of the MOH network, following the dismantling of the Division of Maori Hygiene, led to a significant increase in Native School inspections, particularly in the densely populated North Auckland and East Cape regions. Coverage was further improved when a number of district nurses assumed the dual role as school nurses which had been anticipated by Valintine in 1911.[314] Yet it was not until 1940 that Native Schools adopted the same routine for school inspection as their European equivalents.[315]

In the early 1930s the recently appointed Inspector of Native Schools, D.G. Ball, noted that district nurses had to a large extent relieved teachers of their quasi-medical duties.[316] In 1934 the Director of Education expressed a fear that Native School teachers would be tempted to leave everything to the district nurses if the latter attended each week to provide health instruction.[317] The issue was thrashed out at a meeting between representatives of the Native, Health and Education Departments, when it was agreed that district nurses should visit schools periodically but should not undertake classroom instruction. This was confirmed in an Education Department memorandum for head teachers which set out a health instruction curriculum intended to 'influence more directly the health and living conditions of the Maoris'. Ball (as successor to James Pope) and the Director of School Hygiene also undertook to co-operate in compiling a book on hygiene for distribution through the classrooms.[318]

This was an important concord, since the Native Schools had the potential to make a significant contribution to the monitoring of child health. F.S. Maclean, the MOH for Wellington, had reminded his departmental head in 1932 that Maori did not parade their ill-health, which meant that only Native School teachers and Health Department officials were aware of the 'dreadful' Maori vital statistics. In 1936, not long before her retirement as Director of School Hygiene, Ada Paterson emphasised the importance of co-operation between the Departments of Health and Education in the face of continuing limited access to professional medical facilities.[319] One tangible result was the appointment for six months of Emere Kaa, a public health nurse, to fill some of the gaps in the School

Medical Service coverage in Northland. Although the experiment was apparently a success it appears not to have been repeated.[320]

The fact that Kaa was appointed to work under the Education Department underlines the disparity in the funding of Maori health and education. Lambert calculated in 1937 that the Maori schools had an annual budget of £100,000 compared with the Health Department's total Maori health allocation of around £16,600.[321] The reaffirmation of the schools' health role in the 1930s did not impress all teachers. One commented wryly in 1939 that while health was theoretically a concern of the Health Department, 'whose offices are established in some more or less inaccessible centre', the burden had to be directly shouldered by schoolteachers as 'a somewhat irksome branch of the manifold extraneous duties relegated to them'.[322]

Since the time of James Pope the Native Schools credo had been that any improvement in the Maori race would be 'most readily obtained by the education and training of its children'.[323] Some historians now look back on this policy as a prescriptive ideology; this interpretation is comparable to the criticism of Truby King which has marked much of the academic interest in the activities of the Plunket Society.[324] In both instances the policies were intended to elevate health standards. The extent to which they were politically or racially motivated is open to debate. Policy makers and those charged with implementing health standards and goals in the Maori schools may have displayed 'unwitting arrogance and over-simplified ideas of assimilation'.[325] For the majority of Native School teachers, however, the goal appears to have been a very simple one, that of maintaining or improving the physical well-being of their communities.[326]

The School Dental Service was established in 1921; here, too, services for Maori lagged behind those provided for Europeans. In 1928 parliamentarians criticised the Department's failure to meet Maori dental needs. Health Minister James Young, a dentist by profession, praised the work of the existing clinics and claimed that the government was 'sympathetic to Maori children in every way, and was quite prepared to give them the best possible service'.[327] The first Maori dental graduate, funded through the Maori Purposes Board, completed his studies in May 1928 and was promptly sent to Tikitiki, 'a thickly-populated Maori district' on the East Coast. A second graduate took up the challenge near Whakatane in 1930.[328] These were the exceptions. Few Native Schools were located in areas accessible to the growing network of dental clinics in the mid 1930s. Many Maori communities could not in any case afford to meet the basic requirements for the provision of a local clinic. In 1940 these included the cost of accommodation, non-technical equipment, cleaning, lighting, and a contribution of £30 towards the dental officer's salary.[329] But in that year Harold Turbott stated: 'The School Dental Service is being extended to Maori children, and progress is being achieved.'[330] The tide, it seems, was on the turn.

The story of Maori child health in the inter-war years is essentially one of limited resources and, arguably, missed opportunities. While there was considerable frustration at the inability to reduce the disparities between Maori and European health standards, many officials and observers were slow to acknowledge their existence. By the end of the period there was a greater degree of frankness about these shortcomings. Turbott admitted in

School dental nurse Urquhart and some of her Te Araroa patients, early 1940s. *ATL, F106538 1/2*

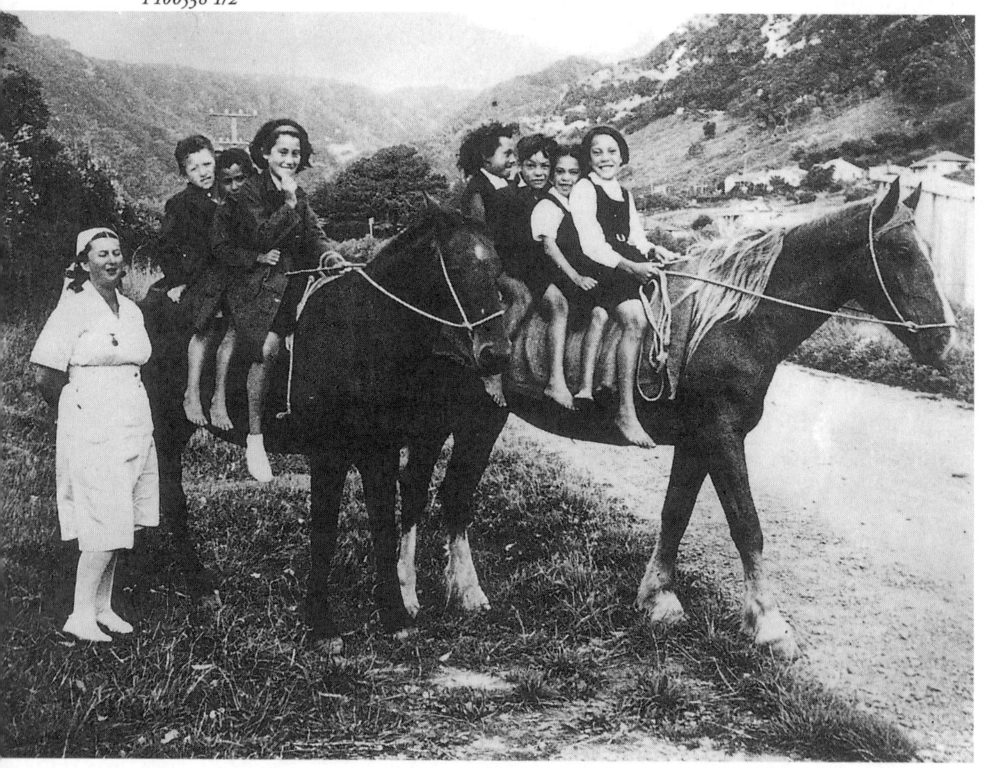

1940: 'During 1938 more than four Maori babies died for every *pakeha* one, surely a disgrace to the country renowned for the lowest European mortality rate and the Plunket system of infant care.'

At the same time Turbott felt it necessary to attribute much of the responsibility to Maori themselves: 'There is defective Maori leadership here, the *tohunga* is often behind the scenes, and the blame mainly rests on the shoulders of the Maori for allowing their babies to die at a heavier rate than the *pakeha*.'[331] Some modern commentators have shifted accountability to the other end of the spectrum,[332] but neither view fairly reflects the complexity of the issues involved.

'More definite information': health research

The inter-war period saw the first systematic attempts to quantify Maori health conditions, and the introduction of formal research projects to define problems and explore solutions. The collection of data on Maori health had long been inadequate. Late nineteenth century scholars had concentrated on physical anthropology,[333] which was also Peter Buck's main area of interest.[334] Dr Thomas Bell had claimed in 1890, without supplying any evidence, that 'many investigations and inquiries' were currently being conducted into Maori health.[335] None, it would seem, had any tangible output in the form of publications or reports. The Maori Councils Act was intended to alter this pattern. Councils were not only to 'collect and tabulate facts and statistics' relating to mortality and health, but were also expected to provide some assessment of 'the progress that may be made towards the adoption of healthier habits and pursuits'.[336] Little was achieved in this regard. Most of the information available to Pomare and Buck before 1910 came from the Native Medical Officers. The analyses based on these data, which related only to parts of the North Island, were hailed by Buck as the start of 'the statistical study of the ailments which afflict the Maori'.[337] The failure to impose strict registration of Maori births and deaths hindered this process; limited registration began in 1913 but as late as 1930 only 60 per cent of Maori deaths were registered.[338]

There were two specific Maori health research initiatives of limited scope just before World War I. One was the Health Department's tuberculin trial at Tuahiwi Park in 1910. The other was an investigation of immunity to dental disease among Urewera Maori. This was undertaken in 1913 by

Drs Henry Pickerill and Sydney Champtaloup of the Otago University Schools of Medicine and Dentistry and was partly funded by the London-based Royal Society of Medicine.[339]

The Health Act of 1920 imposed a new obligation on the Health Department 'to promote or carry out researches and investigations in relation to matters concerning the public health, and the prevention or treatment of disease'. Much of this research was conducted at the Otago Medical School, which received a pound for pound subsidy for the purpose.[340] Very little of this early work targeted Maori. In 1923 the *New Zealand Journal of Science and Technology* published a survey of scientific research in New Zealand. Only one of the fourteen Otago Medical School projects, an investigation of Polynesian blood types, had any obvious relevance to Maori health. The Health Department's only contributions were those attributed to Buck and the Division of Maori Hygiene. These included his Maori somatology and a joint project with Maori Councils and village committees to determine the percentage of full-blooded Maori. The other three were studies of basketry, clothing and fishing nets.[341]

A second survey in 1925 showed little change. Buck's agenda was unchanged, although the departmental entry now listed venereal disease studies (currently being transferred to the hospital boards) and Professor Charles Hercus's study of goitre.[342] Much of this latter research was carried out by the school medical officers, some of whom specifically noted the differences between Europeans and Maori. The Health Department's annual report for 1924 estimated that the incidence of goitre among Maori was only half that found in Europeans. Four years later, the report was less precise: 'Goitre is found among Maoris, but in what extent is not yet defined.'[343]

The author of the first of these reports was Ralph Mecredy, one of the Department's school medical officers. According to the 1924 annual report, Mecredy also verified Pickerill and Champtaloup's 1913 findings that Maori enjoyed superior dental status thanks to their diet.[344] Buck subsequently questioned both Pickerill's basic approach and his conclusion about Maori dental health. He stated that Mecredy's results demonstrated that for most Maori schoolchildren 'the percentage of dental caries is little less than amongst New Zealand children of European stock. It is significant, however, that in Native schools in back areas the percentage is less.' Buck linked this finding to the abandonment by Maori of their pre-European diet.[345] His claim was confirmed in the Department's annual report for 1925, which noted the favourable comparison between the Urewera Maori and the general population but warned that Maori living in cities under the same conditions as Europeans tended to lose their dental superiority.[346] Without Buck's intervention it is possible that the conclusions of Pickerill, Champtaloup and Mecredy might have been used selectively to allocate priorities for the overstretched School Dental Service.

Maori health research, or the lack of it, has to be seen in the context of medical research funding as a whole. From the mid 1920s Peter Fraser, then in opposition, repeatedly urged the government to increase research funding and ensure that money provided in the estimates was fully utilised. The sums involved were not large. In 1925, for example, only £2,800 was allocated in the Health Department estimates; Fraser advocated £20,000. In July 1926 he noted that while the allocation had been raised to £5,000, only £1,982 had actually been spent. None of these discussions made any specific mention of Maori, even in 1925 when Maui Pomare was Minister of Health.[347]

In 1931 Apirana Ngata cast doubts upon the commitment to research of both politicians and officials: 'My experience the last two months as Chairman of the Economy Committee has convinced me that the average Cabinet Minister and Permanent Head are impatient of things labelled scientifically which they label "stunts". Thus scientific research items and Forestry and even Health votes suffer in their mental regard.'[348] His pessimism was perhaps misplaced. In 1928 Turbott had begun a comparative study of Maori and European health, a 'quiet investigation' prompted by 'various persistent and seemingly wild statements as to dangerous health conditions among Maoris'.[349] This initiative gained momentum in the early 1930s, with the annual report of 1931 containing details of two special investigations on Maori health carried out under the aegis of the School Medical Service.[350] These studies on the nutritional value of milk and Maori susceptibility to certain infectious diseases were hailed by the editor of the *NZMJ* as 'medical research work of special interest and importance'.[351]

The predominant focus of Maori health research in the 1930s was on tuberculosis control and treatment. In 1926 the Health Department reported that Maori tuberculosis was being investigated at the Otago Medical School and that Robert Makgill, then based in the Department's head office, was to discuss a possible co-ordination of research with the British Medical Research Council and Ministry of Health.[352] Nothing came of this proposal, at least in the short term.

Two years later the Committee of Inquiry on the Prevention and Treatment of Pulmonary Tuberculosis in New Zealand criticised the lack of commitment to Maori health and recommended that 'more definite information be obtained in regard to the extent of tuberculosis amongst Maoris, and that more active measures be taken for the control of the disease in Maori districts'.[353] Once again the health authorities were slow to act. Ellison conceded in 1929 that 'a good deal of the disease exists' but claimed the position was less serious than formerly. Not long afterwards, however, he expressed concern at the ravages of tuberculosis, describing it as a 'subject calling for the closest investigation with a view to reducing the incidence and staying its propagation.'[354]

Tutere Wi Repa responded to this challenge by drawing up 'Suggestions for the Study of Tuberculosis Amongst the Maoris'. Wi Repa criticised the existing Pakeha model, claiming the Health Department was incapable of providing suitable services for Maori. He believed the solution lay with the Native Department, whose Minister, Apirana Ngata, was already acquainted with the Maori side of the problem. As a further inducement, Wi Repa stated that his research agenda might help revitalise the Maori Councils.[355] Ngata was apparently persuaded by these arguments. Without consulting the Health Department, he provided Wi Repa with a Maori Purposes Board research grant to conduct a tuberculosis survey, restricted by Ngata in the first instance to Matakaoa and East Opotiki. The intention was to combine clinical data, enquiries into economic and social conditions, and information about whakapapa. Informing Buck of this development in January 1931, Ngata explained: 'I have tried to interest the Health Department but it takes too long to argue things out with them, and in the end I know they will look to the Native Department for the money.'[356]

Departmental officials, most notably Gisborne's MOH, Harold Turbott, were incensed by the Native Minister's actions.[357] Turbott's 'preliminary study' of Maori and Pakeha comparative health, undertaken in 1928–9, was appreciated by the public health nurses most involved in Maori health,

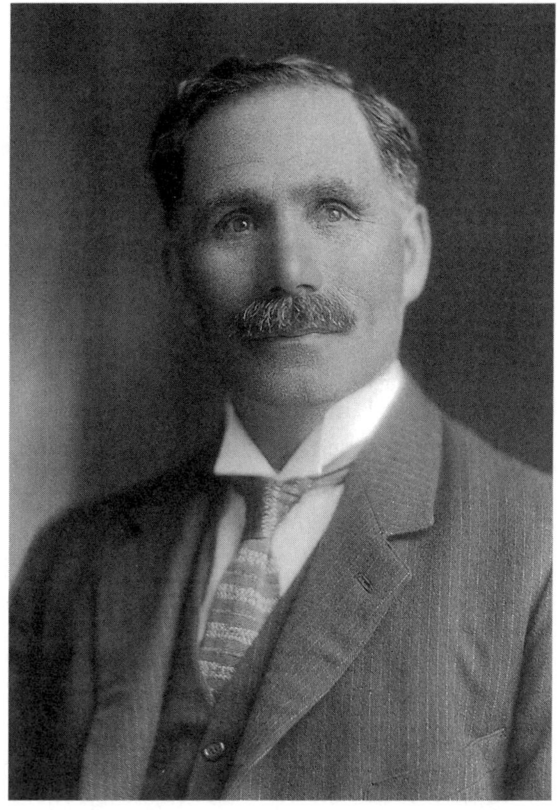

Tutere Wi Repa (1877–1945) graduated MB ChB NZ in 1908. His *NZMJ* obituarist noted: 'He was a Maori of the Maoris. He loved his race and was proud of it.' *ATL, 43315 1/2*

if not by Ngata.[358] By the early 1930s Turbott had begun to quantify the disparity between Maori and European tuberculosis rates. His growing expertise was recognised in 1933 when the British Medical Research Council awarded him a Dorothy Temple Cross Fellowship to further his studies. This was probably a belated response to Makgill's overture in 1926. Like Wi Repa's earlier project, Turbott's work was only partly clinical in focus and looked also at the influence of housing and nutrition. The departmental report of 1934 hailed his report as a potential forerunner to further collaboration on 'medical matters of common interest to Great Britain and New Zealand'.[359]

The interest of the British Medical Research Council seems to have been in the pathology of the disease rather than Turbott's targeting of its impact on New Zealand's indigenous population.[360] New Zealand officials and politicians, on the other hand, valued the project primarily as a contribution to improved understanding of Maori health status. Both David

McMillan MHR, a former GP and the originator of Labour's health policy, and Health Minister Fraser paid tribute in August 1936 to Turbott's achievement.[361] One of the six goals identified by McMillan in his pamphlet, *A National Health Service for New Zealand* (1935), was 'adequate provision for research in all matters relating to health'.[362] Fraser set aside £300 in the Department's supplementary estimates to facilitate Turbott's work on Maori tuberculosis in Waiapu.[363] Health Department officers were equally impressed by Turbott's work. The Director of Public Hygiene, Thomas McKibbin, commented in 1934 that Turbott's special methods and good results had been both interesting and enlightening.[364]

Turbott himself complained in 1936 of lost opportunities as a result of Wi Repa's tuberculosis research.[365] Despite this alleged hindrance most observers recognised the value of Turbott's contribution. In December 1937 the *NZMJ* congratulated both Turbott and the Department for their work on Maori hygiene,[366] and on 25 January 1938 the *Gisborne Times* printed an editorial on tuberculosis among Maori. This described the newly created Medical Research Council of New Zealand as a valuable link in the national health scheme, and one which was 'more than ornamental' since its initial meeting had drawn attention to the 'scourge' inflicted by the disease upon Maori. Turbott was identified as one of the leading players in the battle against tuberculosis. Over the next decade his research was commended by New Zealand health professionals as the only scientific study of its kind, and one on a scale of its own.[367] It also served in many respects as a model for the health surveys of Maori communities that were carried out by Professor Hercus's Otago students in the 1930s.[368]

Wi Repa's criticism in 1930 of the inappropriate nature of Pakeha research into Maori health has been echoed in recent years.[369] However, it is difficult to see how the glaring discrepancies between Maori and European health could have been brought to public attention in the 1930s other than through the endeavours of Turbott and, on a more modest level, the Otago medical students. Dr Golan Maaka was commissioned by the Health Department in the early 1940s to conduct blood surveys among full-blooded Maori for research purposes, but no fully trained Maori health researchers were to emerge until the late 1970s.[370]

The outbreak of war in 1939 hampered the development both of this research output and of Maori health initiatives in general. Despite this,

Harold Turbott, acknowledged as the Health Department expert on Maori health, remained optimistic. He concluded his 1940 contribution to Sutherland's general survey of the Maori people on an upbeat, albeit paternalistic note: 'there has been progress during this last decade, uphill though the preventive struggle has been. . . . all of which should lead towards the goal of hardy, healthy, self-supporting, brown-skinned New Zealanders'.[371] Fulfilment of this goal has remained elusive.

Bibliographical Essay

Problems relating to Maori health have exercised politicians and government officials since the first years of European administration in New Zealand, yet until recent years the history of health care for Maori was a largely neglected topic.[1] This applied equally to both Maori and Pakeha interpretations. Concern about this lack of interest was expressed quite early during the European settlement of New Zealand. In 1863 John Batty Tuke, an Edinburgh medical graduate who had practised in Wanganui for the previous three years, published 'Medical Notes on New Zealand' in the *Edinburgh Medical Journal*. His opening paragraph lamented the cursory level of interest in the decline of the Maori shown by almost all contemporary writers, a state of affairs rendered more urgent by his conviction that the evidence pointed to the 'gradual extermination' of the Maori.[2]

Although Peter Buck's MD thesis (1910) contained sections on ancient Maori medicine, the impact of Western civilisation, and the current health status of the race, his avowed intention was to make a 'small contribution to ethnology' rather than to history per se.[3] It was not until 1932 that Apirana Ngata, then Minister of Native Affairs, revealed his desire to write the story of Maori health reform. Encouraged by Buck's assessment of his paper on Maori land development as a 'masterly exposition', Ngata announced his intention to 'tackle it from the simple basis of old Pope's

"Health for the Maori"'. Nothing came of this proposal.[4]

Three years after this initial spark, the ethnologist Ivan Sutherland, then a university lecturer in Wellington, urged that a Maori historian come forward to tell the truth about the damage done to Maori health since the arrival of Europeans. It was, he warned, a distressing tale and one about which no European could 'fully find out the details'. As with Ngata's earlier proposal, this challenge produced no tangible result.[5]

It was not until the late 1950s that historians began to consider what was dubbed the 'fatal impact' of introduced Western diseases upon Maori. The term was popularised in the mid 1960s by Alan Moorehead.[6] His work followed earlier comments by Harrison Wright, who acknowledged that Maori lacked immunity to imported infection but placed much of the responsibility on Maori themselves, targeting their alleged lack of attention to sanitation and 'absurd methods of cure'.[7]

The debate about the influence of disease and depopulation has been revisited most recently by James Belich, who rejected the 'fatal impact' thesis.[8] Other recent writers have been less sanguine in their assessments. Mason Durie asserted in 1994 that early acceptance by Maori of the new Pakeha order gave way to 'resignation and despair … [as] wave after wave of new diseases swept through the country'.[9] Earlier he had attributed the turnaround in Maori fortunes to 'a relatively small group of youthful Maori leaders who launched a revival movement that in 50 years turned the "dying race" into a highly virile one'.[10] Durie therefore described his 1994 publication as 'a tribute to early Maori leaders and their total rejection of the concept of the dying race'.[11]

As Ivan Sutherland had feared, the tone of Pakeha historical comment on Maori health tended to be uncritical and self-congratulatory; it also focused almost entirely on the twentieth century. The pattern was set as early as 1938 in an MA thesis on public health in New Zealand prior to 1920. Intended as a tribute to the 1900 establishment of the Health Department, D.F.B. Eyres' work relied almost entirely on the Department's own published annual reports. Maori health care was summarised in the following terse statement: 'Here was a piece of work to be done; the officers of the Department did it. It was their duty; they expected no praise and were not disappointed. Yet the work done in raising the standard of Native hygiene is one of the greatest services ever rendered to the country.'[12]

Interestingly, Eyres' interpretation was supported by Peter Buck, the first New Zealand-trained Maori medical graduate and the Health Department's Director of Maori Hygiene from 1920 to 1927. Writing in 1940, at a time when the centennial of the signing of the Treaty of Waitangi encouraged reflection on the past, Buck agreed that there had been no organised effort to protect Maori against introduced diseases until the Department came into being, since when 'the health of Maoris had received great attention'.[13]

This uncritical view of official endeavours continued into the 1960s. J.K. Hunn acknowledged in his 1960 report on the Department of Maori Affairs that Maori and Pakeha health were not yet on a par, 'but in this century the Maoris have the more impressive record of health improvement. There was undoubtedly more room for it.'[14] The first attempt at a comprehensive account of government health policy came four years later with F.S. Maclean's *Challenge for Health*, which incorporated a chapter on Maori health and welfare. The foreword by Charles Hercus, former Professor of Preventive Medicine in the University of Otago, predicted that Maclean's 'brilliantly told' story of European impact on the Maori would be of international interest. Maclean's book, however, was limited in both scope and interpretation; like Eyres and Buck before him, he largely ignored any nineteenth century efforts to ameliorate conditions.[15]

The first academic historian to tackle Maori health was Raeburn Lange, in a pathbreaking MA thesis in 1972. While, in Lange's view, demographers and medical statisticians would have the major role, he perceived a need for an historian to investigate social and group influences. Nominally focused on the period from 1900 to 1918, Lange's thesis ranged more widely. The emphasis remained with Maori, and 'the significance of Maori attitudes to and participation in the reforms'. The role of the Maori Councils which came into being in 1900 was central to his research.[16] Like Maclean and others, Lange regarded 1900 as a watershed: 'At no stage before 1900 did the Government see a need for official action against low standards of Maori health.'[17] This statement has been repeated or endorsed by other historians from the 1970s to the present.[18] The interpretation is one which has been challenged in this book.

In particular, historians tended to underestimate the contribution made to Maori health care by the Native Medical Officers during the nineteenth century. The seeds of this error may have been sown in 1938 when Apirana

Ngata claimed that prior to 1900 'there was no recognition by the State, through the Government, that the health of the Maori was a special problem, that matter being left, very largely, in the hands of the Native school-teachers and subsidized medical men.'[19] The implication that there was no correlation between central government and these subsidised doctors appears to have influenced the thinking of Dr F.S. Maclean, who worked continuously for the Health Department from 1927 until 1957 as a medical officer of health and Director of Public Hygiene; his history of the Department stated that government medical services for Maori in the nineteenth century had been virtually non-existent: 'About this time [c. 1904] subsidies began to be paid to private medical practitioners, working in Maori districts, to provide a medical service. The Maoris, however, were somewhat reluctant to take full advantage of this service.[20]

Maclean's error was partially corrected by Lange, who claimed that the system 'had begun in a small way some time after the Wars',[21] and by Alan Ward, who produced evidence that the service began even earlier in his 1973 history of 'racial "amalgamation"' in New Zealand.[22] Both, however, left many questions unanswered. Their comments were often based on isolated examples, with no analysis of numbers employed or of geographical location. How many remote Maori communities had resident doctors? What was the relationship with European settlement? How much government money was spent on European doctoring at this time? Here answers are provided to some, though not all, of these questions.[23]

Few historians attempted to build on Lange's pioneering work over the next two decades. Geoffrey Rice's examination of the 1920 Health Act referred to the creation of a Division of 'Maori Welfare' but made no further reference to Maori.[24] While the most recent general history, Derek Dow's *Safeguarding the Public Health* (1994), included short summaries of the status of Maori health provision in seven of its eight chapters, these were indicative, with no attempt to present a comprehensive overview. In the early 1990s two Auckland MA students produced case studies of specific aspects of Maori health. Kate Goodfellow wrote about health provision in Native Schools between 1890 and 1940 (expanding on the work of Barrington and Beaglehole),[25] and Alex McKegg assessed government backblocks nursing services and the role of Maori health nurses from 1909 to 1939. Although necessarily limited in scope and range, both have an important part to play in the wider context of Maori health history.[26]

While historians by and large shied away from Maori health, the demographer Ian Pool produced a number of informative analyses which engage with the 'fatal impact' theory. Expressing concern about the partial nature of some studies, he described the source material for 1769–1840 and 1840–1901 as 'highly subjective qualitative data', the validity of which was open to question, and urged scholars not to accept too uncritically the 'seemingly clinical record'. The lack of detailed studies prevented him from arriving at any definitive analysis of mortality, and Pool himself warned readers that his conclusions for the period 1840–1901 'should be seen in terms of proposals for future research'.[27]

Rice, Dow, Goodfellow and McKegg are all non-Maori. In 1988 J.M. Boddy, a Massey University Senior Lecturer in Nursing Studies and herself a Pakeha, noted the growing belief that 'it is only appropriate for Maori people to talk about Maori health'. Boddy concluded: 'From a Maori perspective of health, the present ill-health of Maori people can be understood in relation to the past.'[28] The belief that history is an active part of the political and social process is best displayed in the writings of Professor Mason Durie.

Over the past two decades Durie, initially as Director of Psychiatry at Palmerston North Hospital and latterly as Professor of Maori Studies at Massey University, has become the most influential writer on Maori health. His work answers Sutherland's plea for a Maori version of events and offers a useful corrective to the uncritical views of Eyres and his successors. Durie's history is often provocative and thought-provoking. The tone is set in the preface to his most substantive publication, *Whaiora* (1994): 'Maori health development is about the trials and discoveries of the past, the energies and initiatives of the present, and the priorities and plans for the future. It is also about Maori determination in the face of overwhelming odds'. Durie is essentially concerned with developments since the early 1980s. In writing of earlier historical periods, his rhetoric is commonly unsupported by any evidence other than his own previous writings.[29] The opportunity for trained historians to contribute to the debate about Maori health is just as great now as it was when Lange first explored this topic more than a quarter of a century ago.

A Note on Sources

The starting point for any study of public health in nineteenth century New Zealand is the files of the Colonial Secretary's Office (renamed the Department of Internal Affairs when New Zealand achieved Dominion status in 1907), held at National Archives in Wellington. Until the establishment of the Department of Public Health in 1900, responsibility for health remained with this office. In 1840 the Colonial Secretariat handled 893 items of correspondence. By 1852 this figure had risen to more than 3,000 a year, and it continued to expand for the rest of the century.[1] Identifying relevant material can be time-consuming since few files are arranged by subject. Two exceptions are the outward letterbook covering medical topics in the 1840s and 1850s (IA Series 4.ii.281) and the letterbooks of the Protector of Aborigines 1841–60 (Series 4, 271 & 272). This material is supplemented, and in some instances duplicated, for the middle third of the nineteenth century by the New Zealand volumes in the Irish University Press series of *Great Britain Parliamentary Papers.*

National Archives also houses two other major collections used in the compilation of this book. Maori Affairs files from the mid 1880s contain crucial information on such matters as Maori Councils, sanitation and Native Reserves. These proved especially useful for the first decade of the twentieth century when responsibility for health shifted back and forward between the Departments of Health and Native Affairs.

The Health Department files comprise official reports and correspondence. Correspondents include officials from health and other government agencies, outside bodies, and private individuals. Many files are fleshed out with press cuttings sent to head office by staff from around the country. Unfortunately there are few records extant for the first decade of the Department's existence but thereafter the survival rate is much greater. They are arranged by series, with considerable overlap between subject areas. Although there are some series dedicated to Maori health, there are also numerous references to Maori in, for example, those dealing with hospital care, or infectious diseases.

Justice and Education Department files provide useful material to supplement these major holdings. The former illuminate the involvement of Justice in Maori health between 1893 and 1906, while the latter shed light on the health activities of the Native schools.

Annual and other reports located in the *Appendix to the Journals of the House of Representatives* constitute a second and invaluable source. Prior to the creation of any formal health system the 'Reports from Officers in Native Districts', covering the years 1871 to 1892, furnished an overview of health and welfare issues around the North Island. Initially listed within Series F of the *AJHR*, from 1873 these are contained within Series G. From 1882 onwards the *AJHR* also contains the annual reports of the Inspector-General of Hospitals. These provide a statistical and qualitative overview of individual hospitals and supply some specific information on the use made of these institutions by Maori. They appear in Series H. Information from this source was supplemented by the use of Otago Hospital Board and Dunedin Hospital minutes and annual reports, 1879–1910 (held in the Hocken Library, Dunedin) and Auckland Hospital Board minutes, 1885–1910 (held at National Archives, Auckland).

From 1921 onwards the 'Reports on Hospitals and Charitable Institutions' were incorporated into those of the Director-General of Health. Department of (Public) Health annual reports appear in the *AJHR* from 1901, as H-31. In some years these reports run to several hundred pages. From 1901 to 1909, and again from 1921 to 1930, they contain separate sections on Maori health.

For a brief spell during the period covered by this book the Health

Department published its own monthly journal. This was known as the *Journal of the Department of Public Health, Hospitals, and Charitable Aid* from July 1917 to May 1920, and as the *New Zealand Journal of Health and Hospitals* between June 1920 and December 1921, when government retrenchment brought about its demise.[2]

Only two other journals reported on Maori health with any degree of regularity. The *New Zealand Medical Journal*, the official organ of the New Zealand branch of the British Medical Association, first appeared in 1887. It ceased publication in 1896 but was revived in 1900. For the next five years it was edited by Dr James Mason, Chief Health Officer of the Department of Public Health. The *NZMJ* frequently commented on government health policy as seen through the eyes of the medical profession.[3] *Kai Tiaki* (later the *New Zealand Nursing Journal*) began publication in 1908. Like the *NZMJ* in the early years of the century, it had a quasi-official status from the outset. Its proprietor until 1923 was Hester Maclean, Assistant Inspector of Hospitals from 1906 until 1920, when she became the Health Department's first Director of Nursing. Under her editorship, which lasted until her death in 1932, the journal took a close interest in Maori health.[4]

Notes

Introduction

1 Lester to Johnson, 6 May 1842, IA 1, 1842/757, Johnson to Colonial Secretary, 17 May 1842, IA 1, 1842/864, NA.

2 D.A. Dow, *Safeguarding the Public Health: A History of the New Zealand Department of Health*, Wellington, 1995, pp.42–66. The title Department of Public Health was used until 1909, when it became known as the Department of Public Health, Hospitals and Charitable Institutions, to reflect its expanded role. Under the 1920 Health Act it was renamed the Department of Health, the title which it retained until its replacement by the Ministry of Health in 1993. For the sake of simplicity I have used the term 'Health Department' throughout.

3 Attention was first drawn to the impact of this upon current health practices by Warwick Brunton, a young history graduate who joined the department's new Health Services Research Unit in 1972. See W.A. Brunton, 'Hostages to History', *New Zealand Health Review*, vol.3, no.2, 1983, pp.3–6; and W. Brunton, 'The Place of History in Health Policy-Making: A View from the Inside', in L. Bryder and D.A. Dow (eds), *New Countries and Old Medicine: Proceedings of an International Conference on the History of Medicine and Health*, Auckland, 1995, pp.132–9.

4 Personal communication from Warwick Brunton, who has made an extensive study of New Zealand mental health history. See, for example, [W.A. Brunton], 'Development of Psychiatric Services in New Zealand', in *Royal Commission to Inquire into and Report upon Hospitals and Related Services: Stage II: Psychological Services: Department of Health 1st Submission*, Wellington, 1972, pp.1–21, and W.A. Brunton, 'Deinstitutionalisation: A Romance For All Seasons', in H. Haines & M. Abbott (eds), *The Future of Mental Health Services in New Zealand: Deinstitutionalisation*, Auckland, 1986, pp.44–63.

5 M.P.K. Sorrenson, 'The Purchase of Maori Lands, 1865–1892', MA thesis, Auckland, 1955. This was followed by his

'Land Purchase Methods and Their Effect on Maori Population, 1865–1901', *Journal of the Polynesian Society*, vol.65, no.3, 1956, pp.183–99.

6 See, for example, B.S. Rose, 'Maori Health and European Culture', *NZMJ*, vol.61, 1962, pp.491–5, R.T. Lange, 'The Revival of a Dying Race: A Study of Maori Health Reform 1900–1918 and its Nineteenth Century Background', MA thesis, Auckland, 1972, p.18, and D.I. Pool, *Te Iwi Maori: A New Zealand Population, Past, Present and Projected*, Auckland, 1991, p.62.

7 E. Murchie, 'Preface', in Public Health Commission, *He Matariki: A Strategic Plan for Maori Public Health. He Kaupapa Whainga Roa Mo Te Hauora Tumatanui Maori. The Public Health Commission's Advice to the Minister of Health 1994–1995*, Wellington, 1995, p.ii.

8 M.H. Durie, 'A Maori Perspective of Health', *Social Science and Medicine*, vol.20, no.5, 1985, pp.483–6; M.H. Durie, 'Implications of Policy and Management Decisions on Maori Health: Contemporary Issues and Responses' in M.W. Raffel and N.K. Raffel (eds), *Perspectives on Health Policy: Australia, New Zealand, United States*, New York, 1986, p.206; M.H. Durie, 'The Objectives of the Treaty and the Scope of Its Provisions', in I.H. Kawharu (ed.), *Maori and Pakeha Perspectives of the Treaty of Waitangi*, Auckland, 1989, p.281; M.H. Durie, *Whaiora: Maori Health Development*, Auckland, 1994, p.38.

9 MOH Carlyle Gilberd to Director-General of Health, 2 December 1938, H 1, 121 B.72, National Archives, Wellington (NA).

10 M. Durie, 'The Treaty of Waitangi and Health Care', *NZMJ*, vol.102, 1989, p.203; Durie, 1994, p.82.

11 Public Health Commission, 1995, p.13.

12 M.H. Watt, 'The Rest of the Day to Myself', unpublished autobiography (deposited in Health Department), p.82.

Chapter 1

1 On the work of the colonial surgeons see P.B. Maling, 'How the Canterbury Settlement Obtained its First Medical Officer', *NZMJ*, vol.55, 1956, pp.368–70; A.C. Hayton and H.D. Mullon, 'The Unfortunate Dr McShane of Nelson and New Plymouth', *NZMJ*, vol.87, 1978, pp.20–3; R. Donaldson, 'Dr J.P. Fitzgerald, Pioneer Colonial Surgeon, 1840–1854', *NZMJ*, vol.101, 1988, pp.636–8; G. Lambert, *Peter Wilson: Colonial Surgeon*, Palmerston North, 1981.

2 Colonial Secretary to George Clarke, 5 February 1846, IA 4/271, NA.

3 Earl Grey to Governor Grey, 28 July 1848, *GBPP*, vol.6, 1847–50 [1002], p.180.

4 J. Rutherford, *Sir George Grey: A Study in Colonial Government*, London, 1961, pp.240–1.

5 G.V. Butterworth and H.R. Young, *Maori Affairs: A Department and the People Who Made It*, Wellington, 1990, pp.28–9.

6 R.T. Lange, 'The Revival of a Dying Race: A Study of Maori Health Reform 1900–1918 and its Nineteenth Century Background', MA thesis, Auckland, 1972, pp.86–7, 93.

7 FitzHerbert to Colonial Secretary, 11 July 1854, IA 1, 1854/2586, NA.

8 Memorandum by Grey, 16 May, and reply by Alfred Domett, Colonial Secretary, 18 May 1863, *AJHR*, 1863, E-7A, pp.4–6.

9 The preceding paragraph are based in part on Butterworth and Young, 1990, pp.21, 24–5, 28–9, 38–9, 123–4.

10 'Statement of All Sums Expended Under the "Native Purposes Appropriation, 1862", on Account of the Financial Year 1862–3', *AJHR*, 1863, E-8.

11 *AJHR*, 1863, B-1, pp.17–18.

12 *AJHR*, 1866, B-1, p.3.

13 *AJHR*, 1867, B-1, p.3.

14 *AJHR*, 1870, B-6, pp.6–7.

15 J.M.R. Owens, 'Missionary Medicine and Maori Health: The Record of the

Wesleyan Mission to New Zealand Before 1840', *Journal of the Polynesian Society*, vol.81, 1972, pp.424–6.

16 A.C. Ross, 'The Scottish Missionary Doctor', in D.A. Dow (ed.), *The Influence of Scottish Medicine,* Carnforth, 1988, p.91.

17 W.B. Marshall, *Personal Narrative of Two Visits to New Zealand in HMS* Alligator, London, 1836, p.150, cited in L.K. Gluckman, *Tangiwai: Medical History of New Zealand Prior to 1860*, Auckland, 1976, p.52. For a more analytical account of this early interaction see M. Nicholson, 'Medicine and Racial Politics: Changing Images of the New Zealand Maori in the Nineteenth Century', in D. Arnold (ed.), *Imperial Medicine and Indigenous Societies*, Manchester, 1988, pp.66–104.

18 Owens, 1972, pp.420–1; J.M. Kehoe, 'Medicine, Sexuality and Imperialism: British Medical Discourse Surrounding Venereal Disease in New Zealand and Japan: A Socio-Historical and Comparative Study', PhD thesis, Victoria, 1992, p.153.

19 E.H. Roche, 'Some Medical Pioneers in New Zealand: Part 2', *NZMJ*, vol.71, 1970, p.90.

20 On Ford's presence see New Zealand Waitangi Tribunal, *Muriwhenua Land Report (Waitangi 45)*, Wellington, 1997, pp.70, 91, 93, 99, 147, 183, 221.

21 Kehoe, 1992, p.134. Kehoe omitted to mention Christopher Davies, who succeeded Butt as surgeon to St John's College in 1843 after Butt's ordination.

22 I.D. Beattie (ed.), *Ever Ready, the Life of Arthur Guyan Purchas: Including E.H. Roche's Article on His Grandfather and a Sermon, Some Hymns and Drawings by Dr Purchas*, Auckland, 1993; J.E. Gorst, *New Zealand Revisited: Recollections of the Days of My Youth*, London, 1908, pp.239–40.

23 F. Porter (ed.), *The Turanga Journals, 1840–1850: Letters and Journals of William and Jane Williams Missionaries to Poverty Bay*, Wellington, 1974, *passim.*

24 *Ibid.*, pp.183, 257.

25 *Ibid.*, pp.116, 210.

26 J.M. Barrington and T.H. Beaglehole, *Maori Schools in a Changing Society: An Historical Review*, Wellington, 1974, pp.92–3.

27 For an assessment of Colenso's influence see P. Goldsmith, 'Medicine, Death and the Gospel in Hawke's Bay, 1845–1852', in L. Bryder and D.A. Dow (eds), *New Countries and Old Medicine: Proceedings of an International Conference on the History of Medicine and Health*, Auckland, 1995, pp.354–60. An expanded version of this paper appeared in *NZJH*, vol.30, no.2, 1996, pp.163–81.

28 J.W. Stack, *Early Maoriland Adventures*, Wellington, 1935, pp.51, 117. For the 1841 medical activities of another Wesleyan missionary, the Revd Samuel Ironside, see C.A. MacDonald, *Pages From the Past: Some Chapters in the History of Marlborough*, Blenheim, 1933, pp.143–7.

29 Porter, 1974, p.259. Charles Baker was a CMS catechist, later a deacon.

30 D.M. Stafford, *Te Arawa: A History of the Arawa People,* Wellington, 1967, pp.301, 331.

31 Davis to Colonial Secretary, 13 April 1850, in IA 1, 1850/566, and reply dated 17 April in Medical Outwards Letterbook, IA 4.ii.281 f.89, NA.

32 *NZPD*, 1854–55, 11 September 1855, pp.538–9.

33 'Further Papers Relative to Sir George Grey's Plan of Native Government: Reports of Officers: Section V: East Cape', *AJHR*, 1862, E-9, p.5.

34 J. Watkins, *GBPP*, vol.1, 1837–40 [680], p.13.

35 J.B. Tuke, 'Medical Notes on New Zealand', *Edinburgh Medical Journal*, vol.9, 1863, p.724.

36 The missionary influence did not entirely disappear. Missionary nurses, in particular, continued to serve Maori until the 1940s. See, for example: F. Hayman, *King Country Nurse*, Auckland, 1964; J.H.

Starnes, 'A Pioneer Missionary in the Urewera: Sister Annie Henry MBE 1875–1971', *Historical Review: Bay of Plenty Journal of History*, vol.6, no.3, 1958, pp.84–93; A.J. North, 'Reminiscences of a Missionary Nurse', *Historical Review: Bay of Plenty Journal of History*, vol.14, no.1, 1966, pp.18–21.

37 The map is reproduced in D.A. Dow, *Safeguarding the Public Health: A History of the New Zealand Department of Health*, Wellington, 1995, p.39. The original is held by the Museum of Wellington, City and Sea.

38 Kehoe, 1992, p.115.

39 Quoted in Gluckman, 1976, p.52.

40 Roche, 1970, p.90.

41 D. McMillan, *Byways of History and Medicine: With Special Reference to Canterbury, New Zealand*, Christchurch, 1946, pp.69–70; New Zealand Department of Health, 'Historical Summary', in *A Review of Hospital and Related Services in New Zealand*, Wellington, 1969, p.9.

42 A.S. Thomson, *The Story of New Zealand*, vol.2, London, 1859, p.61.

43 J.L. Campbell, *Poenamo: Sketches of the Early Days of New Zealand*, London, 1881, pp.115–16.

44 Lady Martin, *Our Maoris*, London, 1884, pp.73, 77.

45 *New Zealand Gazette*, 16 May 1840, quoted in W.E. Henley, 'The Early History of the Auckland Hospital', *NZMJ*, vol.71, April 1970, p.201.

46 Colonial Secretary to FitzGerald, 7 September 1843, in IA 4.ii.281 f.13, NA.

47 Bishop of New Zealand to Colonial Secretary, 9 May 1843, IA 1, 1843/953, NA.

48 IA 1, 1844/1694, NA, and memorandum of Colonial Secretary, 7 September 1843, IA 4.ii.281, NA.

49 Lester to Johnson, 6 May 1842, IA 1, 1842/757, NA; Johnson to Colonial Secretary, 17 May 1842, IA 1, 1842/864, NA; Colonial Secretary to Johnson, 10 June 1842, IA 4.ii.281 f.1, NA.

50 Henley, 1970, p.201.

51 Gluckman, 1976, p.103.

52 A.H. McLintock (ed.), *An Encyclopaedia of New Zealand*, vol.2, Wellington, 1966, p.507.

53 Taylor diary, 28 November 1844, quoted in *Historical Record: Journal of the Whanganui Historical Society Inc*, vol.4, no.1, May 1973, p.1.

54 Porter, 1974, pp.298, 397, 402–3, 414.

55 S.H. Selwyn, *Reminiscences 1809–1867*, Auckland, 1961, edited by E.A. Evans, quoted in Porter, 1974, p.428.

56 Porter, 1974, pp.22, 431, 437. Porter repeated claims by some contemporary observers that this was a typhus outbreak, a claim which had been denied at the time by Colonial Surgeon John Johnson. See J.K. Davis, *The History of St John's College*, Auckland, 1911, p.60.

57 Stafford, 1967, pp.314, 320–1, 327.

58 New Zealand Department of Health, 1969, pp.9–22.

59 A. Ward, *A Show of Justice: Racial 'Amalgamation' in Nineteenth Century New Zealand*, Auckland, 1995, pp.ix, 87. Ward's book first appeared in 1973 and was republished in 1995 with only minor corrections to the original text.

60 Nicholson, 1988, pp.67–8, 77–8; Kehoe, 1992, p.137; M. Belgrave, '"Medical Men" and "Lady Doctors": The Making of a New Zealand Profession 1867–1941', PhD thesis, Victoria, 1985, p.212.

61 Quoted in M.B. Brown, 'The Auckland School of Nursing, 1883–1990: The Rise and The Fall', MA thesis, Auckland, 1991, p.23.

62 Governor Grey to Earl Grey, 4 February 1847, *GBPP*, vol.5, 1846–7 [837], pp.92–3.

63 Governor Grey to Earl Grey, 5 April 1848, *GBPP*, vol.6, 1847–50 [1120], p.20.

64 R. Donaldson, 'Dr J.P. FitzGerald: Pioneer Colonial Surgeon, 1840–1854', *NZMJ*, vol.101, 1988, p.637. For an account of the operation see A.J. Newson, 'New Zealand's First General Anaes-

thetic', *Anaesthesia & Intensive Care*, vol.3, 1975, pp.204–8, and D. Dow, 'Ether Ushers In a New Era for Local Surgery', *New Zealand Doctor*, 9 July 1997, p.57.

65 FitzGerald report, 13 November 1841, IA 1, 1841/1526, NA. John Watkins, who visited New Zealand for some weeks in 1833 as surgeon aboard a trading vessel, claimed he had performed the first surgical operation upon a Maori, a female who 'was very anxious for it'. See *GBPP*, vol.1, 1837–40 [680], pp.12, 20.

66 Governor Grey to Earl Grey, 6 February 1851, enclosing FitzGerald's 'very interesting report' on Wellington Hospital 1847–51, *GBPP*, vol.7, 1851 [1420], pp.133–4.

67 'First Annual Report of the New Plymouth Hospital', December 1849, *GBPP*, vol.6, 1847–50 [1280], p.115.

68 Auckland Hospital annual report, *GBPP*, vol.6, 1847–50 [1136], pp.28–31.

69 Kehoe, 1992, p.141.

70 For an account of early Wanganui hospitals, see articles by A.L. Kirk, *Historical Record: Journal of the Whanganui Historical Society Inc*, vol.4, no.1, May 1973, pp.1–18.

71 Lieutenant-Governor Eyre to Governor Grey, 9 June 1849, *GBPP*, vol.6, 1847–50 [1280], pp.86–7; R.E. Wright-St Clair, *Caring for People: A History of the Wanganui Hospital Board*, Wanganui, 1987, p.9.

72 Wright-St Clair, *Caring for People*, 1987, p.10.

73 Governor Grey to Earl Grey, 14 August 1851, *GBPP*, vol.9, 1852–4 [1779], pp.25–33. Rees did not claim, as did Grey in his covering letter, that all 159 were 'cured'.

74 Kehoe, 1992, p.141; Wanganui Hospital returns, 6 February 1854, IA 1, 1854/538, NA.

75 Governor Grey to Earl Grey, 10 March 1849, *GBPP*, vol.6, 1847–50 [1136], p.28.

76 Governor Grey to Earl Grey, 5 April 1848, *GBPP*, vol.6, 1847–50 [1120] p.20, and 10 March 1849, *ibid.*, [1136] pp.28–31.

77 Wellington Hospital Returns, September 1847–March 1849, in *GBPP*, vol.6, 1847–50 [1280], p.166.

78 G. Lambert, 'Colonial Hospital Now Serves the Arts', *Historic Places in New Zealand*, vol.12, March 1986, p.8.

79 L.H. Barber and R.J. Towers, *Wellington Hospital 1847–1976*, Wellington, 1976, p.10.

80 See 'Appendix 3: Mortality in Selected Voluntary Hospitals to 1875', in J. Woodward, *To Do the Sick No Harm: A Study of the British Voluntary Hospital System to 1875*, London, 1974, pp.153–8.

81 Wellington Hospital annual reports for 1847–51, *GBPP*, vol.7, 1851 [1420], p.134, vol.9, 1852–4 [1779], pp.73–4. FitzGerald qualified his comment on outpatient deaths with the rather odd statement that some had 'died at remote cultivations without applying for medical aid'.

82 Enclosed in William FitzHerbert, Provincial Secretary, to Colonial Secretary, 11 July 1854, IA 1, 1854/2586, NA.

83 Annual report of Colonial Surgeon for 1852, dated 11 January 1853, IA 1, 1853/87, NA.

84 Lambert, 1981, pp.183, 185; W.H. Skinner, *Pioneer Medical Men of Taranaki 1834 to 1880*, New Plymouth, 1933, p.117.

85 Taylor's journal, 25 November 1851, cited in *Historical Record: Journal of the Whanganui Historical Society Inc*, vol.4, no.1, May 1973, p.7.

86 Wright-St Clair, *Caring for People*, 1987, p.10.

87 *NZPD*, 1854–55, 8 September 1854, pp.385–6.

88 *NZPD*, 1854–55, 11 September 1854, p.414.

89 *GBPP*, vol.10, 1854–60 [2719], pp.56, 161. These sums were voted for on 14 September 1854. See *NZPD*, 1854–55, 14 September 1854, p.431.

90 *AJHR*, 1860, B-1, p.17.

91 J.H. Angus, *A History of the Otago Hospital Board and its Predecessors*, Dunedin, 1984, pp.15–21.

92 D.I. Pool, *Te Iwi Maori: A New Zealand Population, Past, Present & Projected*, Auckland, 1991, p.61.
93 Colonial Secretary to Dr Wilson, 26 March 1855, IA 4.ii.281, NA.
94 Angus, 1984, p.21.
95 M. Tennant, *Paupers and Providers: Charitable Aid in New Zealand*, Wellington, 1989, pp.12–13.
96 George Rees to Colonial Secretary, 8 February 1853, *GBPP*, vol.9, 1852–4 [1779], pp.192–3.
97 Colonial Secretary to Colonial Surgeon, Wanganui, 12 June 1854, IA 4.ii.281, NA.
98 G. Rees, Remarks on the Sanitary Conditions of his District together with the Hospital Returns, 10 September 1855, IA 1, 1855/2887, NA; Colonial Secretary to Rees, 4 October 1855, IA 4.ii.281, NA.
99 Barber and Towers, 1976, p.16.
100 FitzGerald report of 28 July 1853, *GBPP*, vol.9, 1852–4 [1779], pp.276–7.
101 Thomson, vol.2, 1959, p.323.
102 Governor Grey to Earl Grey, 13 February 1852, *GBPP*, vol.9, 1852–4 [1779], p.73.
103 Quoted in J. Miller, *Early Victorian New Zealand: A Study of Racial Tension and Social Attitudes, 1839–1852*, London, 1958, pp.106–7.
104 Donaldson, 1988, p.636.
105 Doctors who served in this capacity were initially known as 'Native Medical Attendants'. They were more commonly referred to in later years as 'Native Medical Officers'. For the sake of simplicity I have used the latter term throughout.
106 Bishop to Colonial Secretary, 9 May 1843, IA 1, 1843/953, NA; FitzGerald to Colonial Secretary, 1 June 1843, IA 1, 1843/1409, NA.
107 FitzGerald to Colonial Secretary, 4 July 1844, IA 1, 1844/1691, NA.
108 FitzGerald to Colonial Secretary, 17 July 1844, IA 1, 1844/1717, NA.
109 Henry King to Colonial Secretary, 24 August 1844, IA 1, 1844/1937, NA.
110 Butterworth and Young, 1990, p.20.
111 Sinclair to Colonial Secretary, 4 November 1847, IA 1, 1848/20, NA.
112 Sinclair to Colonial Secretary, 26 November 1847 and enclosures, IA 1, 1848/15, NA.
113 McMillan, 1946, p.308.
114 Governor Grey to Earl Grey, 5 April 1848, *GBPP*, vol.6, 1847–50 [1120], p.20.
115 19 June 1849, IA 1, 1849/1383, NA.
116 Colonial Secretary to Bannatine, 19 June 1850, IA 4.ii.281 f.99, NA.
117 See IA 1, 1854/513, and 1855/1364, NA.
118 Report by Rees, 15 June 1854, IA 1, 1854/2056, NA; Colonial Secretary to Rees, 18 July 1854, IA 4.ii.281, NA.
119 FitzHerbert to Colonial Secretary, 11 July 1854, IA 1, 1854/2586, NA.
120 *NZPD*, 1854–55, 11 September 1855, pp.538–9.
121 For an account of Spratt's work see chapter 2, p.81–2.
122 *NZPD*, 1861–63, 3 September 1861, p.363.
123 'Minute by Governor Sir George Grey on the Subject of His Excellency's Plan of Native Government', *AJHR*, 1862, E-2, pp.10–12.
124 Report of meeting held on 3 April 1862, *AJHR*, 1862, E-9, section 2, p.30.
125 *AJHR*, 1862, E-9, p.13.
126 Report of meetings held on 27 January and 12 April 1862, *AJHR*, 1862, E-9, pp.21, 26.
127 Ward, 1995, p.105.
128 'Nominal Roll of the Civil Establishment of New Zealand on the 30th June, 1875', *AJHR*, 1875, H-11.
129 Much of the biographical data on which this analysis is based is taken from Dr R.E. Wright-St Clair's unpublished database of medical practitioners in New Zealand 1840 to 1930.
130 *AJHR*, 1863, E-10, 1864, E-7, 1867, D-2.
131 *AJHR*, 1862, D-17.
132 *AJHR*, 1864, E-7; *Lyttelton Times*, 15 August 1863.
133 *AJHR*, 1862, E-9, pp.26–7.
134 *AJHR*, 1864, E-7.
135 *AJHR*, 1862, E-9, p.18.

136 Ward, 1995, pp.202–3.

137 William L. Williams, quoted in J.A. Mackay, *Historic Poverty Bay and the East Coast*, Gisborne, 1966, p.206.

138 *AJHR*, 1866, D-3. The thirtieth name on the list was Dr Richard Day of Auckland, chairman of the Central Board of Vaccination for the Aborigines of New Zealand.

139 The five were James Tilby (Takaka), Joseph Wilson (Motueka), Samuel Cusack (Nelson), Lewis Horne (Wairau), and Julius Tripe (Queen Charlotte Sound). Only Tilby had no military connection.

140 *AJHR*, 1867, D-3.

142 *NZPD*, Third and Fourth Parliaments, 8 August 1866, p.854.

142 Belgrave, 1985, pp.129–30.

143 Ward, 1995, p.197.

144 Circular issued by W. Rolleston, 15 February 1868, in 'Reports on the Social and Political State of the Natives in Various Districts at the Time of the Arrival of Sir G.F. Bowen', *AJHR*, 1868, A-4, p.1. Bowen was Governor from 5 February 1868 until 19 March 1873.

145 S. Deighton to Under-Secretary, 8 April 1868, and Report by Matthew Scott, *AJHR*, 1868, A-4, pp.17–18. Scott had been in the district for seven years and was acting surgeon with the East Coast Expeditionary Force in 1865.

146 Dow, 1998, p.178.

147 See I. Loudon, *Medical Care and the General Practitioner, 1750–1850*, Oxford, 1986.

148 See, for example, R.E. Wright-St Clair, 'Medical Men in Early New Zealand Politics', *NZMJ*, vol.54, 1955, pp.551–5.

149 A 'certified copy' of the medical register, dated 31 December 1869, was first 'published for general information' in the *New Zealand Gazette*, 22 January 1870, pp.36–9. Like its British counterpart it is updated annually.

150 See, for example, F.S. Maclean, *Challenge for Health: A History of Public Health in New Zealand*, Wellington, 1964, p.145; Lange, 1972, pp.87–91, 141–2.

151 A. Moorehead, *The Fatal Impact: An Account of the Invasion of the South Pacific 1767–1840*, London, 1966. Moorehead concentrated his attention on Tahiti, Australia and the Antarctic.

152 Featherston apparently made the remark at the first meeting of the Wellington Philosophical Society. It seems to have first appeared in print in an article by Walter Buller in the *New Zealand Journal of Science*, vol.2, 1884–5, p.57. Since then it has been repeatedly quoted or misquoted. *An Encyclopaedia of New Zealand* (1966), vol.1, p.634, erroneously claims in the entry on Featherston that he made the speech in Parliament. For an extended discussion of Featherston's comments, see D. Dow, ' "Smoothing their dying pillow": Lingering Longer', *New Zealand Doctor*, 21 January 1998, p.45.

153 Nicholson, 1988, p.85. Interestingly, David Hamer's essay on Featherston in *The Dictionary of New Zealand Biography: Volume 1: 1769–1869*, Wellington, 1990, pp.119–21, made no mention of the 'dying pillow'. He did, however, reveal that Featherston suffered from tuberculosis, left Britain around 1840 in search of improved health, and was troubled by constant ill-health throughout his time in New Zealand.

154 See R.J. Morris, *Cholera 1832*, London, 1976, *passim.*

155 H. Williams, *The Early Journals of Henry Williams Senior Missionary in New Zealand of the Church Missionary Society 1826–1840* (edited by L.M. Rogers), Christchurch, 1961, p.249.

156 Watkins, 1837–8, p.20.

157 J.W. Donovan, 'Measles in Australia and New Zealand 1834–1835', *Medical Journal of Australia*, vol.1, 1970, pp.5–10. Donovan's account is somewhat speculative, with the New Zealand evidence based on early twentieth century secondary sources.

158 H.M. Wright, *New Zealand, 1769–1840: Early Years of Western Contact*, Harvard, 1959, p.64.

159 Maclean, 1964, p.223, states that there were only 9 smallpox deaths between 1872, when these were first recorded, and 1900. He makes no reference to smallpox among Maori before 1913. Occasional references to 'typhus' by nineteenth century doctors were most probably a misdiagnosis of typhoid. A number of public health officials complained about the inability of many local practitioners to distinguish between the two.

160 A.S. Wohl, *Endangered Lives: Public Health in Victorian Britain*, London, 1983, pp.132–3.

161 Dow, 1995, p.28.

162 For an account of the global distribution of the vaccine see J.Z. Bowers, 'The Odyssey of Smallpox Vaccination', *Bulletin of the History of Medicine*, vol.55, 1981, pp.17–33.

163 Watkins, 1837, p.31.

164 Williams diary entries for 13 April and 13 May 1845, quoted in Porter, 1974, pp.333, 338.

165 A.G. Bagnall and G.C. Petersen, *William Colenso . . . His Life and Journeys*, Wellington, 1948, p.308.

166 Extracts from Haswell's report were reprinted in R.A.A. Sherrin and J.H. Wallace, *Early History of New Zealand*, Auckland, 1890, p.591.

167 R. Donaldson, 'Dr John Patrick FitzGerald: Pioneer Colonial Doctor 1840–1860', MPhil thesis, Waikato, 1988, pp.71–6, 107.

168 'First Annual Report of the New Plymouth Hospital', *GBPP*, vol.6, 1847–50 [1280], pp.115–16.

169 Dow, 1995, p.28.

170 *Ibid.*, pp.29–30.

171 *NZPD*, 1854–55, 21 June, 27 June, 14 July 1854, pp.113, 129, 228.

172 See IA 1, 1854/4238, NA for correspondence and reports. The sum of £500 came from the government budget of £36,497 for the period July 1854–June 1855. See *GBPP*, vol.10, 1854–60 [2719], p.56.

173 The appointees were named in the *New Zealand Gazette*. They included H.J. Andrews (1855), T.M. Philson (1858), S.J. Stratford (1858), Richard Matthews (1858) and J.T.W. Bacot (1859).

174 Thomson, vol.2, 1859, p.212.

175 Tuke, 1863, pp.227–8.

176 Ward, 1995, p.197. Ward earlier referred in passing to the work of the 'Vaccination Board' (pp.92, 141).

177 Maclean, 1964, pp.237–43; Dow, 1995, p.29.

178 *AJHR*, 1868, A-4, p.18.

179 'Report by Dr Nicholson, of Auckland, on the Steps Taken by Him to Prevent the Spread of Small-Pox in the Province of Auckland', *AJHR*, 1872, G-32.

180 *AJHR*, 1872, G-3, p.17.

181 W. Harsant to Under-Secretary, 22 April 1873, *AJHR*, 1873, G-1, p.4.

182 H.W. Brabant to Under-Secretary, *AJHR*, 1873, G-1, pp.10–11.

183 See J. Campbell, 'Smallpox in Aboriginal Australia, 1829–31', *Australian Historical Studies*, vol.20, October 1983, pp.536–56, J. Campbell, 'Smallpox in Aboriginal Australia, the Early 1830s', *Australian Historical Studies*, vol.21, April 1985, pp.336–58, and N. Butlin, 'Macassans and Aboriginal Smallpox: The "1789" and "1829" Epidemics', *Australian Historical Studies*, vol.21, April 1985, pp.315–35.

184 Nicholson, 1988, p.70.

Chapter 2

1 *New Zealand Official Yearbook*, 1990, p.158. Pool's 'best estimate' revised figures for Maori are 61,500 in 1857/8 and 47,940 in 1874. See D.I. Pool, *Te Iwi Maori: A New Zealand Population, Past, Present & Projected*, Auckland, 1991, p.76.

2 *AJHR*, 1871, B-9.

3 See table compiled by R.T. Lange, 'The Revival of a Dying Race: A Study of Maori Health Reform 1900–1918 and its

Nineteenth Century Background', Appendix III: Civil List, 1885–1902, MA thesis, Auckland, 1972.

4 *AJHR*, 1875, B-4.

5 A. Ward, *A Show of Justice: Racial 'Amalgamation' in Nineteenth Century New Zealand*, Auckland, 1995, pp.281–2.

6 *AJHR*, 1880, B-5.

7 Ward, 1995, pp.299–300.

8 'Minutes of Evidence Given by T.W. Lewis, Under-Secretary, Native Department', *AJHR*, 1889, I-10, p.11.

9 Otago Hospital Board committee minute book 1885–94, 20 December 1888, Hocken Library, Dunedin; G. Conly, *A Case History: The Hawke's Bay Hospital Board 1876–1989*, Napier, 1992, p.55.

10 G.V. Butterworth and H.R. Young, *Maori Affairs: A Department and the People Who Made It*, Wellington, 1990, p.56.

11 Lange, 1972, pp.86–7. Lange gives annual figures for 1890–4 of between £1,289 and £2,003.

12 The debate can be found in *NZPD*, vol.82, 13 September 1893, pp.240–6.

13 Memorandum by Alexander Mackay, Commissioner of Native Reserves, Nelson, 1872, *AJHR*, 1872, F-3, pp.18–23.

14 G.V. Butterworth and S.M. Butterworth, *The Maori Trustee*, [Wellington], n.d. [1992?], p.10.

15 For comment on tenths see Ward, 1995, pp.88, 89, 192.

16 Butterworth and Butterworth, 1991, p.17.

17 See *AJHR*, 1873, G-2A, 1880, G-3, 1881, G-4, 1882, G-7, 1883, G-7A.

18 *NZPD*, vol.51, 23 June 1885, p.102.

19 New Zealand Department of Health, *A Review of Hospital and Related Services in New Zealand*, Wellington, 1969, pp.9–22; New Zealand Department of Health, *A Health Service for New Zealand*, Wellington, 1974, pp.10–19.

20 I. Hay, *The Caring Commodity: The Provision of Health Care in New Zealand*, Auckland, 1989, p.21.

21 See D.A. Dow, 'Springs of Charity? The Development of the New Zealand Hospital System, 1876–1910', in L. Bryder (ed.), *A Healthy Country: Essays on the Social History of Medicine in New Zealand*, Wellington, 1991, pp.44–64.

22 Memorandum to Colonial Secretary, 27 April 1859, IA 1, 1859/1025, NA.

23 Fox to Armitage, 5 May 1862, *AJHR*, 1862, E-9, section II, p.41.

24 Ward, 1995, pp.148, 150.

25 J.E. Gorst, *New Zealand Revisited: Recollections of the Days of My Youth*, London, 1908, pp.239–40, 277.

26 Preliminary instructions from Sewell to T.H. Smith, 14 December 1861, and Sewell's Further Instructions to Smith, 3 March 1862, *AJHR*, 1862, E-9, section IV, pp.3–4, 18.

27 Second report from Smith to Sewell, 25 January 1862, *AJHR*, 1862, E-9, section IV, p.11.

28 P. Adlam, 'The Story of Medical Practice in Rotorua', in [Rotorua and District Historical Society], *Rotorua 1880–1980*, Rotorua, 1980, p.255 noted the abortive attempts to establish a hospital in the 1840s but made no mention of any 1860s proposal. See also Anon., 'Rotorua Hospital', *New Zealand Hospital*, vol.9, no.3, 1957, pp.29–30.

29 *AJHR*, 1862, E-9, p.6.

30 J.B. Tuke, 'Medical Notes on New Zealand', *Edinburgh Medical Journal*, vol.9, 1863, pp.227–8, 724.

31 Wilson's annual report, co-authored with the Hospital Matron and dated 1 April 1864, is reproduced in D.C. Low, *Salute to the Scalpel: A Medical History of the Nelson Province*, Nelson, 1972, pp.134–7.

32 R.E. Wright-St Clair, *Caring for People: A History of the Wanganui Hospital Board*, Wanganui, 1987, p.10.

33 *Ibid.*, p.12.

34 E.M. Stokes, *Te Raupatu o Tauranga Moana: The Confiscation of Tauranga Lands*, Hamilton, 1990, pp.34–5.

35 Dunedin Hospital Annual Report, 1871/2, *Votes and Proceedings of the Otago Provincial Council*, 1872, Appendix.

36 Lange, 1972, p.55.
37 Mair to Under-Secretary, 2 July 1872, *AJHR*, 1872, F-3, p.8.
38 Mair to Native Minister, 12 June 1873, *AJHR*, 1873, G-1, p.21.
39 R.E. Wright-St Clair, *From Cottage to Regional Base Hospital: Waikato Hospital 1887–1987*, Hamilton, 1987.
40 Clarke to Under-Secretary, 8 May 1874, *AJHR*, 1874, G-2, pp.5–6.
41 Bush to Under-Secretary, 4 June 1883, *AJHR*, 1883, G-1A, p.5. The outbreak was treated by Dr Alexander Reid, the public vaccinator for the district. There were 23 cases, with two fatalities among those attended by Reid.
42 Bush to Under-Secretary, 3 May 1886, *AJHR*, 1886, G-2, pp.12–13.
43 Lange, 1972, pp.43–4.
44 Kemp to Under-Secretary, 28 May 1877, *AJHR*, 1877, G-1, pp.3–4.
45 C. Brown to Under-Secretary, 11 June 1879, *AJHR*, 1879, G-1, p.21.
46 H.W. Brabant to Under-Secretary, 15 May 1880, *AJHR*, 1880, G-4, p.6.
47 Wright-St Clair, *Caring for People*, p.12.
48 Quoted in *ibid.*, p.14.
49 Woon to Under-Secretary, 22 May 1877, *AJHR*, 1877, G-1, p.17.
50 Conly, 1992, pp.19–20, 24, 33.
51 'Notes of Native Meetings', *AJHR*, 1885, G-1, pp.46–50, 56.
52 *AJHR*, 1885, H-18A, p.15.
53 *AJHR*, 1893, H-23, p.25.
54 *AJHR*, 1888, G-1, pp.1, 7.
55 *AJHR*, 1889, I-10, p.2.
56 'Minutes of Evidence', *AJHR*, 1889, I-10, pp.13–15.
57 Annual reports on Hospitals and Charitable Institutions in the Colony were published each year in the *AJHR*.
58 For example, 4 of 1,105 patients in 1892, 5 of 1,095 in 1893, 3 of 1,737 in 1900, 5 of 2,111 in 1904.
59 Dunedin Hospital House Committee minutes, vol.6, 14 May 1902, Hocken Library.
60 Dow, 1991, pp.50–2.
61 *AJHR*, 1882, H-23, p.10.
62 *AJHR*, 1886, H-9, p.4.
63 *AJHR*, 1889, H-3; 1899, 1904, H-22.
64 *AJHR*, 1906, H-22.
65 *AJHR*, H-22, 1898–1900.
66 M. Tennant, *Paupers and Providers: Charitable Aid in New Zealand*, Wellington, 1989, p.12.
67 Wright-St Clair, *From Cottage to Regional Base Hospital*, p.22.
68 M. Belgrave, '"Medical Men" and "Lady Doctors": The Making of a New Zealand Profession 1867–1941', PhD thesis, Victoria, 1985, pp.244, 247.
69 Butterworth and Young, 1990, pp.6, 41–2.
70 Ward, 1995, p.238.
71 *AJHR*, 1875, H-11.
72 Pool, 1991, p.90.
73 The responses were printed in *AJHR*, 1885, G-2A. Originals are in MA 21/19, NA, which nominally contains NMO reports for 1884–90. In fact, some of these date back to the 1870s.
74 Volumes used in this analysis are those for 1888–91 (A 6/2), 1891–4 (A 6/3), 1894–7 (A 6/5) and 1897–1900 (A 6/7). An earlier volume, covering 1884–5, was not used.
75 *AJHR*, 1866, D-3.
76 See, for example, *AJHR*, 1883, G-7A, p.4. The outlay for the year of £93 18s on the medical officer was offset by income of 3s, presumably paid by a grateful patient.
77 'Minutes of Evidence', *AJHR*, 1889, I-10, pp.15, 17.
78 Brabant to Native Minister, 21 February 1871, *AJHR*, 1871, F-6A, p.15.
79 Brabant to Under-Secretary, 23 May 1873, *AJHR*, 1873, G-1, pp.10–11.
80 Brabant to Native Minister, 25 May 1874, *AJHR*, 1874, G-2, p.6.
81 Lewis to Native Minister, 27 July 1886, MA 21/19, NA.
82 *AJHR*, 1885, G-1, p.40. The doctor referred to was Charles Hovell, appointed in 1866 after three years as surgeon to the Waikato Militia.
83 The following account is based on the

correspondence between June and November 1886 which forms part of the Native Medical Officers' Reports 1884–90, MA 21/19, NA.

84 When Donald travelled overseas in 1879 a local Maori wrote proclaiming 'Farewell to you, the skilful healer of diseases among the Maori. No one patient has ever slipped from your grasp all the years past.' The statement was presumably hyperbolic but indicative of the high regard in which he was held. Quoted in D. McMillan, *Byways of History and Medicine: With Special Reference to Canterbury, New Zealand*, Christchurch, 1946, pp.309–10.

85 Pairman's appointment is noted in A 6/5, NA.

86 J.W. Stack to Native Minister, 1 June 1879, AJHR, 1879, G-1, p.21.

87 A. Mackay, Native Commissioner, Nelson to Under-Secretary, 30 April 1881, *AJHR*, 1881, G-3, p.9.

88 Lewis evidence, *AJHR*, 1889, I–10, p.10; Under-Secretary to Native Minister, 4 January 1882, MA 21/19, NA.

89 Education: Native Schools annual report, *AJHR*, 1890, E-2, p.1.

90 Native Department to Fisher, 28 February and reply from Fisher, 14 March 1890, MA 21/19, NA. Fisher was offered £25 per annum, to include both travel and medicines. In declining this offer Fisher stated that return trips from Akaroa to Little River and 'the Kaik' were costed at £30 and £20 respectively.

91 *NZPD*, vol.80, 10 August 1893, p.553.

92 White to Minister, 21 June 1872, *AJHR*, 1872, F-3. Trimnell first held office in May 1859 and served until 1906, with some breaks in continuity.

93 J.H. Campbell to Under-Secretary, 13 June 1874, *AJHR*, 1874, G-2A, p.3.

94 Brabant to Under-Secretary, 31 May 1879, *AJHR*, 1879, G-1, p.18, and 30 May 1882, *AJHR*, 1882, G-1, p.5.

95 On the history of the spa movement in New Zealand see I. Rockel, *Taking the Waters: Early Spas in New Zealand*, Wellington, 1986.

96 This summary of Payne's tenure is based on the correspondence 1880–9 which forms part of the Native Medical Officers' Reports 1884–90, MA 21/19, NA. For a fuller account see D. Dow, 'Rumour Hampers Pioneering Doctor', *New Zealand Doctor*, 18 February 1998, p.36.

97 A.T. Perkins to Native Minister, 4 March 1889, MA 21/19, NA.

98 T.W. Porter, Captain Commanding East Coast District, Gisborne to Under-Secretary, 20 May 1881, *AJHR*, 1880, G-4A, p.13.

99 Internal memo by Morpeth, 2 June 1882, MA 21/19, NA.

100 *NZPD*, vol.51, 10 July 1885, p.515 and 14 July 1885, p.532. Scott was one of the 15 doctors circularised in April 1885. His base in Wairoa was 100 miles south of Tolaga Bay.

101 G. Kelly to Under-Secretary, 9 May 1879, *AJHR*, 1879, G-1, p.1.

102 G.A. Preece to Under-Secretary, 12 May 1880, *AJHR*, 1880, G-4, p.10.

103 Scannell to Under-Secretary, 3 May 1887, *AJHR*, 1887, G-1, p.13.

104 Lewis to Native Minister, 27 July 1886, MA 21/19, NA.

105 'Minutes of Evidence', *AJHR*, 1889, I-10, p.14.

106 F.E. Hamlin to Under-Secretary, 19 June 1874, *AJHR*, 1874, G-2A, p.2.

107 F.E. Hamlin to Under-Secretary, 18 May 1876, *AJHR*, 1876, G-1, p.27.

108 Wilkinson to Under-Secretary, 25 May 1886, *AJHR*, 1886, G-1, p.3, and same to same, 19 May 1887, *AJHR*, 1887, G-1, p.4.

109 Emile Aubin, who was born at Pirongia, qualified in London in 1895 and returned to practice in New Zealand two years later. He was only seventeen years old in 1886. The 'doctor' referred to was probably his father.

110 See 'Reductions in Civil Service: Native', *AJHR*, 1888, H-30, p.2.

111 The following section is based on corre-

spondence dated May 1882–June 1885, MA 21/19, NA.

112 Barr received £25 while De Lowe's salary was £100.

113 C.L. Andrews, 'Aspects of Development, 1870–1890', in I.H. Kawharu (ed.), *Conflict and Compromise: Essays on the Maori Since Colonisation*, Wellington, 1975, p.82.

114 Alexander Mackay, Commissioner of Native Reserves, to Native Minister, 18 July 1872, *AJHR*, 1872, F-3, p.17.

115 Spratt's reports are in MA 21/19, NA. For a more detailed analysis of the 1877 return see D. Dow, 'Revisiting the Life and Times of a Pioneer GP', *New Zealand Doctor*, 1 October 1997, p.51.

116 Payne to Under-Secretary, 17 May 1888, MA 21/19, NA.

117 D. Scannell to Under-Secretary, 21 April 1886, *AJHR*, 1886, G-2, pp.15–16; Scannell's census return for 1886, *AJHR*, 1886, G-12, pp.9–10.

118 J.M. Moore, *New Zealand for the Emigrant, Invalid and Tourist*, London, 1890, p.225. One chapter was 'written for the medical profession alone'.

119 Figures are calculated from Belgrave, 1985, p.257, and Audit Office statistics.

120 Frederick Armitage settled in Tauranga in the late 1860s and remained there until his death in June 1884. His work in supplying attendance and 'medical comforts' was a regular feature of Herbert Brabant's annual reports from 1873 to 1883, though he was not named until 1878. I have found no trace of his name in any published official return.

121 See J. Stenhouse, '"A disappearing race before we came here": Doctor Alfred Kingcome Newman, the Dying Maori, and Victorian Scientific Racism', *NZJH*, vol.30, no.2, 1996, pp.124–40, and Archdeacon Walsh, 'The Passing of the Maori: An Inquiry into the Principal Causes of the Decay of the Race', *Transactions and Proceedings of the New Zealand Institute*, vol.40, 1907, pp.154–75.

122 H.W. Brabant to Native Minister, 25 May 1874, *AJHR*, 1874, G-2, p.6.

123 *Illustrated New Zealand Herald*, 18 February 1869, p.2.

124 *AJHR*, 1881, H-20.

125 J. Ballance, during debate on vaccination of Maori, *NZPD*, vol.48, 10 September 1884, pp.229–30.

126 E.S. Maunsell to Under-Secretary, 9 May 1882, *AJHR*, 1882, G-1, p.13. In 1881 Maunsell stated there were 1,067 Maori in Wairarapa, revising this in 1882 to approximately 800. See *AJHR*, 1881, G-3, p.25.

127 G.T. Wilkinson to Under-Secretary, 17 May 1882, *AJHR*, 1882, G-1, p.4.

128 S. Deighton, Resident Magistrate, Chatham Islands to Under-Secretary, 25 May 1882, *AJHR*, 1882, G-1, p.13.

129 G.A. Preece, Resident Magistrate, Napier to Under-Secretary, 26 June 1882, *AJHR*, 1882, G-1, p.6.

130 Wilkinson to Under-Secretary, 17 May 1882, *AJHR*, 1882, G-1, p.4.

131 T. Jackson, Resident Magistrate, Papakura to Under-Secretary, 21 April 1885, *AJHR*, 1885, G-2, p.8.

132 H.W. Brabant to Under-Secretary, 30 May 1882, *AJHR*, 1882, G-1, p.5.

133 *NZPD*, vol.48, 10 September 1884, pp.229–30.

134 Under-Secretary to Native Minister, 28 May 1885, MA 21/19; G.A. Preece to Under-Secretary, 8 June 1885, *AJHR*, 1885, G-2, p.16.

135 For an account of one such campaigner see D. Dow, 'The Undying Verve of an Anti-Vaccinationist', *New Zealand Doctor*, 2 October 1996, p.51.

136 Similar attitudes were common in Britain at this time. See A. Hardy, *Epidemic Streets: Infectious Disease and The Rise of Preventive Medicine, 1856–1900*, Oxford, 1993.

137 General Report by J.E. Gorst, *AJHR*, 1862, E-9, p.12.

138 Tuke, 1863, pp.222ff.

139 Bishop to Under-Secretary, 24 June 1892,

AJHR, 1892, G-3, p.1. This was the final series of 'Reports from Officers in Native Districts'.

140 F.S. Maclean, *Challenge for Health: A History of Public Health in New Zealand*, Wellington, 1964, pp.246–53.

141 Pool, 1991, p.84.

142 R.S. Bush to Under-Secretary, 4 June 1883, *AJHR*, 1883, G-1A, p.5.

143 D.A. Dow, *Safeguarding the Public Health: A History of the New Zealand Department of Health*, Wellington, 1995, pp.34–5.

144 'Civil List Vote for Native Purposes', *AJHR*, 1895, G-5; 'Civil List, Native', *AJHR*, 1897, G-5.

145 *NZPD*, vol.82, 22 September 1893, p.561.

146 Seddon to Parata, 12 September 1898, MA 21/1, NA.

147 *NZPD*, vol.112, 27 July 1900, p.244.

148 Lange, 1972, p.95; K.S. Goodfellow, 'Health for the Maori? Health and the Maori Village Schools 1890–1940', MA thesis, Auckland, 1991, pp.ii–iii.

149 J.A. Pope, *Health for the Maori: A Manual for Use in Native Schools*, Wellington, 1884, p.82.

150 J.M. Barrington and T.H. Beaglehole, *Maori Schools in a Changing Society: An Historical Review*, Wellington, 1974, pp.101–5, 115.

151 Butterworth and Young, 1990, p.45; Goodfellow, 1991, p.5; Barrington and Beaglehole, 1974, pp.124–5.

152 Lange, 1972, p.95.

153 R.W. Woon to Under-Secretary, 28 May 1878, *AJHR*, 1878, G-1, p.15.

154 See Regulation 2(2), in *AJHR*, 1880, H-1F.

155 H.W. Bishop, Resident Magistrate, Mangonui to Under-Secretary, 30 April 1885, *AJHR*, 1885, G-2, pp.2–3.

156 *AJHR*, 1885, E-2, p.3.

157 See 1892 memorandum from the Inspector-General of Education, cited in Goodfellow, 1991, pp.16–17.

158 'Pakeha and Maori: A Narrative of the Premier's Trip Through the Native Districts of the North Island', *AJHR*, 1895, G-1, pp.71, 83.

159 Pope joined the Education Department in 1879, about the time the Native Schools were transferred. He remained in the post, latterly with the title of chief inspector, until 1903. See W. Renwick, 'Pope, James Henry, 1837–1913', *The Dictionary of New Zealand Biography: Volume 2: 1870–1900*, Wellington, 1993, pp.393–5.

160 Dow, 1995, pp.33–4; Goodfellow, 1991, p.24; Renwick, 1993, p.395.

161 S. von Sturmer, Resident Magistrate, Hokianga to Under-Secretary, 7 May 1880, *AJHR*, 1880, G-4, p.2.

162 Grace's proposal was eventually published. See 'Correspondence Relative to Fever Amongst the Natives at Herekino', *AJHR*, 1890, G-6.

163 See, for example, von Sturmer to Under-Secretary, 20 April 1885, Bishop to same, 30 April 1885, *AJHR*, 1885, G-2, pp.1–3, and Bush to same, 3 May 1886, *AJHR*, 1886, G-2, pp.12–13.

164 'Education: Native Schools', *AJHR*, 1885, G-2, pp.2, 14.

165 Davis, 13 March 1891, *AJHR*, 1891, G-2.

166 J.F. Cody, *Man of Two Worlds: Sir Maui Pomare*, Wellington, 1953, pp.25–9; Lange, 1972, pp.113–16.

167 Letter from Rewiti Morgan, in 'Education: Native Schools', *AJHR*, 1892, E-2, pp.3–4.

168 See M.P.K. Sorrenson, 'Modern Maori: The Young Maori Party to Mana Motuhake', in K. Sinclair (ed.), *The Oxford Illustrated History of New Zealand*, Auckland, 1990, pp.323–31.

169 M.H. Durie, *Whaiora: Maori Health Development*, Auckland, 1994, p.39.

170 For a summary of environmental health in nineteenth century New Zealand see Maclean, 1964, pp.59–90 and Dow, 1995, pp.15–41.

Chapter 3

1 R.T. Lange, 'The Revival of a Dying Race: A Study of Maori Health Reform 1900–1918 and its Nineteenth Century Background', MA thesis, Auckland, 1972, pp.170, 173–4.

2 D.A. Dow, '"Here is my habitation": Dr James Malcolm Mason and Otaki', *Historical Journal/Otaki Historical Society*, vol.20, 1997, pp.54–7.

3 *AJHR*, 1901, H-31, p.14.

4 G.M. Valentine, 'Maui Pomare and the Adventist Connection', in P.H. Ballis (ed.), *In and Out of The World: Seventh-Day Adventists in New Zealand*, Palmerston North, 1985, pp.82–108. The missionary motif was frequently employed in the first decade of the twentieth century.

5 The two had an affinity based partly on nationality. Mason was a Scotsman from Arbroath, an east coast fishing port, while Pomare's maternal grandfather was a Scottish sailor and whaler.

6 *AJHR*, 1904, H-31, p.65.

7 *NZMJ*, vol.3, 1904, pp.236–8.

8 'Reports of Dr Pomare, Health Officer to the Maoris, and of the Native Sanitary Inspectors', *AJHR*, 1907, H-31, p.52.

9 *NZPD*, vol.124, 29 July 1903, p.63.

10 Lange, 1972, Appendix III.

11 See memoranda in H 1, 160/22 (13498), NA.

12 Lange, 1972, p.194.

13 Mason to Under-Secretary, 18 September 1906, MA 21/20, NA.

14 *NZPD*, vol.138, 12 October 1906, p.249.

15 Under-Secretary to Native Minister, 12 October 1906, MA 21/20, NA. Lange, 1972, Appendix III provides a breakdown of the Civil List from 1885 to 1920 under the headings pensioners, medicines and doctors' subsidies, rations, contingencies and others. The sum given over to rations varied from a low of £91 in 1884/5 to a high of £2,947 in 1898/9. There is no correlation between these figures and those for medicines and subsidies.

16 Carroll to Fowlds, 17 October 1906, MA 21/20, NA.

17 Chief Health Officer to Minister of Health, 5 December 1906, and Under-Secretary to Native Minister, 12 December 1906, MA 21/20, NA.

18 *NZPD*, vol.139, 19 July 1907, pp.518–21, 525.

19 D.A. Dow, *Safeguarding the Public Health: A History of the New Zealand Department of Health*, Wellington, 1995, pp.61, 64.

20 Chief Health Officer to Minister of Health, 29 June 1909, MA 21/20, NA.

21 'Report by Dr Pomare on Sanitary Conditions of the Maori', *AJHR*, 1909, H-31, p.60.

22 Chief Health Officer to Pomare, 31 July 1909, and Pomare to Chief Health Officer, 2 August 1909, MA 21/20, NA. The formal wording of the two memos suggests a certain coolness between the two, unlike the warm relationship between Pomare and Mason.

23 Under-Secretary to Acting Prime Minister, 5 August 1909, and Ngata to Acting Prime Minister, 18 August 1909, MA 21/20, NA.

24 *NZPD*, vol.148, 10 December 1909, p.943.

25 The following account is based on correspondence covering the period 27 July 1910 to 29 April 1911, in MA 21/20, NA.

26 Hospitals and Charitable Aid Supply debate, *NZPD*, vol.156, 3 October 1911, pp.317–18.

27 The phrase was used by Hone Heke during the initial parliamentary discussions. See *NZPD*, vol.114, 28 August 1900, p.373.

28 *NZPD*, vol.115, 12 October 1900, pp.201–3.

29 Lange, 1972, pp.186–7.

30 Both accounts were published on 8 May 1901.

31 M. King, *Te Puea: A Biography*, Auckland, 1990, pp.32, 58 (fn.20).

32 Lange, 1972, pp.299–300.

33 Pomare used this title in his evidence for the 'Report of the West Coast Settlement Reserves (North Island) Commission', *AJHR*, 1912, G-2, p.105.
34 *AJHR*, H-31, 1906, pp.73–5, 1907, p.60.
35 Mair to Under-Secretary, 1 August 1906, MA 23/14, NA.
36 Undated memorandum from Edgar to Native Minister, 1906, MA 21/20, NA.
37 Supply debate: Maori Councils, *NZPD*, vol.137, 21 September 1906, p.748.
38 Lange, 1972, p.255.
39 J.A. Williams, 'Maori Society and Politics 1891–1909', PhD thesis, Wisconsin, 1963, pp.147–9, 169ff; F.S. Maclean, *Challenge for Health: A History of Public Health in New Zealand*, Wellington, 1964, p.193.
40 *NZPD*, vol.144, 20 August 1908, p.275.
41 *NZPD*, vol.148, 10 December 1909, p.943.
42 See comments by W. Dinnie (Tokerau), G.H. Woods (Whangarei), W.H. Bowler (Manakau, Thames etc), A. Keefer (Gisborne) and H.W. Bishop (South Island). A dissenting view came from J.W. Browne (Rotorua), who found no evidence to support this view and recommended frequent inspections of kainga by competent advisers. See *AJHR*, 1911, H-14A.
43 Address in Reply, *NZPD*, vol.154, 3 August 1911, p.155.
44 Supply debate: Maori Councils, *NZPD*, vol.164, 5 September 1913, p.447. For other assessments of the work of Maori Councils in this period see Lange, 1972, pp.254–62, and R.J. Martin, 'Aspects of Maori Affairs in the Liberal Period', MA thesis, Auckland, 1956, pp.82–111.
45 Buck made this comment during a discussion on venereal disease. See *Transactions of the Tenth Session of the Australasian Medical Congress*, Auckland, 1916, p.143.
46 J.B. Condliffe, *Te Rangi Hiroa: The Life of Sir Peter Buck*, Christchurch, 1971, p.81.
47 *AJHR*, 1908, H-31, p.130.
48 *AJHR*, 1909, H-31, p.37.
49 The hospital statistics in the following paragraphs are derived from the annual reports in *AJHR*, H-22.
50 *AJHR*, 1908, H-22, p.52.
51 *AJHR*, 1909, H-22, p.40.
52 Supply debate: Health Department, *NZPD*, vol.140, 5 September 1907, pp.720–2.
53 *AJHR*, 1907, H-22, p.37. In 1911 Whangarei had a nominal bed complement of 20 and an average occupancy of 11 patients. These figures were unlikely to have changed greatly in the previous four years.
54 *AJHR*, 1905, H-22, p.25.
55 *NZPD*, vol.156, 3 October 1911, p.318.
56 See G.K. Welch, *Doctor Smith: Hokianga's 'King of the North'*, Hamilton, 1965, *passim*.
57 G.M. Smith, 'Dr Smith and the Jones Baby', in M. Damian (comp.), *Growl You May But Go You Must*, Wellington, 1968, p.40.
58 Auckland Hospital Board minutes, 30 March 1903, A493/35, NA (Auckland). The minutes record that the solicitor's letter was 'received' but give no indication of any resulting discussion.
59 Auckland Hospital Board minutes, 26 February 1900, A493/72, and 28 August 1905, A493/155, NA (Auckland).
60 Auckland Hospital Board minutes, 23 October 1905, A493/155, NA (Auckland). The Costley Block was opened in 1898 and extended in 1905. From the latter year it accepted an increasing number of adult patients. See M. Brown, D. Masters and B. Smith, *Nurses of Auckland: The History of the General Nursing Programme in the Auckland School of Nursing*, Auckland, 1995, pp.38–9.
61 See King, 1990, p.33, and L.A. Ferguson, 'Marae Based Health Initiatives Within the Tainui Iwi From 1970–1995', MA thesis, Auckland, 1997, pp.17–18. King cited his source as F.O.V. Acheson, 'Princess Te Puea Speaks', *New Zealand Mirror*, vol.18, 1940.

62 In her reply Stewart asked Edgar to give her love to his wife with hopes that they might spend an afternoon together if she visited the Exhibition—presumably the forthcoming Christchurch Exhibition.
63 This account is based on the correspondence in MA 21/20, NA. Edgar's comment is reproduced in King, 1990, p.33 and Ferguson, 1997, pp.17–18.
64 See D.A. Dow, 'Springs of Charity? The Development of the New Zealand Hospital System, 1876–1910', in L. Bryder (ed.), *A Healthy Country: Essays on the Social History of Medicine in New Zealand*, Wellington, 1991, pp.52–6; D.A. Dow, 'Up With the World? The New Zealand Hospital System, 1876–1910', in P. Winterton and D. Gurry (eds), *The Impact of the Past Upon the Present: Second National Conference of the Australian Society of the History of Medicine: Perth, July 1991*, Perth, 1992, pp.103–7.
65 *AJHR*, 1907, H-31, pp.2, 52.
66 *NZPD*, vol.140, 5 September 1907, pp.720, 723.
67 'Proposed Amendment of Hospitals and Charitable Institutions Acts: Conference of Delegates of Hospital and Charitable Aid Boards and Separate Institutions, Held at Wellington on the 9th, 10th, and 11th June, 1908', *AJHR*, 1908, H-22A, p.1.
68 Waikato Hospital Board to Joseph Ward, 18 July 1910, quoted in R.E. Wright-St Clair, *From Cottage to Regional Base Hospital: Waikato Hospital 1887–1987*, Hamilton, 1987, p.31.
69 Chief Health Officer to Under-Secretary, 27 October 1910, MA 21/20, NA.
70 'Hospitals and Charitable Institutions in the Colony: Appendix III: Minutes, Reports of Proceedings, etc of the Hospitals Conference, June 1911', *AJHR*, 1911, H-31, p.163. For an assessment of the amalgamation see Dow, 1995, pp.67–72.
71 *AJHR*, 1911, H-31, pp.182–3.
72 Supply debate: Hospitals and Charitable Aid, *NZPD*, vol.156, 3 October 1911, pp.317–18.
73 *AJHR*, 1913, H-31, pp.2–3.
74 *AJHR*, 1902, H-31, p.65.
75 *AJHR*, 1906, H-31, p.74.
76 Wi Repa to Chief Health Officer, 8 July 1911, H 1, 160/14, NA.
77 G.V. Butterworth and H.R. Young, *Maori Affairs: A Department and the People Who Made It*, Wellington, 1990, pp.61–2.
78 Supply debate: Justice: Maori Councils, *NZPD*, vol.125, 8 September 1903, p.381.
79 *NZPD*, vol.129, 10 August 1904, p.344.
80 *NZPD*, vol.135, 20 September 1905, p.25.
81 Report of Waaka Te Huia, Sanitary Inspector, Dargaville, *AJHR*, 1908, H-31, p.134. The Dargaville project may have been compromised by the erection of the Northern Wairoa Hospital at Te Kopuru in 1903.
82 *AJHR*, 1905, H-31, pp.57–8.
83 *AJHR*, 1907, H-31, pp.55–6. Mokonuiarangi made no reference to Ballance's 1885 promise of a hospital in return for ceding the Ohinemutu lands.
84 *AJHR*, 1907, H-31, p.60.
85 A.H. McKegg, '"Ministering Angels": The Government Backblock Nursing Service and the Maori Health Nurses, 1909–1939', MA thesis, Auckland, 1991, p.171.
86 *New Zealand Official Yearbook*, 1990, p.158.
87 M. Belgrave, '"Medical Men" and "Lady Doctors": The Making of a New Zealand Profession 1867–1941', PhD thesis, Victoria, 1985, pp.244, 247.
88 *NZPD*, vol.80, 28 July 1893, p.305.
89 *NZPD*, vol.111, 6 July 1900, pp.316–17.
90 *NZPD*, vol.126, 7 October 1903, p.262.
91 *NZPD*, vol.133, 16 August 1905, p.674.
92 *NZPD*, vol.135, 20 September 1905, pp.25–6.
93 *NZPD*, vol.140, 21 August 1907, p.342.
94 *AJHR*, 1906, H-22, p.14.
95 *NZPD*, vol.140, 11 September 1907, p.816.
96 *NZPD*, vol.124, 4 August 1903, p.184.
97 *NZPD*, vol.125, 1 September 1903, pp.196, 198, 16 September 1903, p.563.

98 *NZPD*, vol.129, 19 August 1904, pp.581–3.

99 See M. Tennant, *Paupers and Providers: Charitable Aid in New Zealand*, Wellington, 1989, *passim*.

100 *AJHR*, 1902, H-31, pp.62–3.

101 *AJHR*, 1907, H-31, pp.iv–v.

102 Chief Health Officer to Mercer, 8 January 1913, H 1, 160/5, NA.

103 *AJHR*, 1913, H-31, pp.2–3.

104 H. Chesson to Chief Health Officer, 7 February 1919, H 1, 160/17 (13496), NA.

105 Under-Secretary to Bishop, 23 June 1906, and Bishop to Under-Secretary, 30 June 1906, MA 21/20, NA. Bishop joined the Native Department in 1873 and was Resident Magistrate in the Bay of Islands (1882–93) before his removal to Christchurch. See *Cyclopedia of New Zealand: Volume 3: Canterbury Provincial District*, Christchurch, 1903, p.243.

106 Mair to Under-Secretary, 1 August 1906, MA 23/14, NA.

107 *NZPD*, vol.138, 12 October 1906, p.249, 29 October 1906, pp.714–15. On 29 October Health Minister George Fowlds informed Parliament that the Health Department takeover of the NMOs had only occurred within the previous week.

108 Under-Secretary to Chief Health Officer, 26 October 1906, MA 21/20, NA; 'Medical Attendance on Maoris (Return Relative to)', *AJHR*, 1906, Session II, G-4. The North Island locations (in the order listed) were Mangonui, Kaitaia, Rawene, Ohaeawai, Kawakawa, Dargaville, Huntly, Raglan, Kawhia, Otorohanga and Taumarunui, Te Kuiti, Taupo, Te Puke, Whakatane, Waipiro Bay, Tolago Bay, Wairoa, New Plymouth, Waipawa, Pahiatua, Hutt. Those in the South Island were Kaikoura, Kaiapoi, Akaroa, Little River, Southbridge, Rapaki, Temuka, Palmerston, Oamaru, Waimate, Westport, Port Chalmers, Taieri, Balclutha, Riverton, Bluff. Peter Webster's claim that there were about 30 doctors 'scattered over the North Island' resulted from a misreading of the printed return laid before Parliament in September 1906. The 30 names represented just 21 locations (all in the North Island), with nine replacements listed alongside their predecessors. See P. Webster, *Rua and the Maori Millennium*, Wellington, 1979, p.144; *NZPD*, vol.137, 29 August 1906, p.195.

109 *AJHR*, 1911, H-14A, p.2.

110 *AJHR*, 1907, H-31, pp.iv–v.

111 *NZPD*, vol.139, 19 July 1907, pp.518–21.

112 *NZPD*, vol.140, 20 and 21 August 1907, pp.302–3, 371–2, vol.144, 28 August 1908, pp.506–7.

113 *NZPD*, vol.140, 7 August 1907, pp.87–8.

114 *AJHR*, 1903, H-31, p.71.

115 Buck to Chief Health Officer, 15 August 1907, Minister to Chief Health Officer, 6 January 1909, and Buck to Chief Health Officer, 30 January 1909, H 1, 160/32, NA.

116 *AJHR*, 1909, H-31, p.61.

117 Chief Health Officer to Minister of Health, 29 June 1909, MA 21/20, NA.

118 Chief Health Officer to District Health Officer John Purdy, 16 June 1909, MA 21/21, NA.

119 Purdy to Chief Health Officer, 2 July 1909, MA 21/20, NA.

120 I.S. Ewing, 'Public Service Reform in New Zealand, 1866–1912', MA thesis, Auckland, 1979, p.43. For an assessment of the impact on one government department see J.E. Martin, *Holding the Balance: A History of New Zealand's Department of Labour, 1891–1995*, Christchurch, 1996, pp.80–2, 102–3.

121 *NZPD*, vol.148, 8 December 1909, p.748.

122 The memo was typed on unheaded paper and it is not clear which department prepared it. The full list, in the order in which it appeared, was NGAPUHI: Kaitaia, Kawakawa, Dargaville, Whangaroa, Otamatea, Whangarei, Ohaeawai, Hokianga, Mangonui; WAIKATO: Huntly, Raglan, Taumarunui, Te Kuiti, Tuakau, Otorohanga, Morrinsville,

Kawhia, Thames, Coromandel, Paeroa, Hukanui; BAY OF PLENTY: Tauranga, Te Puke, Whakatane, Opotiki; TAUPO: Tapueharuru; EAST COAST: Waiapu, Tolago Bay, Te Karaka, Wairoa, Takapau, Te Hauke, Pahiatua, Masterton, Hutt; WEST COAST: Hawera, Patea, Manaia, New Plymouth, Opunake, Foxton, Oroua and Manawatu, Wanganui; SOUTH ISLAND: Picton, Havelock, Henley, Hokitika, Temuka, Oamaru, Nelson, Rapaki, Marlborough, Kaiapoi, Riverton, Waihao, Westport, Port Chalmers, Kaikoura, Moeraki, Southbridge, Motueka, Banks Peninsula, Akaroa, Bluff and Stewart Island, Balclutha, Takaka.

123 See, for example, King, 1990, p.33 which claims that few Waikato doctors would attend Maori patients and that in 1906 only four Waikato doctors received payment from the Native Department.

124 *NZPD*, vol.149, 13 July 1910, p.445.

125 *NZPD*, vol.154, 9 August 1911, pp.305–6, 320. It appears the former NMO, Herbert Barclay, was one of those dispensed with in 1909.

126 *NZPD*, vol.163, 30 July 1913, pp.219–20.

127 *AJHR*, H-31, 1914, p.3, 1915, p.4.

128 *AJHR*, 1915, H-31, pp.26–7, 28. The four were George McCall Smith (Rawene), Harry Phippen (Wellsford), Alexander Macfarlane (Te Puke) and Arthur Latchmore (Taupo).

129 The following paragraphs are based on files relating to the Native medical attendants at Kaitaia (H 1, 160/24, NA) and Whangaroa (H 1, 160/5, NA).

130 The doctor on this occasion was Percy Lunn, the apparently alcoholic son of an English brewer. See Dow, 1995, p.82.

131 W.A. Brunton, 'Hostages to History', *New Zealand Health Review*, vol.3, no.2, 1983, pp.3, 6.

132 *NZPD*, vol.139, 19 July 1907, pp.524–5.

133 *NZPD*, vol.124, 29 July 1903, p.63.

134 Barclay to Carroll, 8 October 1903, H 1, 160/34, NA.

135 Makgill to Under-Secretary, 27 July 1910, and Makgill to Chief Health Officer, 28 July 1907, MA 21/20, NA.

136 Lange, 1972, pp.48–9.

137 Teichelmann to Acting Chief Health Officer, 18 August 1914, H 1, 160/7, NA.

138 M.H. Durie, 'Implications of Policy and Management Decisions on Maori Health: Contemporary Issues and Responses', in M.W. Raffel and N.K. Raffel (eds), *Perspectives on Health Policy: Australia, New Zealand, United States*, New York, 1986, p.207.

139 Lange, 1972, p.161.

140 Te Rangi Hiroa, *The Coming of the Maori*, Wellington, 1949, pp.410–12.

141 Ngata to Buck, 30 January 1899, in M.P.K. Sorrenson (ed.), *Na To Hoa Aroha: From Your Dear Friend: The Correspondence Between Sir Apirana Ngata and Sir Peter Buck*, Auckland, 1986, vol.1, pp.15–16.

142 O.T.J. Alpers, 'The Young Maori Party', 1903, reprinted in P.M. Jackson (ed.), *Maori and Education or, the Education of Natives in New Zealand and its Dependencies*, Wellington, 1931, pp.144–61.

143 *AJHR*, 1903, H-31, p.67; *NZPD*, vol.125, 15 September 1903, p.549.

144 Dunedin Hospital Annual Report, 1906–7. The Dunedin Hospital Trustees Minute Book 1895–1907, Hocken Library, Dunedin, which recorded his appointment on 19 February 1907, made no comment on the fact that he was a Maori.

145 District Health Officer, memorandum to Valintine, 10 July 1913, following interview with Wi Repa, H 1, 160/14, NA. Wi Repa's bitterness was recorded in R.R. Alexander, *The Story of Te Aute College*, Wellington, 1951, p.247, and Lange, 1972, p.246.

146 Lange, 1972, p.246.

147 Chief Health Officer to Minister of Health, 18 July 1913, H 1, 160/14, NA. My assessment is based on the contents of this file and another, H 1, 184/250, NA,

entitled 'Medical Registration: Wi Repa 1908–46'.

148 *AJHR*, 1906, Session II, H-31, pp.67–8.
149 Undated memorandum from Edgar to Native Minister, 1906, MA 21/20, NA.
150 *NZPD*, vol.139, 19 July 1907, pp.518–21.
151 D. Colquhoun, 'The History of a Medical School', *NZMJ*, vol.8, no.35, 1910, pp.1–11.
152 Lange, 1972, p.46.
153 *NZPD*, vol.156, 3 October 1911, p.318.
154 'Report of the Conference on Administrative Control and Treatment of Tuberculosis', *AJHR*, 1913, H-31A, p.9.
155 *NZPD*, vol.167, 13 December 1913, p.1153.
156 *AJHR*, 1901, B-7, p.15.
157 J.F. Cody, *Man of Two Worlds: Sir Maui Pomare*, Wellington, 1953, pp.73–4.
158 *AJHR*, 1903, H-31, pp.v, 66.
159 Supply debate: Justice Department (Maori Councils), *NZPD*, vol.125, 8 September 1903, p.380.
160 *AJHR*, 1905, H-31, pp.56–62. When Tutere Wi Repa was struggling to complete his medical course in 1905–6 it was suggested he might become a Maori sanitary officer. See Lange, 1972, pp.137–9.
161 *AJHR*, 1907, H-31, p.60.
162 See lists and tables in MA 21/20 and MA 23/14, NA.
163 Supply debate: Health Department, *NZPD*, vol.144, 28 August 1908, pp.506–7.
164 *NZPD*, vol.154, 3 August 1911, p.155, 9 August 1911, p.305.
165 Maori Councils: Minutes of General Conference 1903–11, MA-MC 3/2, NA.
166 *NZPD*, vol.156, 26 September 1911, p.126.
167 Cody, 1953, pp.73–4.
168 *AJHR*, 1908, H-31, pp.119–20.
169 Maori Councils: Minutes of General Conference 1903–11, 20 July 1908, MA-MC 3/2, NA.
170 *AJHR*, 1907, H-31, p.60; Condliffe, 1971, p.83.
171 *AJHR*, 1909, H-31, p.61.
172 Williams' Journal, 15 November 1847, in F. Porter (ed.), *The Turanga Journals, 1840–1850: Letters and Journals of William and Jane Williams Missionaries to Poverty Bay*, Wellington, 1974, p.456.
173 Wilkinson to Under-Secretary, 28 June 1892, *AJHR*, 1892, G-3, p.2.
174 J.A. Pope, *Health for the Maori: A Manual for Use in Native Schools*, Wellington, 1884, pp.96–7.
175 McLean, 1964, Foreword.
176 *AJHR*, 1902, H-31, pp.61–4.
177 *NZPD*, vol.135, 22 September 1905, pp.146–7.
178 *AJHR*, 1907, H-31, pp.55–6, 61.
179 The phrase was Carroll's. See *NZPD*, vol.139, 19 July 1907, p.510.
180 *NZPD*, vol.139, 19 July 1907, pp.510–25.
181 For analysis of the Act and its effect see R.T. Lange, 'The Tohunga and the Government in the Twentieth Century', *Annual: University of Auckland History Society*, 1968, pp.12–38; M. Voyce, 'Maori Healers in New Zealand: the Tohunga Suppression Act 1907', *Oceania: A Journal Devoted to the Study of the Native Peoples of Australia, New Guinea, and Other Islands of the Pacific Ocean*, vol.60, no.2, 1989, pp.99–123.
182 *AJHR*, 1908, H-31, pp.132–3.
183 *NZPD*, vol.139, 19 July 1907, p.513
184 See J.M. Gray, 'Potions, Pills and Poisons: Quackery in New Zealand, circa 1900–1915', BA(Hons) thesis, Otago, 1980, and L. May, 'Medical Malversations: Quacks, the Quackery Prevention Act 1908, and the Orthodox Medical Profession's Push for Power', BA(Hons) thesis, Otago, 1994.
185 T. Bevan, *Reminiscences of an Old Colonist*, Otaki, 1911, p.11.
186 *NZPD*, vol.165, 26 September 1913, p.267.
187 *AJHR*, 1898, E-2, p.12. For critiques of this initial proposal see P.J. Wood, 'Efficient Preachers of the Gospel of Health: The 1898 Scheme for Educating Maori Nurses', *Nursing Praxis in New Zealand*, vol.7, no.1, 1992, pp.12–21; M. Holdaway, 'Where Are the Maori Nurses

Who Were to Become Those "efficient preachers of the gospel of health"?', *Nursing Praxis in New Zealand*, vol.8, no.1, 1993, pp.25–34.

188 G. Conly, *A Case History: The Hawke's Bay Hospital Board 1876–1989*, Napier, 1992, p.48.

189 Stewart to Under-Secretary, 19 July 1906, MA 21/20, NA.

190 Auckland Hospital Board minutes, 18 December 1905, 12 March, 7 May, 27 August, 10 September, 22 October 1906, 3 June, 1 July, 28 August, 7 October 1907, A493/155, NA (Auckland).

191 Auckland Hospital Board minutes, 13 January, 9 March 1908, A493/155, NA (Auckland). The parameters of this revised scheme had been worked out at a meeting in November 1908 between George Fowlds, Minister for both Health and Education, Drs Mason, Valintine and Pomare, and the Secretary for Education. See McKegg, 1991, pp.65–6.

192 *NZMJ*, vol.3, 1904, pp.236–8.

193 *AJHR*, 1908, H-31, p.119.

194 *AJHR*, 1907, H-31, p.54.

195 *Kai Tiaki*, January 1909, pp.4–5.

196 Chief Health Officer to J. Purdy, 16 June 1909, MA 21/21, NA.

197 'Medical Attendance on Natives', Circular 295, MA 21/20, NA.

198 McKegg, 1991, pp.78–9.

199 *AJHR*, 1911, H-31, p.4.

200 *Ibid.*, pp.160–1, 163–5, 182–5.

201 *NZMJ*, vol.10, 1911, pp.46–52.

202 *NZPD*, vol.156, 3 October 1911, pp.317–18.

203 *AJHR*, 1912, H-31, pp.9, 77. For Makgill's status and influence see G.W. Rice, 'The Making of New Zealand's 1920 Health Act', *NZJH*, April 1988, pp.3–22.

204 *NZMJ*, vol.11, 1912, p.59.

205 *NZPD*, vol.163, 30 July 1913, pp.219–20.

206 McKegg, 1991, p.123.

207 See, for example, *Kai Tiaki*, July 1911, pp.108–10, 125, January 1912, pp.25–7, October 1912, p.99, October 1913, pp.146, 152–3.

208 *Kai Tiaki*, April 1917, p.117.

209 *NZPD*, vol.149, 20 July 1910, pp.690, 706, vol.155, 6 September 1911, pp.337, 340, vol.156, 3 October 1911, pp.317–18. See tribute to Collins, *NZPD*, vol.239, 10 August 1934, pp.141–3.

210 McKegg, 1991, pp.62–3; Wood, 1992, p.12.

211 McKegg, 1991, p.74; *Kai Tiaki*, July 1909, pp.104–5, July 1910, pp.103–4.

212 For Hei's obituary see *Kai Tiaki*, January 1911, pp.37–8. For a more detailed account of her career see '"Efficient Preachers of the Gospel of Health": Akinihi Hei (1882?–1910) and the Maori Health Nursing Scheme', in P.A. Sargison, *Notable Women in New Zealand Health/Te Hauora ki Aotearoa: Ona Wahine Rongonui*, Wellington, 1993, pp.21–4, and P.A. Sargison, 'Hei, Akenehi, 1877/78?–1910', in *The Dictionary of New Zealand Biography: Volume 3: 1900–1920*, Wellington, 1996, pp.204–5.

213 *AJHR*, 1911, H-31, p.183.

214 McKegg, 1991, pp.71–5.

215 *Kai Tiaki*, April 1912, p.38.

216 *AJHR*, 1923, H-31, pp.31–2.

217 *AJHR*, 1906, H-31, p.67.

218 One of Mason's mentors, Sir James Crichton-Browne, was Vice President of the 1902 Imperial Vaccination League. See D. Dow, 'The Undying Verve of an Anti-Vaccinationist', *New Zealand Doctor*, 2 October 1996, p.51.

219 Lange, 1972, p.213. On the 1904 campaign see Dow, 1995, pp.51–3.

220 *AJHR*, 1903, H-31, p.v.

221 *Ibid.*, H-31, pp.68, 72–3.

222 *AJHR*, 1904, H-31, pp.60–4.

223 *NZMJ*, vol.4, 1905, pp.338–44.

224 G.T. Bloomfield, *New Zealand: A Handbook of Historical Statistics*, Boston, 1984, p.82.

225 *AJHR*, 1906, H-31, pp.78, 80.

226 On the activities of the anti-vaccinationists see Dow, 1995, pp.51–2, and Dow, 1996, p.51.

227 *New Zealand Observer*, 18 January 1908, p.4.

228 Quoted in *New Zealand Observer*, 24 October 1908, p.4.

229 Maclean, 1964, pp.232–6 estimated there were 1,978 Maori cases and 55 deaths, compared with 116 European cases and no deaths. For a detailed account of the epidemic see A.S. Day, '"The Maori Malady": The 1913 Smallpox Epidemic and Its Nineteenth Century Background', MA thesis, Auckland, 1998. Day's thesis was not available when I compiled this section.

230 In a speech by A.M. Myers (Auckland), *NZPD*, vol.162, 8 July 1913, p.241.

231 This initial debate appears in *NZPD*, vol.162, 11 July 1913, pp.454–8.

232 See, for instance, *NZPD*, vol.162, 23 July 1913, pp.724–5, vol.163, 6 August 1913, pp.443–4, and P. Buck's contribution to discussion on venereal disease, *Transactions of the Tenth Session of the Australasian Medical Congress, Auckland*, Wellington, 1916, pp.141–2.

233 *NZPD*, vol.163, 24 July, 6 August 1913, pp.14–21, 442–8.

234 *NZPD*, vol.164, 21 August 1913, pp.1–2.

235 *Ibid.*, 29 August 1913, pp.206–9.

236 *NZPD*, vol.165, 16 October 1913, pp.764, 779–80.

237 P. Buck, 'The Smallpox Epidemic Amongst the Maoris in the Northern District', *Transactions of the Tenth Session of the Australasian Medical Congress, Auckland*, Wellington, 1916, pp.212–23.

238 'Smallpox Epidemic (Particulars Relative to the)', *AJHR*, 1914, H-33.

239 *AJHR*, 1914, H-31, pp.60–1.

240 *NZPD*, vol.165, 26 September, 1 October 1913, pp.262, 360, 374.

241 See Maclean, 1964, pp.246–81.

242 See Health Department annual reports in *AJHR*, H-31.

243 Barclay to Carroll, 8 October 1903, H 1, 160/34, NA.

244 P.H. Buck, 'Foreword', in I.L.G. Sutherland (ed.), *The Maori People Today: A General Survey*, Oxford, 1940, pp.8–9.

245 Buck's report, *AJHR*, 1907, H-31, p.61.

246 Buck's report, *AJHR*, 1906, H-31, pp. 73–4.

247 Makgill to Dr C.C. Jenkins, 20 January 1911, H 1, 162/16, NA.

248 Makgill to Under-Secretary, 21 January 1911, MA 21/20, NA. This has sometimes been cited as proof of Makgill's racist antagonism to Maori. See, for example, Lange, 1972, p.201, and Webster, 1979, pp.145–6. In fact Makgill's uncompromising criticism of insanitary conditions in 1890s Auckland had been even more damning and made him hugely unpopular with its European inhabitants.

249 *AJHR*, 1918, H-31, p.5.

250 See, for example, comments by G.F. Powell (Waipiro), C. Gray (Gisborne) and F.M. Mackay (Auckland), *AJHR*, 1911, H-31, pp.8, 182–5.

251 *AJHR*, 1912, H-31, pp.76–7.

252 *Journal of the Department of Public Health, Hospitals, and Charitable Aid*, June 1918, p.175.

253 *Kai Tiaki*, October 1916, p.234.

254 *AJHR*, 1920, H-31, p.14.

255 *AJHR*, 1915, H-31, pp.26–7.

256 J.W. Butcher, 'Cancer Mortality in New Zealand', *New Zealand Official Yearbook*, 1917, p.776.

257 *NZMJ*, vol.4, pp.25–31.

258 *AJHR*, 1911, H-31, pp.169–82; 'Report of the Conference on Administrative Control and Treatment of Tuberculosis', *AJHR*, 1913, H-31A.

259 *NZPD*, vol.186, 28 July 1920, p.770; *NZMJ*, vol.19, 1920, pp.101–11.

260 L. Bryder, 'Tuberculosis and the Maori, 1900–1960', in P. Winterton and D. Gurry (eds), *The Impact of the Past Upon the Present: Second National Conference of the Australian Society of the History of Medicine: Perth, July 1991*, Perth, 1992, pp.191–4.

261 E. Chill, 'Phthisis and Superstition Among the Maories', *British Medical Journal*, 18 August 1906, p.376.

262 *AJHR*, 1903, H-31, p.72.

263 *AJHR*, 1904, H-31, p.65.

264 *AJHR*, 1908, H-31, pp.124, 130–1.
265 *AJHR*, 1909, H-31, pp.37–8.
266 See reports by Drs Sydney Champtaloup and Hugh Finch, *AJHR*, 1912, H-31, pp.76–7.
267 J.H. Crawshaw, 'Some Remarks on the Treatment of Tuberculosis Amongst the Maoris at Tuahiwi Park', *NZMJ*, vol.13, 1914, pp.346–8.
268 For the procedures involved see report by Christchurch's District Health Officer, *AJHR*, 1914, H-31, p.62.
269 *AJHR*, 1915, H–31, p.28.
270 *AJHR*, 1920, H-31, p.15.
271 G.W. Rice, *Black November: The 1918 Influenza Epidemic in New Zealand*, Wellington, 1988, pp.1, 3; L. Bryder, '"Lessons" of the 1918 Influenza Epidemic in Auckland', *NZJH*, vol.16, no.2, 1982, pp.116–17.
272 Chill, 1906, p.376.
273 *NZPD*, vol.138, 17 October 1906, p.304.
274 *NZPD*, vol.131, 2 November 1904, p.758.
275 *NZPD*, vol.154, 3 August 1911, p.156.
276 Health Department circular no.251, 7 April 1908, MA 21/21, NA. For comments on supplying adults see K.S. Goodfellow, 'Health for the Maori? Health and the Maori Village Schools 1890–1940', MA thesis, Auckland, 1991, pp.16–17.
277 Chief Health Officer to J. Purdy, 16 June 1909, MA 21/21, NA.
278 *AJHR*, 1911, H-31, p.183.
279 Cited in J.M. Barrington and T.H. Beaglehole, *Maori Schools in a Changing Society: An Historical Review*, Wellington, 1974, p.154.
280 *NZPD*, vol.165, 1 October 1913, pp.356, 360.
281 Native school teacher to 'Principal Medical Officer', 25 March 1919, H 1, 162/78 (12634), NA.
282 District Health Officer Robert Makgill to Chief Health Officer, 27 April 1915, H 1, 162/43 (12619), NA. For other evidence of such clashes see Goodfellow, 1991, p.29.
283 Goodfellow, 1991, pp.22–3.

Chapter 4

1 L. Bryder, '"Lessons" of the 1918 Influenza Epidemic in Auckland', *NZJH*, vol.16, no.2, 1982, p.106.
2 *AJHR*, 1919, H-31A, p.10.
3 The correspondence relating to this campaign is in H 1/36 (13303), NA.
4 In 1912 Pomare was appointed as a member of the Executive Council representing the 'Native race' and placed in charge of Maori Councils. According to Butterworth he was 'able to accomplish little in these minor posts'. See G. Butterworth, 'Pomare, Maui Wiremu Piti Naera 1875/76?–1930', in *The Dictionary of New Zealand Biography: Volume 3: 1900–1920*, Wellington, 1996, pp.404–7. The Native Minister at this time was W.H. Herries.
5 J.B. Condliffe, *Te Rangi Hiroa: The Life of Sir Peter Buck*, Christchurch, 1971, p.152.
6 H 1/36 (13303), NA.
7 *AJHR*, 1919, H-31A, p.37.
8 The comments of the two men were reprinted in the *Journal of the Department of Public Health, Hospitals, and Charitable Aid*, July 1919, vol.2, no.7, pp.186–91.
9 *AJHR*, 1919, H-31, p.5.
10 *AJHR*, 1920, H-31, p.14.
11 Both Bryder and Rice mistakenly refer to the Division of Maori Welfare, a title which bears quite different implications from Hygiene. See Bryder, 1982, pp.102, 118, and G.W. Rice, 'The Making of New Zealand's 1920 Health Act', *NZJH*, vol.22, no.1, April 1988, p.18. Rice's analysis of the Act contains no further reference to Maori.
12 Valintine to Buck, 7 September 1920, H 1, 121 B.75, NA.
13 See correspondence between Under-Secretary, Native Department and Director of Maori Hygiene, 3 and 5 August 1922, H 1, 121 B.72, NA.
14 *AJHR*, 1921, H-31, p.33.
15 *AJHR*, 1923, H-31, p.43.
16 *AJHR*, 1929, H-31, p.31, and Director of

Maori Hygiene to Director-General of Health, 9 December 1929, H 1, 160 (12038), NA.
17 Leaf to Chesson, 28 July, Chesson to Director-General of Health, 1 August 1930, H 1, 121/12, NA.
18 E.P. Ellison, 'The Maori and Hygiene', in P.M. Jackson (ed.), *Maori and Education or, the Education of Natives in New Zealand and its Dependencies*, Wellington, 1931, pp.293–4.
19 Tamihana Tikitere to Pomare, 22 November 1920, H 1, 121/13 B.74, NA.
20 Memo dated 2 September 1921, H 1, 121 B.72, NA.
21 *AJHR*, 1928, H-31, p.36.
22 Kaa to MOH, 20 August 1938, H 1, 121 B.75, NA. For Kaa's career in the Health Department see E.M. Ellis and H.M. Harte, 'A Maori Health Nurse', in S. Coney (ed.), *Standing In The Sunshine: A History of New Zealand Women Since They Won The Vote*, Auckland, 1993, pp.102–3, and D.A. Dow, *Safeguarding the Public Health: A History of the New Zealand Department of Health*, Wellington, 1995, pp.136–7.
23 *AJHR*, 1922, H-31, p.34.
24 *AJHR*, 1924, H-31, p.41.
25 Chairman to Director of Maori Hygiene, 29 October 1929, H 1, 121/17 B.75, NA.
26 Ritchie to Director-General of Health, 25 July 1931, H 1, 121/21, NA.
27 Minute of meeting of 7 January 1938, H 1, 194/1/4 (13923), NA.
28 Maori Councils Act 1900, section 16(7).
29 Quoted in R.T. Lange, 'The Revival of a Dying Race: A Study of Maori Health Reform 1900–1918 and its Nineteenth Century Background', MA Thesis, Auckland, 1972, p.259.
30 Under-Secretary to Director of Maori Hygiene, 7 April 1923, and reply dated 18 April 1923, H 1, 121 B.72, NA.
31 *AJHR*, 1930, H-31, p.40; Ellison, 1931, pp.293–4.
32 Ritchie to Director-General of Health, 24 December 1930 and 17 December 1932, H 1, 121/21, NA.
33 Details of the conference were forwarded by Carlyle Gilberd, Auckland's MOH. See Gilberd to Director-General of Health, 2 December 1938, H 1, 121 B.72, NA.
34 Buck to Under-Secretary, 17 May 1921, H 1, 121/10 B.74, NA.
35 See 'Sanitation of Maori Settlements: Ratana Pa 1925–40', H 1, 36/26 (13306), NA.
36 Buck to T. McKibbin, Director of Public Hygiene, 24 November 1926, H 1, 36/26, NA.
37 Ellison to Mayor of Marton, 1 July 1928, H 1, 194/1/19 (7960), NA.
38 Buck to Director-General of Health, 1 November 1921, H 1, 194/1/20 (8456), NA.
39 Buck to Director-General of Health, 15 June 1922, H 1, 194/1/21, NA; Buck to Gordon Smith, 4 July 1922, H 1, 36/26, NA.
40 Correspondence between Chesson and Buck, 14 and 21 July 1922, H 1, 194/1/21, NA.
41 Hooper to Buck, 31 October 1925, H 1, 121/25, NA.
42 *AJHR*, 1926, H-31, p.44.
43 Hooper to Buck, 12 May 1926, H 1, 121/22, NA.
44 Correspondence between Buck, Director-General of Health and Hooper, 26 June–29 September 1926, H 1, 36/26, NA.
45 Ellison, 1931, p.294.
46 See, for example, Director-General of Health to MOH, Napier, 19 October 1931, H 1, 121/23, NA.
47 I.L.G. Sutherland, *The Maori Situation*, Wellington, 1935, pp.103–4, 44.
48 *AJHR*, 1934, H-31, p.8.
49 Director-General of Health to Fraser, 14 February 1936, H 1, 194/8 B.125, NA.
50 S.M. Lambert, 'A Survey of the Maori Situation', unpublished report, 1937, p.53.
51 H.B. Turbott, 'Health and Social Welfare' in I.L.G. Sutherland (ed.), *The Maori People Today: A General Survey*,

Oxford, 1940, pp.262–3. Section 16(19) of the Maori Councils Act 1900 authorised councils to levy fines for 'non-compliance with or breach of all or any of the by-laws' relating to sanitation and public health, sly-grogging, the sale of tobacco, etc.

52 *AJHR*, 1921, B-7, p.121.

53 *AJHR*, 1929, B-1, p.267.

54 Valintine to Minister of Health, 29 February 1929, H 1, 54/24 B.19, NA.

55 Stallworthy to H.G. Dickie, Hawera, 12 December 1929, H 1, 160 (12038), NA.

56 Watt's words were almost a direct quote from Valintine's comments in 1911 on the benefits resulting from the 1909 amalgamation of the Hospitals and Health Departments.

57 M.H. Watt, 'The Rest of the Day to Myself', unpublished autobiography (deposited in Health Department), pp.83–4.

58 Lambert, 1937, pp.31–2.

59 *AJHR*, 1925, H-31, p.9.

60 *AJHR*, 1923, H-31, p.43, 1924, H-31, p.42. In 1922 Buck had published his survey of 814 officers and men of the Maori Battalion, modelled on the 1919 *Report of the Committee of the British Association on Anthropomorphic Investigation*. See Te Rangi Hiroa, 'Maori Somatology: Racial Averages', *Journal of the Polynesian Society*, vol.31, 1922, pp.37–44, 145–53, 159–70, vol.32, 1923, pp.21–8, 189–99.

61 Valintine to Buck, 19 May 1924, H 1, 172/21/52 (12197), NA.

62 Buck to Ngata, 8 March 1927, in M.P.K. Sorrenson (ed.), *Na To Hoa Aroha: From Your Dear Friend: The Correspondence Between Sir Apirana Ngata and Sir Peter Buck*, Auckland, vol.1, 1986, pp.47–9.

63 *AJHR*, 1927, H-31; 1928, H-31, p.4.

64 Correspondence between Ngata and Buck, 9 February, 28 August and 24 September 1928, in Sorrenson, vol.1, 1986, pp.66, 128, 135–6.

65 Ellison, 1931, pp.292–3.

66 F.S. Maclean, *Challenge for Health: A History of Public Health in New Zealand*, Wellington, 1964, pp.203–4.

67 M.H. Watt, summary of the Maori health situation, in Lambert, 1937, pp.31–2; Ngata to Buck, 15 May 1931, in Sorrenson, vol.2, 1987, p.140.

68 Watt, in Lambert, 1937, p.37.

69 Director-General of Health to Health Minister Peter Fraser, 14 February 1936, H 1, 194/8, NA.

70 *AJHR*, 1920, H-31, p.8.

71 Sorrenson, vol.1, 1986, pp.34–5. He provided no evidence to support this contention.

72 M.H. Durie, *Whaiora: Maori Health Development*, Auckland, 1994, p.45.

73 By 1930 there were still only four Maori medical graduates in New Zealand: Pomare, Buck, Ellison and Wi Repa. They were joined in that year by Louis Potaka.

74 Te Rangi Hiroa, *The Coming of the Maori*, Wellington, 1949, p.414.

75 Lambert, 1937, pp.8–10, 50–1. Lambert repeated his praise of the four men in his autobiography, *A Doctor in Paradise*, London, 1942, pp.263–4.

76 The article was reprinted in the *Journal of the Department of Public Health, Hospitals, and Charitable Aid*, May 1919, p.131.

77 The original Bay of Islands board was subdivided from 1 April 1920 into the Bay of Islands, Mangonui, Whangaroa and Hokianga hospital boards. See *Journal of the Department of Public Health, Hospitals, and Charitable Aid*, March 1920, p.89.

78 *Journal of the Department of Public Health, Hospitals, and Charitable Aid*, June 1920, p.181; *New Zealand Journal of Health and Hospitals*, July 1920, p.187. The change of name did not signify any major changes in direction or content.

79 *New Zealand Journal of Health and Hospitals*, July 1920, pp.189–91.

80 Dow, 1995, pp.97–100, 172–5.

81 'Hospitals Commission', *AJHR*, 1921, H-31A, p.11.

82 Frengley to Minister of Health, 19 September 1922, H 1, 54/24 B.19, NA.
83 Director-General of Health to Minister of Health, 5 September 1923, H 1, 54/24, NA.
84 Conference of Delegates of Hospital Boards, 7 October 1924, H 1, 44/41/7 (2328), NA.
85 Correspondence between Director-General of Health and Under-Secretary, Native Department, 26 February and 14 April 1926, H 1, 54/24, NA.
86 Killick to Director-General of Health, 19 July 1927, H 1, 160 (12038), NA.
87 Notes of meeting held on 27 April 1927, 'Native Medical Services General 1927–39', H 1, 160 (12038), NA
88 Deputy Native Trustee to Director-General of Health, 1 August 1927, H 1, 160 (12038), NA.
89 See correspondence between Minister of Health and Matamata Town Board, 18, 27 May 1927, H 1, 160 (12038), NA.
90 'Maoris in Hospitals: Hospital Boards Confer', *Waikato Times*, 27 August 1929; *Dominion*, 28 August 1929.
91 Notes prepared by A. Peebles, chairman of Bay of Plenty Hospital Board, 5 September 1929, H 1, 54/24, NA; *Dominion*, 6 September 1929.
92 Ngata to Ward, 16 September 1929, H 1, 54/24, NA.
93 Correspondence between New Zealand Farmers' Union, Prime Minister and Minister of Health, 15 July, 12 September, 15 September 1930, H 1, 54/24, NA. The NZFU later challenged the Minister's claim as unproved. See *Dominion*, 8 July 1931.
94 R.E. Wright-St Clair, *From Cottage to Regional Base Hospital: Waikato Hospital 1887–1987*, Hamilton, 1987, pp.57–8.
95 'Hospital Boards Association Executive Committee Report on Hospital Treatment and Relief of Maoris', 7 October 1932, H 1, 54/24, NA.
96 'Report of Committee on Rating of Native Land', *AJHR*, 1933, G-11, p.3.
97 Memorandum by Director-General of Health, 8 December 1933, H 1, 54/24, NA.
98 A.M. Finlay, *Social Security in New Zealand: A Simple Guide for the People*, Christchurch, 1944, pp.27, 31–2.
99 Turbott, 1940, p.235.
100 *New Zealand Journal of Health and Hospitals*, September 1920, p.241.
101 *AJHR*, 1924, H-31, p.5.
102 G.K. Welch, *Doctor Smith: Hokianga's 'King of the North'*, Hamilton, 1965, pp.78–9.
103 Notes of Hokitika deputation to Minister of Health, 4 April 1927, H 1, 160 (12038), NA.
104 *Waikato Times*, 27 August 1929.
105 Cook Hospital Board to Director-General of Health, 19 July 1935, H 1 54/24, NA. Hospital data used in this and later paragraphs has been abstracted from the appendices to the Health Department's annual reports.
106 Waiapu Hospital Board to Acting Native Minister Langstone, 19 March 1937, H 1, 53/73 (42437), NA
107 Killick to Director-General of Health, 19 July 1927, H 1, 160 (12038), NA.
108 *Dominion*, 28 August 1929.
109 W.N. Dane to Director of Maori Hygiene, 3 October 1927, H 1, 194/1/21, NA.
110 Ellison to Director-General of Health, 6 July 1928, H 1, 54/24, NA.
111 Maclean to Director-General of Health, 13 October 1932, H 1, 194/1/24 (8458), NA.
112 Watt, in Lambert, 1937, p.35.
113 *Waikato Times*, 27 August 1929. For Ngata's land development policy see G.V. Butterworth and S.M. Butterworth, *The Maori Trustee*, [Wellington] n.d. [1992?], pp.28–9, 34, and Ellison, 1931, p.291.
114 Mangonui Hospital Board to Director-General of Health, 1 July 1932, H 1, 54/24, NA. In 1936 the Hokianga Hospital Board suggested a similar scheme involving a levy on cream cheques at a confer-

ence of the four Northland boards. See Welch, 1965, p.163.

115 Hospital Boards Association Executive Committee Report on Hospital Treatment and Relief of Maoris, 7 October 1932, H 1, 54/24, NA.

116 *AJHR*, 1935, H-31, p.9.

117 MOH to Director of Maori Hygiene, 29 September 1921, H 1, 194/1/5, NA.

118 See, for example, R.H. Dawson and G.I. Louisson, 'The Taranaki Maoris; Their Public Health and Hygiene (With Special Reference to Housing', DPH thesis, Otago, 1938, p.34, and T.C. Trott, 'The Maoris of the Northern King Country: The Relationship of Housing to Health', DPH thesis, Otago, 1940, p.22.

119 See Deputy Director-General of Health to Opotiki Hospital Board on financial assistance towards proposed Apanui Medical Association, 16 September 1930, H 1, 160/14, NA.

120 *Dominion*, 6 September 1929.

121 Bay of Plenty Sub-province of the New Zealand Farmers' Union to Prime Minister, 15 July 1930, H 1, 54/24, NA.

122 *AJHR*, 1933, G-11, p.3.

123 Director-General of Health to Ron Ritchie, Wanganui, 24 November 1931, H 1, 121/21, NA.

124 B.T.W. Irwin to Director-General of Health, 12 February 1936, H 1, 131/4/72 (16904), NA.

125 Correspondence between Valintine, Bennett and Health Minister James Young, March 1928, H 1, 160 (12038), NA. Bennett was consecrated as the first Bishop of the Maori diocese of Aotearoa in December 1928.

126 *Waikato Times*, 27 August 1929.

127 Correspondence and memoranda between Waiapu Hospital Board and Acting Native Minister Langstone, 19 March and 16 April 1937, H 1, 53/73, NA.

128 Welch, 1965, p.163.

129 Bay of Islands Hospital Board Secretary to Director-General of Health, 4 May 1937, H 1, 53/73, NA.

130 Cook Hospital Board to Director-General of Health, 19 July 1935.

131 Dawson and Louisson, 1938, p.35.

132 M. Beedie and N. Hunter, 'Health Survey of Maoris of Southern Hawke's Bay', DPH thesis, Otago, 1942, p.18.

133 B.d'E. Barclay, 'A Public Health Survey of the Wanganui River Pahs and the Wanganui Maoris', DPH thesis, Otago, 1933, pp.246, 255.

134 Beedie and Hunter, 1942, p.18.

135 Dawson and Louisson, 1938, pp.32–3.

136 Rough notes, dated 26 August 1936, of discussion in Auckland which preceded conference on Maori welfare, H 1, 194/8, NA; *Dominion* report on Maori health conference, 3 September 1936. In a memorandum of 31 August Dr Dawson of New Plymouth, who had recently transferred from the Christchurch office, likened changed Maori attitudes to the disappearance of objections to hospitals by London slum dwellers of the early 1900s.

137 Correspondence between Wairoa Hospital Board, Health Department and Native Department, August–October 1938, H 1, 160 (12038), NA.

138 Turbott, 1940, p.235.

139 The figures in this paragraph are derived from M. Belgrave, "Medical Men" and "Lady Doctors": The Making of a New Zealand Profession 1867–1941', PhD thesis, Victoria, 1985, p.257; *New Zealand Official Yearbook*, 1990, p.158.

140 *NZPD*, vol.111, 13 July 1900, pp.541–2.

141 *NZPD*, vol.140, 5 September 1907, pp.719–20.

142 *AJHR*, 1912, H-31, p.9.

143 David Buddo, MHR for Kaiapoi in North Canterbury, was Minister of Public Health from 1909 to 1912. Dow, 1995, p.93.

144 *Journal of the Department of Public Health, Hospitals, and Charitable Aid*, July 1917, p.4.

145 *Ibid.*, November 1919, p.344.

146 Bryder, 1982, p.103.

147 *NZMJ*, vol.21, 1922, p.87.
148 Cited in M. Holdaway, 'Where Are the Maori Nurses Who Were to Become Those "efficient preachers of the gospel of health"?', *Nursing Praxis in New Zealand*, vol.8, no.1, 1993, p.32.
149 *AJHR*, 1920, H-31, p.14.
150 *AJHR*, 1921–22, H-31, pp.5, 33.
151 *AJHR*, 1922, H-31, p.35.
152 Frengley memorandum, 19 September 1922, H 1, 54/24, NA.
153 In March 1928 the Department employed 20 district nurses for Maori, 28 NMOs and four Maori health inspectors. See departmental telegram to Health Minister James Young, 7 March 1928, H 1, 160 (12038), NA.
154 *AJHR*, 1929, H-31, p.32.
155 Annotation by Ellison on letter from Native Trustee, 17 October 1930, H 1, 160/175, NA.
156 *AJHR*, 1931, H-31, pp.292, 306; Ellison, 1931, p.306. Ellison seemed unaware of the pre-1900 doctors.
157 Maclean to Director-General of Health, 16 December 1932, H 1, 160/175, NA. See also Simmons' obituary, *NZMJ*, vol.53, 1954, p.80.
158 Maclean to Director-General of Health, 16 December 1932, H 1, 160/175, NA. Maclean based his analysis on the 1926 census figures.
159 Cook to Director-General of Health, 7 February 1933, H 1, 160/175, NA.
160 Maclean to Director-General of Health, 13 October 1932, H 1, 194/1/24, NA.
161 Maclean to Director-General of Health, 16 December 1932, H 1, 160/175, NA.
162 Mercer to Director-General of Health, 11 June 1928, H 1, 160/12 (13461), NA.
163 Correspondence between Buck and CHO, 15 October and 3 November, 1920, H 1, 121 B.75, NA.
164 'Patients' Payments', in *New Zealand Journal of Health and Hospitals*, vol.4, no.12, December 1921, pp.348–9.
165 Findlay to Director-General of Health, 22 December 1932, H 1, 160/175, NA. D. McMillan, *Byways of History and Medicine: With Special Reference to Canterbury, New Zealand, Christchurch,* 1946, pp.170, 235, 255–6.
166 Cook to Director-General of Health, 7 February 1933, H 1, 160/175, NA.
167 Director-General of Health to MOsH, 16 June 1933, and replies from Turbott, 27 July 1933, and Boyd, 11 July 1933, H 1, 160/175, NA.
168 Director-General of Health to NZMBA, 13 December 1933, H 1, 160/175, NA.
169 Report on Maori Hygiene conference, 9–10 May 1934, and Director-General of Health to Minister of Health, 26 May 1934, H 1, 194/8, NA. See also *AJHR*, 1937, H-31, p.6 for summary of issues.
170 *NZMJ*, vol.33, 1934, p.312.
171 Director-General of Health to Minister of Health, 22 April 1936, and Director-General of Health to MOsH, 1 June 1936, H 1, 160/175, NA.
172 McKibbin to Director-General of Health, 20 August 1936, and Maclean to Director-General of Health, 16 December 1932, H 1, 160/175, NA.
173 MOH to Director-General of Health, 22 May 1936, H 1, 160/31 (12982), NA; Director-General of Health to MOH, 26 June 1936, H 1, 160/175, NA.
174 Irwin to Director-General of Health, 17 September 1936, H 1, 160/175, NA.
175 Details of the 1936 arrangements were reiterated in a memorandum of 12 August 1940 by Acting Director-General Robert Shore, H 1, 160/175, NA.
176 Turbott to Director-General of Health, 14 December 1932, H 1, 160/175, NA.
177 Wadmore to Gisborne MOH, 4 December 1936, H 1, 160/175, NA.
178 Wadmore to Hultquist, 23 February 1937, H 1, 160/175, NA.
179 Minister of Health to Hultquist, 16 March 1937, H 1, 160/175, NA.
180 *NZPD*, vol.249, 5 November 1937, p.203.
181 Correspondence between Director-General of Health and Whangaroa Hospital

Board, 17 May and 17 June 1938, H 1, 160/175, NA.

182 Gilberd to Director-General of Health, 1 September 1938, H 1, 160/175, NA.

183 B. Haami, *Dr Golan Maaka: Maori Doctor*, Birkenhead, 1995, pp.91ff, 108–9.

184 See Director-General of Health memorandum and replies, October 1940, H 1, 160/175, NA.

185 List of Medical Officers, 4 March 1941, H 1, 160/88, NA. The scheme seems to have ended in 1942, when the file was closed.

186 Correspondence between Health Department, Native Trustee and McClymont, June 1922–November 1923, H 1, 160/52 (13506), NA.

187 See, for example, report from District Health Officer to Chief Health Officer on problems at Akaroa, 11 March 1915, H 1, 160/41 (13503), NA.

188 Correspondence 2 December 1924–20 April 1925, H 1, 160/12 (13461), NA.

189 *NZMJ*, vol.24, 1925, p.219.

190 Correspondence 14 May 1932–9 October 1936, H 1, 160/19 (13497), NA. Potaka died in Nelson Hospital after overdosing on morphine while in a state of depression.

191 Corban to Minister of Health, 20 July 1929, H 1, 160 (12038), NA.

192 Durie, 1994, pp.51–3.

193 See 'Medical Registration: Wi Repa 1908–46', H 1, 184/250 (24164), NA.

194 C.J. Orange, 'A Kind of Equality: Labour and the Maori People 1934–49', MA thesis, Auckland, 1977, pp.237–8.

195 Beedie and Hunter, 1942, p.47.

196 Director-General of Health to Minister of Health, 14 February 1936, H 1, 194/8, NA.

197 *AJHR*, 1920, H-31, p.14.

198 See *AJHR*, 1920, H-31, p.14, and correspondence between Ngata and Buck, 26 June and 13 July 1932, in Sorrenson, vol.2, 1987, pp.276, 282.

199 *AJHR*, 1920, H-31, p.7.

200 *AJHR*, 1921, H-31, p.33.

201 See, for example, Buck to Chairman of Takitimu Maori Council, 5 July 1921, H 1, 121/16 B.133, NA, and Pomare to C.J. Parr, 16 October 1922, H 1, 121/21 B.76, NA.

202 *AJHR*, 1924, H-31, p.42.

203 *AJHR*, 1926, H-31, p.44.

204 MOH Robert Shore to Director-General of Health, 10 August 1927, H 1/36 (13303), NA.

205 *New Zealand Herald* report on Native School Teachers' Association, 21 January 1928; Ellison, 1931, pp.292, 306.

206 See Hooper to Ellison, 3 February 1929, H 1, 194/1/19, NA.

207 Hooper to Buck, 14 June 1926, H 1, 36/26, NA. For an overview of the work of the Maori inspectors see 'Maori Hygiene: Monthly Reports: General 1925–7', H 1, 194/2 (13938), NA, which includes summaries of itineraries and work done.

208 Lambert, 1937, pp.31–2.

209 D.F.B. Eyres, 'An Account of the Maintenance of the Public Health in New Zealand Prior to 1920', MA Thesis, Victoria, 1938, p.119.

210 Matahiwi Maori to Taite te Tomo MP, 8 April 1932, H 1, 194/1/19, NA.

211 See obituary notice, *Public Health*, 1967, p.6.

212 L. Bryder, 'The 1918 Influenza Epidemic in Auckland', MA thesis, Auckland, 1980, pp.149–50.

213 See Buck's annual reports, *AJHR*, 1923–7, H-31.

214 See 'Maori Model Villages', *AJHR*, 1926, G-7, 1927, H-31, p.27.

215 *Opotiki Herald*, 2 and 19 December 1921.

216 See Ellison's first two reports, on plans for Te Kuiti and Ngaruawahia pa, *AJHR*, H-31, 1928, p.36, 1929, p.31.

217 Acting Director-General of Health to Native Department Under-Secretary, 21 June 1929, and Ellison to Director-General of Health, 22 July 1929, H 1/36 (13303), NA.

218 Ngata to Buck, 6 February 1931, in Sorrenson, vol.2, 1987, p.111.

219 Ngata to Buck, 23 January and 11 June

1933, in Sorrenson, vol.3, 1987, pp.58, 91.

220 M.P.K. Sorrenson, 'Ngata, Apirana Turupa 1874–1950', in *The Dictionary of New Zealand Biography*, vol.3, pp.359–63.

221 Lambert, 1937, pp.26–7, 37.

222 Watt to Under-Secretary, Native Department, 25 November 1937, H 1/36 (13303), NA. For Ngata's speech see *NZPD*, vol.249, 15 November 1937, pp.403–4.

223 *AJHR*, H-31, 1929, p.60, 1930, p.76.

224 Turbott, 1940, pp.244–5.

225 K.R. Taylor, 'Public Health Administration in New Zealand', MCom thesis, Canterbury, 1939, p.41. For an assessment of these studies see D.A. Dow, '"To set our medical history into order": A Historiography of Health in New Zealand', *Archifacts*, April 1996, p.22.

226 *NZPD*, vol.191, 11 October 1921, pp.390–1, and *New Zealand Herald*, 12 October 1921.

227 F.I. Preston, *Lady Doctor Vintage Model*, Wellington, 1974, pp.82–3. See also *Journal of the Department of Public Health, Hospitals, and Charitable Aid*, January 1918, p.101, June 1921, p.175.

228 See report on typhoid at Te Mingi, Northland, *AJHR*, 1924, H-31, p.40.

229 See, for example, *Journal of the Department of Public Health, Hospitals, and Charitable Aid*, April 1918, p.144, and *AJHR*, 1921, H-31, p.14. Welch, 1965, pp.146–7, names Hokianga district nurse Ella Leslie, appointed in 1925, as one who had a marked influence.

230 J. Frengley to Minister of Health, 19 September 1922, H 1, 54/24, NA.

231 Welch, 1965, p.83.

232 Correspondence between Health Department and Nelson Hospital Board, March–April 1934, H 1, 131/4, NA.

233 Buck to H. Chesson, 24 July 1922, H 1, 194/1/21, NA. Sylvester Lambert noted in 1937 that typhoid among Maori was controlled by vaccine rather than soil sanitation, the more common strategy. See Lambert, 1937, p.28.

234 *AJHR*, 1923, H-31, p.43.

235 See, for example, *AJHR*, H-31, 1922, p.34, 1927, p.27, and *New Zealand Herald* report on Native School Teachers' Association, 21 January 1928.

236 See, for example, *AJHR*, H-31, 1927, pp.4, 43, 44, 1928, p.37, 1929, p.31, 1930, pp.40, 62.

237 Circular dated 5 July 1922, H 1, 131/4, NA.

238 Cited in K.S. Goodfellow, 'Health for the Maori? Health and the Maori Village Schools 1890–1940', MA thesis, Auckland, 1991, p.45.

239 Turbott, 1940, p.247; H.B. Turbott, 'Progress in Prevention of Typhoid Fever in Maoris', *AJHR*, 1933, H-31, Appendix B, p.51.

240 *AJHR*, 1926, H-31, pp.42–3.

241 See, for example, G.J. Blackmore, 'Pulmonary Tuberculosis in Young Children', *Australasian Medical Congress (British Medical Association): Transactions of the Second Session, Dunedin, February 3 to 10, 1927*, Sydney, 1927, pp.234–7, 241.

242 C.E. Hercus, 'The Incidence, Aetiology and Prevention of Goitre in New Zealand', *Australasian Medical Congress (British Medical Association): Transactions of the Second Session, Dunedin, February 3 to 10, 1927*, Sydney, 1927, p.12.

243 See *AJHR*, 1929, H-31, p.9. The claim was repeated verbatim in the next three annual reports.

244 *AJHR*, 1928, H-31A, pp.4–6.

245 W. Aitken, 'Tuberculosis Reduction in New Zealand', *NZMJ*, vol.27, 1928, pp.185–96.

246 *AJHR*, 1930, pp.24, 62, 79.

247 Director-General of Health to Minister of Native Affairs, 7 April 1930, H 1, 194/1/20, NA.

248 Sutherland, 1935, p.116.

249 Minutes of meetings of 5 August 1937, H 1, 160 (12038), NA, and 10 March 1938, H 1, 54/56/1 (11751A), NA. Some of this rise was attributed to more accurate reporting. See Taylor, 1939, p.39.

250 See, for example, *AJHR*, 1932, H-31, p.5, Sutherland, 1935, p.116, and Report by

Colonel Allen Bell on Maori Problem at Te Hapua, 1 March 1935, H 1, 194/1/1, NA.

251 Lambert, 1937, p.24.

252 *NZPD*, vol.249, 5 November 1937, p.203.

253 Turbott, 1940, pp.249–51. The original plan to construct cottages rather than huts had been opposed by Ngata on the grounds that the former were five times as expensive.

254 Ngata to Fraser, 7 July 1939, H 1, 131/3, NA; *AJHR*, 1940, H-31, p.3.

255 *AJHR*, 1928, H-31A, p.25.

256 N.L. Edson, 'Mortality from Tuberculosis in the Maori Race', *NZMJ*, vol.42, 1943, pp.102–10.

257 C.A. Taylor, 'Notification of Tuberculosis in New Zealand', *NZMJ*, vol.42, 1943, pp.151–5.

258 J.H. Crawshaw, 'Some Remarks on the Treatment of Tuberculosis Amongst the Maoris at Tuahiwi Park', *NZMJ*, vol.13, 1914, p.248.

259 Blackmore, 1927, pp.234–7.

260 L. Bryder, 'BCG Vaccination: Comparative Perspectives', in H. Attwood, R. Gillespie and M. Lewis (eds), *New Perspectives on the History of Medicine: First National Conference of The Australian Society of the History of Medicine 1989*, Melbourne, 1990, pp.193–9.

261 Director-General of Health to Robert Francis, 13 August 1936, H 1, 13/7/3, NA.

262 Correspondence between Ngata and Fraser, 27 July and 5 September 1938, 7 July 1939, H 1, 131/3, NA. On the introduction of BCG to New Zealand see Dow, 1995, pp.166–7.

263 V. Heiser, *An American Doctor's Odyssey: Adventures in Forty-five Countries*, New York, 1936, pp.356–7.

264 See, for example, M.H. Watt, 'Infant Mortality in New Zealand', *New Zealand Journal of Health and Hospitals*, vol.4, no.4, 1921, p.88, 'New Zealand', in A. Balfour and H.H. Scott (eds), *Health Problems of the Empire: Past Present and Future*, London, 1924, p.182, and J.B. Condliffe, *New Zealand in the Making*, London, 1930, pp.369–72.

265 *AJHR*, H-31, 1927, p.1, 1929, p.14.

266 Statistics used in this analysis are derived from Health Department annual reports for the 1920s and 1930s.

267 *AJHR*, 1903, H-31, p.71.

268 *AJHR*, 1908, H-31, p.122.

269 Ellison, 1931, pp.298–300.

270 *AJHR*, 1934, H-31, p.8.

271 For details from 1939 to 1958 see Maclean, 1964, p.217.

272 A.S. Thomson, *The Story of New Zealand*, London, 1859, vol.2, p.285.

273 Report by Williams dated 1 June 1868, *AJHR*, 1868, A-4, p.23.

274 See Pomare's annual reports in *AJHR*, H-31, 1902, pp.64–5, 1903, p.71, 1904, pp.57–8, 1905, p.57, 1908, p.122. These reports contradict Mason Durie's 1986 claim that 'Within health circles, westernization was considered a reasonable destiny for Maori people. New child-rearing techniques were promoted: breast feeding being regarded as less reliable than a milk formula'. See M.H. Durie, 'Implications of Policy and Management Decisions on Maori Health: Contemporary Issues and Responses' in M.W. Raffel and N.K. Raffel (eds), *Perspectives on Health Policy: Australia, New Zealand, United States*, New York, 1986, p.203.

275 M. Pomare, *Nga Kohungahunga Me Nga Kai Ma Ratou*, Turanga, 1909, comprised 10 pages. *Ko Nga Tamaririki Me Nga Kai Ma Ratou: Infants and Their Foods: With Additions by District Nurses for Maoris*, Wellington, 1916, had expanded to 31 pages. For the history of these publications see H 1, 127/30 (3415).

276 *AJHR*, 1908, H-31, pp.129, 133.

277 See comments by Buck, Field and James Carroll, *NZPD*, vol.152, 7 October 1910, pp.315–16, and *AJHR*, 1911, H-31, p.78.

278 *AJHR*, 1911, H-31A, pp.148, 183.

279 W.N. Dane to Director of Maori Hygiene, 3 October 1927, H 1, 194/1/21, NA.

280 *AJHR*, 1932, H-31, p.35.

281 See Health Department to Wairoa Maori Council, 8 January 1932, H 1, 121/10, NA.
282 Maclean to Director-General of Health, 16 December 1932, H 1, 160/175, NA.
283 Lambert, 1937, p.17.
284 Director of Education to Director-General of Health, 9 May 1934, H 1, 194/8, NA.
285 H. Grieve, *Sketches from Maoriland*, London, 1939, pp.47–8.
286 Lambert, 1937, p.17.
287 Grieve, 1939, p.54.
288 See correspondence from 1 June 1932 to 4 August 1932, H 1, 194/1/12, NA.
289 *AJHR*, 1906, H-31, p.75.
290 Editorial, *NZMJ*, vol.7, 1908, p.22.
291 Personal communication from Linda Bryder, who is currently researching the history of Plunket.
292 *AJHR*, 1930, H-31, p.41.
293 Ellison, 1931, p.292.
294 *AJHR*, 1933, H-31, p.6.
295 See Mary Lambie, Director of Nursing, to Anne Pattrick, Plunket Society Director of Nursing, 31 July 1934, H 1, 23/1, NA, and 'Maori Hygiene: Conference on Native Health 1933–6', H 1, 194/8, NA. For the introduction to schools see Goodfellow, 1991, p.52.
296 Maclean to Director-General of Health, 16 December 1932, H 1, 160/175, NA.
297 See correspondence between Director-General of Health and New Plymouth MOH, November 1937, H 1, 160/175, NA.
298 Grieve, 1939, pp.55–7.
299 New Zealand Country Women's Institute, *Portrait of Change: A Record of Country Women's Institute in New Zealand*, Wellington, 1996, pp.7, 10, 18, 90–1.
300 Sutherland, 1935, p.115.
301 Lambert, 1937, p.22.
302 See correspondence September–December 1937, H 1, 194/1/5, NA.
303 Turbott, 1940, p.266.
304 *Rotorua Post*, 2 October 1937, reproduced in 'Erihapeti', *The Binding of Te Arawa*, Rotorua, 1952, p.21.
305 See correspondence between MOH Dr Gilberd and Director-General of Health, September–December 1940, H 1, 21/124 (23049), NA. For the history of the Women's Health League see M. White (ed.), *The Unfolding Years 1937–1987: Women's Health League*, Rotorua, 1988.
306 *Portrait of Change*, 1996, p.91. For a summary of the League's work see M. King, *Whina: A Biography of Whina Cooper*, Auckland, 1983, pp.166–87, and A. Rogers and M. Simpson (eds), *Te Timatanga Tatau Tatau: Early Stories From Founding Members of the Maori Women's Welfare League*, Wellington, 1993.
307 For an overview of developments, and the underlying ideologies, see M. Tennant, "Missionaries of health": The School Medical Service During the Inter-war Period', in L. Bryder (ed.), *A Healthy Country: Essays on the Social History of Medicine in New Zealand*, Wellington, 1991, pp.129–48, and M. Tennant, 'The Origins of School Medicine in New Zealand' in P. Winterton and D. Gurry (eds), *The Impact of the Past Upon the Present: Second National Conference of the Australian Society of the History of Medicine: Perth, July 1991*, Perth, 1992, pp.175–9.
308 Goodfellow, 1991, pp.ii–iii; *AJHR*, 1908, H-31, p.133.
309 *AJHR*, 1909, H-31, p.60.
310 *AJHR*, 1923, H-31, pp.25–6.
311 Director-General of Health to Director of Education, 17 July 1923, H 1, 162 (11667), NA.
312 See correspondence from 25 July to 10 October 1925, H 1, 35/1/4, NA.
313 *New Zealand Herald* report on Native School Teachers' Association, 21 January 1928; *AJHR*, 1929, H-31, p.23. The 1929 statistics are cited in J.M. Barrington and T.H. Beaglehole, *Maori Schools in a Changing Society: An Historical Review*, Wellington, 1974, p.155.
314 *AJHR*, H-31, 1933, pp.6, 24, 1934, pp.22–3, 44.

315 Director of School Hygiene to Director of Education, 23 August 1940, H 1/35, NA.
316 Barrington and Beaglehole, 1974, p.211.
317 Director of Education to Director of School Hygiene, 28 March 1934, H 1, 194/8, NA.
318 See minutes of meeting, 11 May 1934, H 1, 194/8, NA. The 10-page Health Instruction memorandum was dated 1 February 1934.
319 *New Zealand Education Gazette*, vol.11, no.2, February 1936, p.11, cited in Goodfellow, 1991, p.45.
320 Goodfellow, 1991, pp.44–5.
321 Lambert, 1937, p.47. Lambert estimated the total expenditure on Maori for 1936–7 to be £641,200.
322 Grieve, 1939, p.47.
323 *AJHR*, 1928, H-31, p.25.
324 Goodfellow, 1991, pp.57–8. For the debate about Plunket see E. Olssen, 'Truby King and the Plunket Society: An Analysis of a Prescriptive Ideology', *NZJH*, vol.15, no.1, 1981, pp.3–23, and L. Bryder, 'Perceptions of Plunket: Time to Review Historians' Interpretations?', in L. Bryder and D.A. Dow (eds), *New Countries and Old Medicine: Proceedings of an International Conference on the History of Medicine and Health*, Auckland, 1995, pp.97–103.
325 Barrington and Beaglehole, 1974, p.6.
326 For an overview of teachers' attitudes and Maori responses see J. Simon (ed.), *Nga Kura Maori: The Native Schools System 1867–1969*, Auckland, 1998. This book makes extensive use of oral testimony and photographs but offers little in the way of analysis.
327 *Dominion*, 10 August 1928.
328 Ngata to Buck, 9 February 1928, in Sorrenson, vol.1, 1986, p.66; Ellison, 1931, p.307; *AJHR*, 1934, H-31, pp.34, 36.
329 Goodfellow, 1991, p.44; New Zealand Department of Health, *The New Zealand School Dental Service: The Policy Regarding the Establishment, Maintenance, and Functions of School Dental Clinics*, Wellington, 1940.
330 Turbott, 1940, p.259.
331 *Ibid.*, p.253.
332 Philippa Mein Smith, historian of New Zealand's maternity services during the inter-war years, claimed in 1985 that the maternal and child health problems of Maori society were ignored until the Labour Party came to power in 1935. P. Mein Smith, *Maternity in Dispute: New Zealand 1920–1939*, Wellington, 1986, p.3.
333 See, for example, J.H. Scott, 'Contribution to the Osteology of the Aborigines of New Zealand and of the Chatham Islands', *Transactions and Proceedings of the New Zealand Institute*, vol.26, 1893, pp.1–64; T.W. Bell, 'Medical Notes on New Zealand', *NZMJ*, vol.3, 1890, pp.67–83, 129–45. Bell's paper included an extensive subsection headed 'Medical Notes on the New Zealanders [i.e. Maori] in so far as these are interesting medically'.
334 For an assessment of Buck's interlocking medical and anthropological interests see J.S. Allen, 'Te Rangi Hiroa's Physical Anthropology', *Journal of the Polynesian Society*, vol.103, no.1, 1994, pp.11–27.
335 See Bell, 1890, pp.75–6.
336 Maori Councils Act 1900, section 15.
337 *AJHR*, 1908, H-31, pp.130–2.
338 Lange, 1972, pp.319–20.
339 *British Medical Journal*, 5 December 1913, pp.1482–3.
340 Health Act 1920, section 12(d); Editorial: 'Medical Research in New Zealand', *NZMJ*, vol.60, 1961, pp.408–10.
341 J.A. Thomson and G.M. Thomson, 'Scientific Research in New Zealand', *New Zealand Journal of Science and Technology*, vol.6, December 1923, pp.244, 246, 253–4.
342 G.M. Thomson, 'Scientific Research in New Zealand', *New Zealand Journal of Science and Technology*, vol.8, September 1925, p.62.
343 *AJHR*, H-31, 1924, p.36, 1928, p.28. See also Hercus, 1927, pp.12–23.

344 *AJHR*, 1924, H-31, p.35.
345 Buck, 'The Pre-European Diet of the Maori', *New Zealand Dental Journal*, May 1925, pp.203, 215.
346 *AJHR*, 1925, H-31, p.43.
347 See *NZPD*, vol.207, 19 August 1925, p.448, vol.208, 11 September 1925, pp.275–6, vol.209, 30 July 1926, pp.1211–15.
348 Ngata to Buck, 8 March 1931, in Sorrenson, vol.2, 1987, p.121.
349 H.B. Turbott, 'Maori and Pakeha: A Preliminary Study in Comparative Health', *AJHR*, 1929, H-31, p.23. Turbott's report was not concluded until the following year. See H.B. Turbott, 'Maori and Pakeha: Comparative Health of School-Children', *AJHR*, 1930, H-31, pp.89–90.
350 *AJHR*, 1931, H-31, pp.17–18, 36–8. See also H.B. Turbott and A.F. Rolland, 'The Nutritional Value of Milk: Experimental Evidence from Maori Schoolchildren', *NZMJ*, vol.31, 1932, pp.109–11.
351 Editorial, *NZMJ*, vol.30, 1931, pp.316–17.
352 *AJHR*, 1926, H-31, p.4. The Otago reference must have been to the public health dissertation of J.A. Paterson and W.J. Edgington, 'Tuberculosis in Moeraki Maoris', DPH thesis, Otago, 1924.
353 *AJHR*, 1928, H-31A, p.25.
354 *AJHR*, 1929, H-31, p.32; Ellison, 1931, p.297.
355 Wi Repa to Ngata, n.d. [1930], H 1, 131/3/136 (9151), NA.
356 Ngata to Buck, 11 January 1931, in Sorrenson, vol.2, 1987, p.99.
357 Turbott to Deputy Director-General of Health, 28 January, and reply, 21 February 1931, H 1, 131/3/136, NA.
358 See report of round-table conference on public health nursing, *New Zealand Nursing Journal*, November 1929, pp.191–200.
359 *AJHR*, 1934, H-31, p.8.
360 Personal communication from L. Bryder, 23 April 1998.
361 *NZPD*, vol.246, 13 August 1936, pp.477–8.
362 See J.B. Lovell-Smith, *The New Zealand Doctor and the Welfare State*, Auckland, 1966, p.37.
363 *NZPD*, vol.247, 9 October 1936, p.737. Fraser repeatedly praised Turbott's contribution in Parliament. See *NZPD*, vol.246, 28 August 1936, p.763, and vol.249, 5 November 1937, p.204.
364 McKibbin to Director-General of Health, 16 May 1934, H 1, 194/8, NA.
365 Turbott to Director-General of Health, 7 July 1936, H 1, 160/175, NA.
366 *NZMJ*, vol.37, 1937, pp.349–51.
367 See Edson, 1943, p.110, and T.C. Lonie, 'Some Social Factors in Relation to Tuberculosis', *NZMJ*, vol.46, 1947, pp.25–31.
368 See, for example, DPH theses by Maaka (1930), Barclay (1935), Murray (1937), Dawson and Louisson (1938), Simpson (1940), Trott (1940), Duthie (1940), Beedie and Hunter (1942), Paewai (1945).
369 See Durie, 1986, p.204.
370 Haami, 1995, pp.110, 122.
371 Turbott, 1940, p.268.

Bibliographical Essay

1 See D.A. Dow, '"To set our medical history into order": A Historiography of Health in New Zealand', *Archifacts*, April 1996, pp.27–8; and D.A. Dow (comp.), *Annotated Bibliography for the History of Medicine and Health in Mew Zealand*, Dunedin, 1994, especially pp.84–99.
2 J.B. Tuke, 'Medical Notes on New Zealand', *Edinburgh Medical Journal*, vol.9, September 1863, p.220.
3 P.H. Buck, 'Medicine Amongst the Maoris, in Ancient and Modern Times', MD thesis, University of New Zealand, 1910.
4 M.P.K. Sorrenson (ed.), *Na To Hoa Aroha: From Your Dear Friend: The Correspondence Between Sir Apirana Ngata and Sir Peter Buck*, Auckland, 1987, vol.2, pp.251–2.
5 I.L.G. Sutherland, *The Maori Situation*, Wellington, 1935, p.114.

6 A. Moorehead, *The Fatal Impact: An Account of the Invasion of the South Pacific 1767–1840*, London, 1966. Moorehead concentrated his attention on Tahiti, Australia and the Antarctic.

7 H.M. Wright, *New Zealand, 1769–1840: Early Years of Western Contract*, Harvard, 1969, pp.57–62.

8 J. Belich, *Making Peoples: A History of the New Zealanders from Polynesian Settlement to the End of the Nineteenth Century*, Auckland, 1996, pp.173–8. For a recent overview of the international literature see S.J. Kunitz, *Disease and Social Diversity: The European Impact on the Health of Non-Europeans*, New York, 1994.

9 M.H. Durie, *Whaiora: Maori Health Development*, Auckland, 1994, p.27.

10 M.H. Durie, 'Implications of Policy and Management Decisions on Maori Health: Contemporary Issues and Responses', in M.W. Raffel and N.K. Raffel (eds), *Perspectives on Health Policy: Australia, New Zealand, United States*, New York, 1986, p.201.

11 Durie, 1994, p.vii.

12 D.F.B. Eyres, 'An Account of the Maintenance of the Public Health in New Zealand Prior to 1920', MA thesis, Victoria, 1938, pp.123–4.

13 P.H. Buck, 'Foreword', in I.L.G. Sutherland (ed.), *The Maori People Today: A General Survey*, Oxford, 1940, p.9.

14 J.K. Hunn, Report on Department of Maori Affairs with Statistical Supplement, 24 August 1960, *AJHR*, 1961, G-10, p.19.

15 F.S. Maclean, *Challenge for Health: A History of Public Health in New Zealand*, Wellington, 1964, pp.189–220.

16 R.T. Lange, 'The Revival of a Dying Race: A Study of Maori Health Reform 1900–1918 and its Nineteenth Century Background', MA thesis, Auckland, 1972, pp.ii, 87–91, 243–5. For an assessment of the role of demographers and statisticians see Dow, 1996, pp.17, 27–8, 35.

17 Lange, 1972, pp.82–3, 315, 345–6.

18 See, for example, C.J. Orange, 'A Kind of Equality: Labour and the Maori People 1934–49', MA thesis, Auckland, 1977, p.20; and A.H. McKegg, '"Ministering Angels": The Government Backblock Nursing Service and the Maori Health Nurses, 1909–1939', MA thesis, Auckland, 1991, p.55.

19 *NZPD*, vol.251, 28 July 1938, p.811.

20 Maclean, 1964, p.195.

21 Lange, 1972, pp.87–91, 141–2.

22 A. Ward, *A Show of Justice: Racial 'Amalgamation' in Nineteenth Century New Zealand*, Auckland, 1995, pp.130, 142.

23 For a concise appraisal of the NMOs see D. Dow, '"Specially suitable men?" Subsidized Medical Services for Maori, 1840–1940', *NZJH*, vol.32, no.2, 1998, pp.163–88.

24 G.W. Rice, 'The Making of New Zealand's 1920 Health Act', *NZJH*, vol.22, no.1, 1988, p.18.

25 J.M. Barrington and T.H. Beaglehole, *Maori Schools in a Changing Society: An Historical Review*, Wellington, 1974.

26 K.S. Goodfellow, 'Health for the Maori? Health and the Maori Village Schools 1890–1940', MA thesis, Auckland, 1991; McKegg, 1991. Goodfellow's work remains unpublished, but a summary of McKegg's thesis appeared as 'The Maori Health Nursing Scheme: An Experiment in Autonomous Health Care', *NZJH*, vol.26, no.2, 1992, pp.145–60.

27 D.I. Pool, *Te Iwi Maori: A New Zealand Population, Past, Present & Projected*, Auckland, 1991, pp.xii–xiii, 103. Poole's earlier works include 'The Maori Population of New Zealand' PhD thesis, Australian National University, 1964; and *The Maori Population of New Zealand*, Auckland, 1976,

28 J.M. Boddy, 'Maori Health: Is the Future Determined by the Past?', in J.M. Morse (ed.), *Recent Advances in Nursing: Issues in Cross-Cultural Nursing*, vol.20, 1988, pp.27, 37.

29 See, for example, Durie, 1994, p.38, n.35. Relatively few medical historical works are included in Durie's bibliographies, which are almost entirely devoid of reference to primary sources.

A Note on Sources

1 M. Bassett, *The Mother of All Departments: The History of the Department of Internal Affairs*, Auckland, 1997, pp.22, 39, 54.

2 'Morituri Te Salutamus', *New Zealand Journal of Health and Hospitals*, November 1921, vol.4 no.7, p.307.

3 For the relationship between the NZBMA, the *NZMJ* and the Department prior to 1940 see D.A. Dow, *Safeguarding the Public Health: A History of the New Zealand Department of Health*, Wellington, 1995, chapters 2–5.

4 P.A. Sargison, 'Maclean, Hester, 1859–1932', in *The Dictionary of New Zealand Biography: Volume 3: 1900–1920*, Wellington, 1996, pp.309–11.

Bibliography

PRIMARY SOURCES

Manuscript

Lambert, S.M., 'A Survey of the Maori Situation', unpublished report dated 28 May 1937 (copy held in Health Department Library)

James M. Mason, uncatalogued papers, Alexander Turnbull Library, Wellington

Turbott, H.B., 'A N.Z. Doctor—Peripatetic', unpublished autobiography (deposited in Health Department)

Watt, M.H., 'The Rest of the Day to Myself', unpublished autobiography (deposited in Health Department)

Appendix to the Journals of the House of Representatives

'Appointments Made by the General Government from 1st January to 12th July 1862', *AJHR*, 1862, D-17

'Census of the Maori Population, 1881', *AJHR*, 1881, G-3

'Census of the Maori Population (Papers relating to the)', *AJHR*, 1886, G-12

'Census of the Maori Population', *AJHR*, 1891, G-2

'Census of the Maori Population', *AJHR*, 1911, H-14A

'Fever Amongst the Natives of Herekino', *AJHR*, 1890, G-6

'Further Papers Relative to Sir George Grey's Plan of Native Government', *AJHR*, 1862, E-9

'Hospitals and Charitable Institutions in the Colony: Appendix III: Minutes, Reports of Proceedings, etc of the Hospitals Conference, June 1911', *AJHR*, 1911, H-31

'Hospitals Commission', *AJHR*, 1921, H-31A

Hunn, J.K., Report on Department of Maori Affairs with Statistical Supplement, 24 August 1960, *AJHR*, 1961, G-10

'Maori Model Villages', *AJHR*, 1926, G-7

'Maternal Mortality in New Zealand (Report of Special Committee)', *AJHR*, 1921, H-31A

'Medical Attendance on Maoris (Return Relative to)', *AJHR*, 1906, G-4

'Middle Island Native Claims', *AJHR*, 1889, I-10

'Middle Island Native Land Question', *AJHR*, 1888, G-1

'Minute by Governor Sir George Grey on the Subject of His Excellency's Plan of Na-

tive Government', *AJHR*, 1862, E-2
'Native Population in South and Stewart Island', *AJHR*, 1877, G-9
'Native Reserves, Middle Island (report by Mr. Alex. Mackay)', *AJHR*, 1873, G-2A
'Nominal Roll of the Civil Establishment of New Zealand on the 30th June, 1875', *AJHR*, 1875, H-11
'Notes of Native Meetings', *AJHR*, 1885, G-1
'Pakeha and Maori: A Narrative of the Premier's Trip Through the Native Districts of the North Island', *AJHR*, 1895, G-1
'Prevention and Treatment of Pulmonary Tuberculosis in New Zealand (Report of the Committee of Inquiry)', *AJHR*, 1928, H-31A
'Proposed Amendment of Hospitals and Charitable Institutions Acts: Conference of Delegates of Hospital and Charitable Aid Boards and Separate Institutions, Held at Wellington on the 9th, 10th, and 11th June, 1908', *AJHR*, 1908, H-22A
'Rating of Native Land', *AJHR*, 1933, G-11
'Report by Dr Nicholson, of Auckland, on the Steps Taken by Him to Prevent the Spread of Small-Pox in the Province of Auckland', *AJHR*, 1872, G-32
'Report of the Conference on Administrative Control and Treatment of Tuberculosis', *AJHR*, 1913, H-31A
'Reports on the Social and Political State of the Natives in Various Districts at the Time of the Arrival of Sir G.F. Bowen', *AJHR*, 1868, A-4
'Return of All Officers Employed in Native Districts in January 1864', *AJHR*, 1864, E-7
'Return of Expenditure of Native Department For The Last Three Years', *AJHR*, 1870, B-8
'Return of Officers in the Employ of the Government: Native Lands: Medical Attendants:', *AJHR*, 1866, D-3
'Return of Officers Who Have Ceased to be in the Service of the New Zealand Government Since the 30th June 1865', *AJHR*, 1867, D-2
'Return of Officers Who Have Ceased to be in the Service of the New Zealand Government Since the 30th June 1867', *AJHR*, 1868, D-8
'Smallpox Epidemic (Particulars Relative to the)', *AJHR*, 1914, H-33
'Statement of All Sums Expended Under the "Native Purposes Appropriation, 1862", on Account of the Financial Year 1862–3', *AJHR*, 1863, E-8
Turbott, H.B., 'Maori and Pakeha: A Preliminary Study in Comparative Health', *AJHR*, 1929, H-31, pp.73–4
Turbott, H.B., 'Maori and Pakeha: Comparative Health of School-Children', *AJHR*, 1930, H-31, pp.89–90
Turbott, H.B., 'Progress in Prevention of Typhoid Fever in Maoris', *AJHR*, 1933, H-31, Appendix B, p.51

Books, pamphlets

Bevan, T., *Reminiscences of an Old Colonist*, Otaki, 1911
Campbell, J.L., *Poenamo: Sketches of the Early Days of New Zealand*, London, 1881
Condliffe, J.B., *New Zealand in the Making*, London, 1930
Gorst, J.E., *New Zealand Revisited: Recollections of the Days of My Youth*, London, 1908
Grieve, H., *Sketches from Maoriland*, London, 1939
Hayman, F., *King Country Nurse*, Auckland, 1964
Heiser, V., *An American Doctor's Odyssey: Adventures in Forty-five Countries*, New York, 1936
Lambert, S.M., *A Doctor in Paradise*, London, 1942
Martin, Lady, *Our Maoris*, London, 1884
Moore, J.M., *New Zealand for the Emigrant, Invalid and Tourist*, London, 1890
New Zealand Department of Health, *A Health Service for New Zealand*, Wellington, 1974
New Zealand Department of Health, 'Historical Summary', in *A Review of Hospital and Related Services in New Zealand*, Wellington, 1969, pp.9–22

New Zealand Department of Health, *The New Zealand School Dental Service: The Policy Regarding the Establishment, Maintenance, and Functions of School Dental Clinics*, Wellington, 1940

Pope, J.A., *Health for the Maori: A Manual for Use in Native Schools*, Wellington, 1884

Porter, F. (ed.), *The Turanga Journals, 1840–1850: Letters and Journals of William and Jane Williams Missionaries to Poverty Bay*, Wellington, 1974

Preston, F.I., *Lady Doctor Vintage Model*, Wellington, 1974

Sorrenson, M.P.K. (ed.), *Na To Hoa Aroha: From Your Dear Friend: The Correspondence Between Sir Apirana Ngata and Sir Peter Buck*, 3 vols, Auckland, 1986–8

Stack, J.W., *Early Maoriland Adventures*, Wellington, 1935

Sutherland, I.L.G., *The Maori Situation*, Wellington, 1935

Sutherland, I.L.G. (ed.), *The Maori People Today: A General Survey*, Oxford, 1940

Te Rangi Hiroa, *The Coming of the Maori*, Wellington, 1949

Thomson, A.S., *The Story of New Zealand*, London, 1859

Williams, H. (edited by L.M. Rogers), *The Early Journals of Henry Williams Senior Missionary in New Zealand of the Church Missionary Society 1826–1840*, Christchurch, 1961

Articles

Aitken, W., 'Tuberculosis Reduction in New Zealand', *NZMJ*, vol.27, 1928, pp.185–96

Alpers, O.T.J., 'The Young Maori Party', 1903, reprinted in P.M. Jackson (ed.), *Maori and Education or, the Education of Natives in New Zealand and its Dependencies*, Wellington, 1931, pp.144–61

Bell, T.W., 'Medical Notes on New Zealand', *NZMJ*, vol.3, 1890, pp.67–83, 129–45

Blackmore, G.J., 'Pulmonary Tuberculosis in Young Children', *Australasian Medical Congress (British Medical Association): Transactions of the Second Session, Dunedin, February 3 to 10, 1927*, Sydney, 1927, pp.234–7

Buck, P., 'The Pre-European Diet of the Maori', *New Zealand Dental Journal*, May 1925, pp.203–17

Buck, P., 'The Smallpox Epidemic Amongst the Maoris in the Northern District', *Transactions of the Tenth Session of the Australasian Medical Congress, Auckland*, Wellington, 1916, pp.212–23

Butcher, J.W., 'Cancer Mortality in New Zealand', *New Zealand Official Yearbook*, 1917, pp.776–809

Chill, E., 'Phthisis and Superstition Among the Maories', *British Medical Journal*, 18 August 1906, p.376

Colquhoun, D., 'The History of a Medical School', *NZMJ*, vol.8, 1910, pp.4–11

Crawshaw, J.H., 'Some Remarks on the Treatment of Tuberculosis Amongst the Maoris at Tuahiwi Park', *NZMJ*, vol.13, 1914, pp.346–8

Edson, N.L., 'Mortality from Tuberculosis in the Maori Race', *NZMJ*, vol.42, 1943, pp.102–10

Ellison, E.P., 'The Maori and Hygiene', in P.M. Jackson (ed.), *Maori and Education or, the Education of Natives in New Zealand and its Dependencies*, Wellington, 1931, pp.282–308

Hercus, C., 'The Incidence, Aetiology and Prevention of Goitre in New Zealand', *Australasian Medical Congress (British Medical Association): Transactions of the Second Session, Dunedin, February 3 to 10, 1927*, Sydney, 1927, 12–23

Lonie, T.C., 'Some Social Factors in Relation to Tuberculosis', *NZMJ*, vol.46, 1947, pp.25–31

Maclean, H., 'New Zealand', in L.L. Dock (ed.), *A History of Nursing*, vol.4, New York, 1910, pp.189–222

'New Zealand', in A. Balfour and H.H. Scott (eds.), *Health Problems of the Empire: Past Present and Future*, London, 1924

North, A.J., 'Reminiscences of a Missionary Nurse', *Historical Review: Bay of Plenty Journal of History*, vol.14, no.1, 1966, pp.18–21

Prior, I., 'Health', in E. Schwimmer (ed.), *The Maori People in the Nineteen-Sixties: A Symposium*, Auckland, 1968, pp.270–87

Scott, J.H., 'Contribution to the Osteology of the Aborigines of New Zealand and of the Chatham Islands', *Transactions and Proceedings of the New Zealand Institute*, vol.26, 1893, pp.1–64

Smith, G.M., 'Dr Smith and the Jones Baby', in M. Damian (comp.), *Growl You May But Go You Must*, Wellington, 1968, pp.40–9

Taylor, C.A., 'Notification of Tuberculosis in New Zealand', *NZMJ*, vol.31, 1943, pp.151–5

Te Rangi Hiroa, 'Maori Somatology: Racial Averages', *Journal of the Polynesian Society*, vol.31, 1922, pp.37–44, 145–53, 159–70, vol.32, 1923, pp.21–8, 189–99

Thomson, G.M., 'Scientific Research in New Zealand', *New Zealand Journal of Science and Technology*, vol.8, September 1925, pp.41–62

Thomson, J.A., and G.M. Thomson, 'Scientific Research in New Zealand', *New Zealand Journal of Science and Technology*, vol.6, December 1923, pp.234–56

Tuke, J.B., 'Medical Notes on New Zealand', *Edinburgh Medical Journal*, vol.9, 1863, pp.220–9, 721–8

Turbott, H.B., 'Health and Social Welfare', in I.L.G. Sutherland (ed.), *The Maori People Today: A General Survey*, Oxford, 1940, pp.229–68

Turbott, H.B., and A.F. Rolland, 'The Nutritional Value of Milk: Experimental Evidence from Maori Schoolchildren', *NZMJ*, vol.31, 1932, pp.109–11

Walsh, Archdeacon, 'The Passing of the Maori: An Inquiry into the Principal Causes of the Decay of the Race', *Transactions and Proceedings of the New Zealand Institute*, vol.40, 1907, pp.154–75

Watt, M.H., 'Infant Mortality in New Zealand', *New Zealand Journal of Health and Hospitals*, vol.4, no.4, 1921, pp.88–94

SECONDARY SOURCES

Books, pamphlets

Alexander, R.R., *The Story of Te Aute College*, Wellington, 1951

Angus, J.H., *A History of the Otago Hospital Board and its Predecessors*, Dunedin, 1984

Bagnall, A.G., and G.C. Petersen, *William Colenso . . . His Life and Journeys*, Wellington, 1948

Barber, L.H., and R.J. Towers, *Wellington Hospital 1847–1976*, Wellington, 1976

Barrington, J.M., and T.H. Beaglehole, *Maori Schools in a Changing Society: An Historical Review*, Wellington, 1974

Bassett, M., *The Mother of All Departments: The History of the Department of Internal Affairs*, Auckland, 1997

Beattie, I.D. (ed.), *Ever Ready, the Life of Arthur Guyan Purchas: Including E.H. Roche's Article on His Grandfather and a Sermon, Some Hymns and Drawings by Dr Purchas*, Auckland, 1993

Belich, J., *Making Peoples: A History of the New Zealanders from Polynesian Settlement to the End of the Nineteenth Century*, Auckland, 1996

Bloomfield, G.T., *New Zealand: A Handbook of Historical Statistics*, Boston, 1984

Brown, M., D. Masters and B. Smith, *Nurses of Auckland: The History of the General Nursing Programme in the Auckland School of Nursing*, Auckland, 1995

Butterworth, G.V., and S.M. Butterworth, *The Maori Trustee*, [Wellington], n.d. [1992?]

Butterworth, G.V., and H.R. Young, *Maori Affairs: A Department and the People Who Made It*, Wellington, 1990

Cody, J.F., *Man of Two Worlds: Sir Maui Pomare*, Wellington, 1953

Condliffe, J.B., *Te Rangi Hiroa: The Life of Sir Peter Buck*, Christchurch, 1971

Conly, G., *A Case History: The Hawke's Bay Hospital Board 1876–1989*, Napier, 1992

Davis, J.K., *The History of St John's College*, Auckland, 1911

Dow, D.A., *Safeguarding the Public Health:*

A History of the New Zealand Department of Health, Wellington, 1995

Dow, D.A. (comp.), *Annotated Bibliography for the History of Medicine and Health in New Zealand*, Dunedin, 1994

Durie, M.H., *Whaiora: Maori Health Development*, Auckland, 1994

'Erihapeti', *The Binding of Te Arawa*, Rotorua, 1952

Finlay, A.M., *Social Security in New Zealand: A Simple Guide for the People*, Christchurch, 1944

Gluckman, L.K., *Tangiwai: Medical History of New Zealand Prior to 1860*, Auckland, 1976

Haami, B., *Dr Golan Maaka: Maori Doctor*, Birkenhead, 1995

Hardy, A., *Epidemic Streets: Infectious Disease and The Rise of Preventive Medicine, 1856–1900*, Oxford, 1993

Hay, I., *The Caring Commodity: The Provision of Health Care in New Zealand*, Auckland, 1989

King, M., *Te Puea: A Biography*, Auckland, 1990

King, M., *Whina: A Biography of Whina Cooper*, Auckland, 1983

Kunitz, S.J., *Disease and Social Diversity: The European Impact on the Health of Non-Europeans*, New York, 1994

Lambert, G., *Peter Wilson: Colonial Surgeon*, Palmerston North, 1981

Loudon, I., *Medical Care and the General Practitioner, 1750–1850*, Oxford, 1986

Lovell-Smith, J.B., *The New Zealand Doctor and the Welfare State*, Auckland, 1966

Low, D.C., *Salute to the Scalpel: A Medical History of the Nelson Province*, Nelson, 1972

MacDonald, C.A., *Pages From the Past: Some Chapters in the History of Marlborough*, Blenheim, 1933

Mackay, J.A., *Historic Poverty Bay and the East Coast*, Gisborne, 1966

Maclean, F.S., *Challenge for Health: A History of Public Health in New Zealand*, Wellington, 1964

McLintock, A.H. (ed.), *An Encyclopaedia of New Zealand*, Wellington, 1966

McMillan, D., *Byways of History and Medicine: With Special Reference to Canterbury, New Zealand*, Christchurch, 1946

Martin, J.E., *Holding the Balance: A History of New Zealand's Department of Labour, 1891–1995*, Christchurch, 1996

Mein Smith, P., *Maternity in Dispute: New Zealand 1920–1939*, Wellington, 1986

Miller, J., *Early Victorian New Zealand: A Study of Racial Tension and Social Attitudes, 1839–1852*, London, 1958

Moorehead, A., *The Fatal Impact: An Account of the Invasion of the South Pacific 1767–1840*, London, 1966

Morris, R.J., *Cholera 1832*, London, 1976

New Zealand Country Women's Institute, *Portrait of Change: A Record of Country Women's Institute in New Zealand*, Wellington, 1996

New Zealand Waitangi Tribunal, *Muriwhenua Land Report (Wai 45)*, Wellington, 1997

Pomare, E.W., *Maori Standards of Health: A Study of the 20 Year Period 1955–1975*, Wellington, 1980

Pool, D.I., *Te Iwi Maori: A New Zealand Population, Past, Present and Projected*, Auckland, 1991

Pool, D.I., *The Maori Population of New Zealand*, Auckland, 1976

Rice, G.W., *Black November: The 1918 Influenza Epidemic in New Zealand*, Wellington, 1988

Rockel, I., *Taking the Waters: Early Spas in New Zealand*, Wellington, 1986

Rogers, A., and M. Simpson (eds), *Early Stories From Founding Members of the Maori Women's Welfare League: Te Timatanga Tatau Tatau: Te Ropu Wahine Maori Toko i te Ora*, Wellington, 1993

Rutherford, J., *Sir George Grey: A Study in Colonial Government*, London, 1961

Sherrin, R.A.A., and J.H. Wallace, *Early History of New Zealand*, Auckland, 1890

Simon, J. (ed.), *Nga Kura Maori: The Native Schools System 1867–1969*, Auckland, 1998

Skinner, W.H., *Pioneer Medical Men of*

Taranaki 1834 to 1880, New Plymouth, 1933

Stafford, D.M., *Te Arawa: A History of the Arawa People*, Wellington, 1967

Stokes, E.M., *Te Raupatu o Tauranga Moana: The Confiscation of Tauranga Lands*, Hamilton, 1990

Tennant, M., *Paupers and Providers: Charitable Aid in New Zealand*, Wellington, 1989

Ward, A., *A Show of Justice: Racial 'Amalgamation' in Nineteenth Century New Zealand*, Auckland, 1995

Welch, G.K., *Doctor Smith: Hokianga's 'King of the North'*, Hamilton, 1965

White, M. (ed.), *The Unfolding Years 1937–1987: Women's Health League*, Rotorua, 1988

Wohl, A.S., *Endangered Lives: Public Health in Victorian Britain*, London, 1983

Woodward, J., *To Do the Sick No Harm: A Study of the British Voluntary Hospital System to 1875*, London, 1974

Wright, H.M., *New Zealand, 1769–1840: Early Years of Western Contact*, Harvard, 1959

Wright-St Clair, R.E., *Caring for People: A History of the Wanganui Hospital Board*, Wanganui, 1987

Wright-St Clair, R.E., *From Cottage to Regional Base Hospital: Waikato Hospital 1887–1987*, Hamilton, 1987

Articles

Adlam, P., 'The Story of Medical Practice in Rotorua', in [Rotorua and District Historical Society], *Rotorua 1880–1980*, Rotorua, 1980, pp.253–65

Allen, J.S., 'Te Rangi Hiroa's Physical Anthropology', *Journal of the Polynesian Society*, vol.103, no.1, 1994, pp.11–27

Andrews, C.L., 'Aspects of Development, 1870–1890', in I.H. Kawharu (ed.), *Conflict and Compromise: Essays on the Maori Since Colonisation*, Wellington, 1975, pp.80–95

Anon., 'Rotorua Hospital', *New Zealand Hospital*, vol.9, no.3, 1957, pp.29–30

Boddy, J.M., 'Maori Health: Is the Future Determined by the Past?', in J.M. Morse (ed.) *Recent Advances in Nursing: Issues in Cross-Cultural Nursing*, vol.20, 1988, pp.27–38

Bowers, J.Z., 'The Odyssey of Smallpox Vaccination', *Bulletin of the History of Medicine*, vol.55, 1981, pp.17–33

Brunton, W.A., 'Deinstitutionalisation: A Romance For All Seasons', in H. Haines and M. Abbott (eds), *The Future of Mental Health Services in New Zealand: Deinstitutionalisation*, Auckland, 1986, pp.44–63

[Brunton, W.A.], 'Development of Psychiatric Services in New Zealand', in *Royal Commission to Inquire into and Report upon Hospitals and Related Services: Stage II: Psychological Services: Department of Health 1st Submission*, Wellington, 1972, pp.1–21

Brunton, W.A., 'Hostages to History', *New Zealand Health Review*, vol.3, no.2, 1983, pp.3–6

Brunton, W., 'The Place of History in Health Policy-Making: A View from the Inside', in L. Bryder and D.A. Dow (eds), *New Countries and Old Medicine: Proceedings of an International Conference on the History of Medicine and Health*, Auckland, 1995, pp.132–9

Bryder, L., '"Lessons" of the 1918 Influenza Epidemic in Auckland', *NZJH*, vol.16, no.2, 1982, pp.97–121

Bryder, L., 'Tuberculosis and the Maori, 1900–1960', in P. Winterton and D. Gurry (eds), *The Impact of the Past Upon the Present: Second National Conference of the Australian Society of the History of Medicine: Perth, July 1991*, Perth, 1992, pp.191–4

Butlin, N.G., 'Macassans and Aboriginal Smallpox: The "1789" and "1829" Epidemics', *Australian Historical Studies*, vol.21, no.84, April 1985, pp.315–35

Butterworth, G., 'Pomare, Maui Wiremu Piti Naera 1875/76? –1930', in *The Dictionary of New Zealand Biography: Volume 3: 1900–1920*, Wellington, 1996, pp.404–7

Campbell, J., 'Smallpox in Aboriginal Australia, 1829–31', *Australian Historical Studies*, vol.20, no.81, October 1983, pp.536–56

Campbell, J., 'Smallpox in Aboriginal Australia, the Early 1830s', *Australian Historical Studies*, vol.21, no.84, April 1985, pp.336–58

Cassel, J., 'Public Health in Canada', in D. Porter (ed.), *The History of Public Health and the Modern State*, Amsterdam and Atlanta, 1994, pp.276–312

Doms, J., 'The Treaty of Waitangi as a Health Document', *Nursing Praxis in New Zealand*, vol.4, no.2, 1989, pp.16–19

Donaldson, R., 'Dr J.P. FitzGerald: Pioneer Colonial Surgeon, 1840–1854', *NZMJ*, vol.101, 1988, pp.636–8

Donovan, J.W., 'Measles in Australia and New Zealand 1834–1835', *Medical Journal of Australia*, vol.1, 1970, pp.5–10

Dow, D., 'Ether Ushers In a New Era for Local Surgery', *New Zealand Doctor*, 9 July 1997, p.57

Dow, D.A., '"Here is my habitation": Dr James Malcolm Mason and Otaki', *Historical Journal/Otaki Historical Society*, vol.20, 1997, pp.54–7

Dow, D., 'Revisiting the Life and Times of a Pioneer GP', *New Zealand Doctor*, 1 October 1997, p.51

Dow, D., 'Rumour Hampers Pioneering Doctor', *New Zealand Doctor*, 18 February 1998, p.36

Dow, D., '"Smoothing their dying pillow": Lingering Longer', *New Zealand Doctor*, 21 January 1998, p.45

Dow, D., '"Specially suitable men?" Subsidised Medical Services for Maori, 1840–1940, *NZJH*, vol.32, no.2, 1998, pp.163–88

Dow, D.A., 'Springs of Charity? The Development of the New Zealand Hospital System, 1876–1910', in L. Bryder (ed.), *A Healthy Country: Essays on the Social History of Medicine in New Zealand*, Wellington, 1991, pp.44–64

Dow, D., 'The Undying Verve of an Anti-Vaccinationist', *New Zealand Doctor*, 2 October 1996, p.51

Dow, D.A., '"To set our medical history into order": An Historiography of Health in New Zealand', *Archifacts*, April 1996, pp.15–40

Dow, D.A., 'Up With the World? The New Zealand Hospital System, 1876–1910', in P. Winterton and D. Gurry (eds), *The Impact of the Past Upon the Present: Second National Conference of the Australian Society of the History of Medicine: Perth, July 1991*, Perth, 1992, pp.103–7

Durie, M.H., 'A Maori Perspective of Health', *Social Science and Medicine*, vol.20, no.5, 1985, pp.483–6

Durie, M.H., 'Implications of Policy and Management Decisions on Maori Health: Contemporary Issues and Responses', in M.W. Raffel and N.K. Raffel (eds), *Perspectives on Health Policy: Australia, New Zealand, United States*, New York, 1986, pp.201–13

Durie, M.H., 'The Objectives of the Treaty and the Scope of its Provisions', in I.H. Kawharu (ed.), *Maori and Pakeha Perspectives of the Treaty of Waitangi*, Auckland, 1989, pp.280–99

Durie, M., 'The Treaty of Waitangi and Health Care', *NZMJ*, vol.102, 1989, pp.203–5

Editorial, 'Medical Research in New Zealand', *NZMJ*, vol.60, 1961, pp.408–10

Ellis, E.M., and H.M. Harte, 'A Maori Health Nurse', in S. Coney (ed.), *Standing In The Sunshine: A History of New Zealand Women Since They Won The Vote*, Auckland, 1993, pp.102–3

Goldsmith, P., 'Medicine, Death and the Gospel in Hawke's Bay, 1845–1852', in L. Bryder and D.A. Dow (eds), *New Countries and Old Medicine: Proceedings of an International Conference on the History of Medicine and Health*, Auckland, 1995, pp.354–60

Goldsmith, P. 'Medicine, Death and the Gospel in Wairarapa and Hawke's Bay, 1845–1852', *NZJH*, vol.30, no.2, 1996, pp.163–81

Hayton, A.C., and H.D. Mullon, 'The Unfortunate Dr McShane of Nelson and New Plymouth', *NZMJ*, vol.87, 1978, pp.20–3

Henley, W.E., 'The Early History of the Auckland Hospital' *NZMJ*, vol.71, 1970, pp.201–8

Holdaway, M., 'Where Are the Maori Nurses Who Were to Become Those "efficient preachers of the gospel of health"?', *Nursing Praxis in New Zealand*, vol.8, no.1, 1993, pp.25–34

Lambert, G., 'Colonial Hospital Now Serves the Arts', *Historic Places in New Zealand*, vol.12, March 1986, pp.8–10

Lange, R.T., 'The Tohunga and the Government in the Twentieth Century', *Annual: University of Auckland History Society*, 1968, pp.12–38

McKegg, A.H., 'The Maori Health Nursing Scheme: An Experiment in Autonomous Health Care', *NZJH*, vol.26, no.2, 1992, pp.145–60

Maling, P.B., 'How the Canterbury Settlement Obtained its First Medical Officer', *NZMJ*, vol.55, 1956, pp.368–70

Murchie, E., 'Preface', in Public Health Commission, *He Matariki: A Strategic Plan for Maori Public Health: He Kaupapa Whainga Roa Mo Te Hauora Tumatanui Maori: The Public Health Commission's Advice to the Minister of Health 1994–1995*, Wellington, 1995

Newson, A.J., 'New Zealand's First General Anaesthetic', *Anaesthesia & Intensive Care*, vol.3, 1975, pp.204–8

Nicholson, M., 'Medicine and Racial Politics: Changing Images of the New Zealand Maori in the Nineteenth Century', in D. Arnold (ed.), *Imperial Medicine and Indigenous Societies*, Manchester, 1988, pp.66–104

Owens, J.M.R., 'Missionary Medicine and Maori Health: The Record of the Wesleyan Mission to New Zealand Before 1840', *Journal of the Polynesian Society*, vol.81, 1972, pp.418–36

Pomare, E.W., 'A Historical Perspective: "The Changing World"', *New Zealand Health Review*, Spring 1984, p.6

Renwick, W., 'Pope, James Henry, 1837–1913', in *The Dictionary of New Zealand Biography: Volume 2: 1870–1900*, Wellington, 1993, pp.393–5

Rice, G.W., 'The Making of New Zealand's 1920 Health Act', *NZJH*, vol.22, no.1, 1988, pp.3–22

Roche, E.H., 'Some Medical Pioneers in New Zealand: Part 2', *NZMJ*, vol.71, 1970, pp.29–32, 90–3

Rose, B.S., 'Maori Health and European Culture', *NZMJ*, vol.61, 1962, pp.491–5

Ross, A.C., 'The Scottish Missionary Doctor', in D.A. Dow (ed.), *The Influence of Scottish Medicine*, Carnforth, 1988, pp.87–101

Sargison, P.A., '"Efficient Preachers of the Gospel of Health": Akinihi Hei (1882?–1910) and the Maori Health Nursing Scheme', in P.A. Sargison, *Notable Women in New Zealand Health/Te Hauora ki Aotearoa: Ona Wahine Rongonui*, Wellington, 1993, pp.21–4

Sargison, P.A., 'Hei, Akenehi, 1877/78?–1910', in *The Dictionary of New Zealand Biography: Volume 3: 1900–1920*, Wellington, 1996, pp.204–5

Sargison, P.A., 'Maclean, Hester, 1859–1932', in *The Dictionary of New Zealand Biography: Volume 3: 1900–1920*, Wellington, 1996, pp.309–11

Sorrenson, M.P.K., 'Land Purchase Methods and Their Effect on Maori Population, 1865–1901', *Journal of the Polynesian Society*, vol.65, no.3, 1956, pp.183–99

Sorrenson, M.P.K., 'Modern Maori: The Young Maori Party to Mana Motuhake', in K. Sinclair (ed.), *The Oxford Illustrated History of New Zealand*, Auckland, 1990, pp.323–31

Sorrenson, M.P.K., 'Ngata, Apirana Turupa 1874–1950', in *The Dictionary of New Zealand Biography: Volume 3: 1900–1920*, Wellington, 1996, pp.359–63

Starnes, J.H., 'A Pioneer Missionary in the Urewera: Sister Annie Henry MBE 1875–

1971', *Historical Review: Bay of Plenty Journal of History*, vol.6, no.3, 1958, pp.84–93

Stenhouse, J., '"A disappearing race before we came here": Doctor Alfred Kingcome Newman, the Dying Maori, and Victorian Scientific Racism', *NZJH*, vol.30, no.2, 1996, pp.124–40

Tennant, M., '"Missionaries of health": The School Medical Service During the Inter-war Period', in L. Bryder (ed.), *A Healthy Country: Essays on the Social History of Medicine in New Zealand*, Wellington, 1991, pp.129–48

Tennant, M., 'The Origins of School Medicine in New Zealand', in P. Winterton and D. Gurry (eds), *The Impact of the Past Upon the Present: Second National Conference of the Australian Society of the History of Medicine: Perth, July 1991*, Perth, 1992, pp.175–9

Valentine, G.M., 'Maui Pomare and the Adventist Connection', in P.H. Ballis (ed.), *In and Out of The World: Seventh-Day Adventists in New Zealand*, Palmerston North, 1985, pp.82–108

Voyce, M., 'Maori Healers in New Zealand: The Tohunga Suppression Act 1907', *Oceania: A Journal Devoted to the Study of the Native Peoples of Australia, New Guinea, and Other Islands of the Pacific Ocean*, vol.60, no.2, 1989, pp.99–123

Wood, P.J., 'Efficient Preachers of the Gospel of Health: The 1898 Scheme for Educating Maori Nurses', *Nursing Praxis in New Zealand*, vol.7, no.1, 1992, pp.12–21

Wright-St Clair, R.E., 'Medical Men in Early New Zealand Politics', *NZMJ*, vol.54, 1955, pp.551–5

Theses and research essays

Barclay, B.d'E., 'A Public Health Survey of the Wanganui River Pahs and the Wanganui Maoris', DPH thesis, Otago, 1933

Beedie, M., and N. Hunter, 'Health Survey of Maoris of Southern Hawke's Bay', DPH thesis, Otago, 1942

Belgrave, M., '"Medical Men" and "Lady Doctors": The Making of a New Zealand Profession 1867–1941', PhD thesis, Victoria, 1985

Brown, M.B., 'The Auckland School of Nursing, 1883–1990: The Rise and The Fall', MA thesis, Auckland, 1991

Bryder, L., 'The 1918 Influenza Epidemic in Auckland', MA thesis, Auckland, 1980

Buck, P.H., 'Medicine Amongst the Maoris, in Ancient and Modern Times', MD thesis, University of New Zealand, 1910

Dawson, R.H., and G.I. Louisson, 'The Taranaki Maoris; Their Public Health and Hygiene (With Special Reference to Housing)', DPH thesis, Otago, 1938

Day, A.S., '"The Maori Malady": The 1913 Smallpox Epidemic and Its Nineteenth Century Background', MA thesis, Auckland, 1998

Donaldson, R., 'Dr John Patrick Fitzgerald: Pioneer Colonial Doctor 1840–1860', MPhil thesis, Waikato, 1988

Duthie, J.A., 'A Social Study of the Maoris on the Wanganui River', DPH thesis, Otago, 1940

Ewing, I.S., 'Public Service Reform in New Zealand, 1866–1912', MA thesis, Auckland, 1979

Eyres, D.F.B., 'An Account of the Maintenance of the Public Health in New Zealand Prior to 1920', MA thesis, Victoria, 1938

Ferguson, L.A., 'Marae Based Health Initiatives Within the Tainui Iwi From 1970–1995', MA thesis, Auckland, 1997

Goodfellow, K.S., 'Health for the Maori? Health and the Maori Village Schools 1890–1940', MA thesis, Auckland, 1991

Gray, J.M., 'Potions, Pills and Poisons: Quackery in New Zealand, circa 1900–1915', BA(Hons) thesis, Otago, 1980

Kehoe, J.M., 'Medicine, Sexuality, and Imperialism: British Medical Discourse Surrounding Venereal Disease in New Zealand and Japan: a Socio-Historical and Comparative Study', PhD thesis, Victoria, 1992

Lange, R.T., 'The Revival of a Dying Race: A Study of Maori Health Reform 1900–1918 and its Nineteenth Century Background', MA thesis, Auckland, 1972

McKegg, A.H., '"Ministering Angels": The Government Backblock Nursing Service and the Maori Health Nurses, 1909–1939', MA thesis, Auckland, 1991

Maaka, G.H., 'General Survey of Ratana Pa', DPH thesis, Otago, 1930

Martin, R.J., 'Aspects of Maori Affairs in the Liberal Period', MA thesis, Auckland, 1956

May, L., 'Medical Malversations: Quacks, the Quackery Prevention Act 1908, and the Orthodox Medical Profession's Push for Power', BA(Hons) thesis, Otago, 1994

Murray, G., 'A Survey of the Health and Housing Conditions of the Maoris on the East Coast of the North Island and in the Wanganui District', DPH thesis, Otago, 1937

Orange, C.J., 'A Kind of Equality: Labour and the Maori People 1934–49', MA thesis, Auckland, 1977

Paewai, M.N., 'A Social Study of the Southern Hawke's Bay Maori', DPH thesis, Otago, 1945

Paterson, J.A., and W.J. Edgington, 'Tuberculosis in Moeraki Maoris', DPH thesis, Otago, 1924

Simpson, L.H., 'Health Contrast Between Maoris of Pahs and Country Areas: Rotorua District', DPH thesis, Otago, 1940

Sorrenson, M.P.K., 'The Purchase of Maori Lands, 1865–1892', MA thesis, Auckland, 1955

Taylor, K.R., 'Public Health Administration in New Zealand', MCom thesis, Canterbury, 1939

Trott, T.C., 'The Maoris of the Northern King Country: The Relationship of Housing to Health', DPH thesis, Otago, 1940

Williams, J.A., 'Maori Society and Politics 1891–1909', PhD thesis, Wisconsin, 1963

Index

Page references to illustrations and captions have been *italicised*.